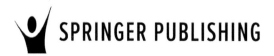 SPRINGER PUBLISHING

MW00648381

GET THE MOST FROM YOUR BOOK

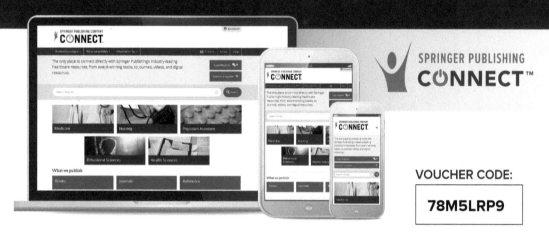

SPRINGER PUBLISHING
CONNECT™

VOUCHER CODE:

78M5LRP9

Online Access

Your print purchase of *Clinical Teaching Strategies in Nursing,
Sixth Edition*, includes **online access via Springer Publishing
Connect**™ to increase accessibility, portability, and searchability.

Insert the code at http://connect.springerpub.com/content/
book/978-0-8261-6705-7 today!

Having trouble? Contact our customer service department at cs@springerpub.com

Instructor Resource Access for Adopters

**Let us do some of the heavy lifting to create an engaging classroom experience with a variety of
instructor resources included in most textbooks SUCH AS:**

**INSTRUCTOR'S
MANUAL**

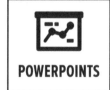

POWERPOINTS

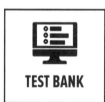

TEST BANK

Visit **https://connect.springerpub.com/** and look for the **"Show Supplementary"** button on your **book homepage** to see
what is available to instructors! First time using Springer Publishing Connect?

Email **textbook@springerpub.com** to create an account and start unlocking valuable resources.

Clinical Teaching Strategies in Nursing

Marilyn H. Oermann, PhD, RN, ANEF, FAAN, is the Thelma M. Ingles Professor of Nursing at Duke University School of Nursing, Durham, North Carolina. She is author or coauthor of 25 books and many articles on teaching and writing for publication in nursing. She is the editor-in-chief of *Nurse Educator* and the *Journal of Nursing Care Quality* and past editor of the *Annual Review of Nursing Education*. Dr. Oermann received the National League for Nursing (NLN) Award for Excellence in Nursing Education Research, NLN President's Award, Sigma Theta Tau International Elizabeth Russell Belford Award for Excellence in Education, American Association of Colleges of Nursing Scholarship of Teaching and Learning Excellence Award, and Margaret Comerford Freda Award for Editorial Leadership from the International Academy of Nursing Editors.

Teresa Shellenbarger, PhD, RN, CNE, CNEcl, ANEF, is executive director, National League for Nursing Commission for Nursing Education Accreditation. She was previously a Distinguished University Professor and Doctoral Nursing Program Coordinator, Indiana University of Pennsylvania, Indiana, Pennsylvania. During her 30 years of classroom and clinical teaching, she has established a reputation as an expert educator, mentor, and respected leader in academia. She was an invited member of the National League for Nursing (NLN) workgroup that developed the Academic Clinical Nurse Educator competencies that serve as the basis for the NLN clinical nurse educator certification exam. Dr. Shellenbarger recently published two books, *Clinical Nurse Educator Competencies: Creating an Evidence-Based Practice for Academic Clinical Nurse Educators* and *Academic Clinical Nurse Educator Review*. Dr. Shellenbarger frequently presents and publishes on topics related to innovative teaching, faculty role development, clinical teaching, and technology in nursing education.

Kathleen B. Gaberson, PhD, RN, CNOR, CNE, ANEF, is the owner of and principal nursing education consultant for OWK Consulting, Pittsburgh, Pennsylvania. She has over 35 years of teaching and administrative experience in graduate and undergraduate nursing programs. She is a coauthor of 12 nursing education books and an author or coauthor of numerous articles on nursing education topics. Dr. Gaberson presents and consults extensively on nursing curriculum revision, assessment and evaluation, and teaching methods.

Clinical Teaching Strategies in Nursing

Sixth Edition

Marilyn H. Oermann, PhD, RN, ANEF, FAAN

Teresa Shellenbarger, PhD, RN, CNE, CNEcl, ANEF

Kathleen B. Gaberson, PhD, RN, CNOR, CNE, ANEF

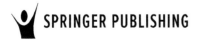

SPRINGER PUBLISHING

Springer Publishing Company, LLC
11 West 42nd Street, New York, NY 10036
www.springerpub.com
connect.springerpub.com/

Acquisitions Editor: Joseph Morita
Compositor: diacriTech

ISBN: 978-0-8261-6704-0
ebook ISBN: 978-0-8261-6705-7
DOI: 10.1891/9780826167057

SUPPLEMENTS:
Instructor Materials:

A robust set of instructor resources designed to supplement this text is located at **http://connect.springerpub.com/content/book/978-0-8261-6705-7**. Qualifying instructors may request access by emailing **textbook@springerpub.com**.

Instructor's Manual ISBN: 978-0-8261-6706-4
Instructor's PowerPoints ISBN: 978-0-8261-6707-1

21 22 23 24 / 5 4 3 2 1

The author and the publisher of this Work have made every effort to use sources believed to be reliable to provide information that is accurate and compatible with the standards generally accepted at the time of publication. The author and publisher shall not be liable for any special, consequential, or exemplary damages resulting, in whole or in part, from the readers' use of, or reliance on, the information contained in this book. The publisher has no responsibility for the persistence or accuracy of URLs for external or third-party Internet websites referred to in this publication and does not guarantee that any content on such websites is, or will remain, accurate or appropriate.

LCCN: 2021920785

Contact sales@springerpub.com to receive discount rates on bulk purchases.

Publisher's Note: **New and used products purchased from third-party sellers are not guaranteed for quality, authenticity, or access to any included digital components.**

Printed in the United States of America by Gasch Printing.

Contents

SECTION III: EVALUATION STRATEGIES IN CLINICAL TEACHING

Contributors to Previous Editions

Eric Bauman, PhD, RN

Suzanne Hetzel Campbell, PhD, WHNP-BC, IBCLC

Kimberly Day, DNP, RN

Mickey Gilmore-Kahn, CNM, MN

Debra Hagler, PhD, RN, ACNS-BC, CNE, CHSE, ANEF, FAAN

Elizabeth Speakman, EdD, RN, FNAP, ANEF, FAAN

Susan E. Stone, DNSc, CNM, FACNM

Diane M. Wink, EdD, FNP, ARNP

Contributors to the Sixth Edition

Christine Lind Colella, DNP, APRN-CNP, FAANP Professor, Interim Associate Dean, and Executive Director, Graduate Programs, College of Nursing, University of Cincinnati, Cincinnati, Ohio

Katie Anne Haerling, PhD, RN, CHSE Professor, School of Nursing and Healthcare Leadership, University of Washington Tacoma, Tacoma, Washington

Meigan Robb, PhD, RN Assistant Professor, Department of Nursing and Allied Health Professions, Indiana University of Pennsylvania, Indiana, Pennsylvania

Preface

Teaching in clinical settings presents nurse educators with challenges that are different from those encountered in the classroom and in online environments. In nursing education, the classroom and clinical environments are linked because students apply in clinical practice what they have learned in the classroom, online, and through other experiences. However, clinical settings require different approaches to teaching. The clinical environment is complex and rapidly changing, with a variety of new settings and roles in which nurses must be prepared to practice.

The sixth edition of *Clinical Teaching Strategies in Nursing* examines concepts of clinical teaching and provides a comprehensive framework for planning, guiding, and evaluating learning activities for prelicensure and graduate nursing students. It is a comprehensive source of information for full- and part-time faculty members whose responsibilities center largely on clinical teaching, for adjuncts and clinical nurse educators whose sole responsibility is clinical teaching, and for preceptors. The book also is useful when teaching nurses and other healthcare providers in the clinical setting. Although the focus of the book is clinical teaching in nursing, the content is applicable to teaching students in other healthcare professions.

The book describes clinical teaching strategies that are effective and practical in a rapidly changing healthcare environment. It presents a range of teaching strategies useful for courses in which the teacher is on site with students, in courses using preceptors and similar models, and in distance education environments. The book also examines innovative uses of technologies for clinical teaching.

Each chapter includes a list of the content from the Certified Nurse Educator (CNE®) and the Certified Academic Clinical Nurse Educator (CNE®cl) Examination Test Blueprints that relate to the chapter content. In addition to the book, we have prepared Instructor Materials with a course syllabus; a complete online course (with modules for each chapter that include a chapter summary, student learning activities, discussion questions, online resources for students, and assessment strategies); and chapter-based PowerPoint presentations (for use in an online course or in-person classes). To obtain an electronic copy of these teaching materials, contact Springer Publishing Company (textbook@springerpub.com).

The book is organized into three sections. The first section, Foundations of Clinical Teaching, comprises six chapters that provide a background for clinical teaching and guide the teacher's planning for clinical learning activities. Chapter 1 discusses the context for clinical teaching and presents a philosophy that provides a framework for planning, guiding, and evaluating clinical learning activities. Chapter 2 discusses outcomes of clinical teaching; it emphasizes the importance of cognitive, psychomotor, and affective outcomes that guide clinical teaching and evaluation.

Clinical education can be provided in a wide variety of clinical sites, as explained in Chapter 3. Examples are provided of clinical learning opportunities in specialized patient care areas not used regularly for clinical learning, community-based settings such as camps and wellness centers, clinical learning at distant sites, and international settings. Chapter 4 describes selecting clinical sites; the roles and responsibilities of faculty members, adjunct and part-time clinical teachers, staff members, preceptors, and others involved in clinical teaching; and methods of preparing educators and students for clinical learning activities.

Chapter 5 discusses the process of clinical teaching—identifying clinical competencies, assessing learning needs, planning learning activities, guiding students, and evaluating performance. Various clinical teaching models are described, including traditional, in which one teacher guides the learning of a small group of students; preceptor; and dedicated education units and other partnerships. This chapter also addresses important qualities of clinical teachers. Chapter 6 addresses ethical and legal issues inherent in clinical teaching, including the use of a service setting for learning activities, the effects of academic dishonesty in clinical learning, incivility between students and clinical teachers, and appropriate accommodations for students with disabilities.

The second section of the book focuses on clinical teaching strategies. One of the most important responsibilities of the clinical educator is selecting teaching methods and crafting clinical assignments that are related to the competencies to be developed, appropriate to students' levels of knowledge and skill, and challenging enough to motivate learning. Chapter 7 presents clinical teaching methods—clinical assignments and options for these assignments (skill vs. total care focus, student–patient ratio options, management activities, guided observation, and service learning); discussion; clinical conferences; and written assignments. The chapter provides a framework for planning clinical assignments for learners.

In Chapter 8, cases, case studies, and unfolding cases are examined. Cases can be used to guide the development of problem-solving and clinical-judgment skills. Chapter 9 is on clinical simulation. The chapter includes discussion about replacing clinical practice with simulation and presents essential content and guidelines for using simulation as a teaching strategy. Fidelity, preparing for simulation, creating or selecting a scenario, implementing and evaluating simulation, debriefing, and standards for simulation are explained in the chapter. Chapter 10 examines different technologies that can be used in clinical education, including simulated electronic health records, telepresence, telehealth, electronic escape rooms, and other technology-related approaches. This chapter also includes virtual clinical learning experiences and how educators responded to COVID-19 with technology use. The chapter includes suggestions for selecting these technologies and the importance of matching the choice of technology to the intended type of learning. Chapter 11 is devoted to the use of preceptors in clinical teaching in prelicensure and advanced practice nursing programs. The selection, preparation, role, and evaluation of preceptors, and the advantages and disadvantages of using preceptors, are discussed.

The final section has two chapters. Chapter 12 describes the process of clinical evaluation in nursing, rating scales, and other methods for evaluating clinical performance. Examples of clinical evaluation tools (rating scales) are included in the chapter and also in Appendix B. Grading systems for clinical courses and addressing students' performance problems are explored in the chapter. Chapter 13 examines distance learning; clinical teaching in distance learning environments; developing partnerships with preceptors and clinical sites; and roles and responsibilities of the faculty member, preceptor, and student. The chapter includes strategies for evaluating students' clinical performance such as site visits, on-campus intensives, and virtual site visits using technology, and for preceptor and clinical site evaluation.

We acknowledge Joseph Morita, Executive Acquisitions Editor at Springer Publishing Company, for his continued support. We also thank Springer Publishing Company for its commitment to nursing education and for publishing our books for many years.

Marilyn H. Oermann
Teresa Shellenbarger
Kathleen B. Gaberson

 A robust set of instructor resources designed to supplement this text is located at **http://connect.springerpub.com/content/book/978-0-8261-6705-7**. Qualifying instructors may request access by emailing **textbook@springerpub.com**.

Instructor Resources

Clinical Teaching Strategies in Nursing, Sixth Edition, includes quality resources for the instructor, located at http://connect.springerpub.com/content/book/978-0-8261-6705-7. Faculty who have adopted the text may gain access to these resources by emailing textbook@springerpub.com.

Instructor resources include:

- Sample Course Syllabus
- 13 Course Modules
- Each Module Includes:
    - Chapter Summary
    - Student Learning Activities
    - Discussion Questions
    - Online Resources
    - Assessment Strategies
- PowerPoint Presentations for Each Module

Foundations of Clinical Teaching

Contextual Factors Affecting Clinical Teaching

Effective clinical teaching and learning are influenced by several factors. Clinical teaching is performed by a faculty within a curriculum that is planned and offered in response to professional, societal, environmental, and educational expectations and demands, using available human, intellectual, physical, and financial resources—the context of the curriculum.

However, considering that educational context is not enough for clinical teachers, they must also consider the healthcare context so that they are adequately preparing qualified nurses to be capable of responding to the needs and challenges of a rapidly changing healthcare environment. Clinical teaching is also impacted by trends and issues beyond the clinical setting and the nursing program. Issues such as diversity, healthcare financing, globalization, technology development, and other trends also influence healthcare and clinical teaching. Curricula must be aligned with the ever-changing practice setting (DeBoor, 2022). Faculty members face a rapidly changing healthcare system burdened with financial pressures, consumption of services by patients with complex needs, delivery of care with expanding technology, and staff shortages. The context of the higher education environment is also a consideration for nursing faculty. Within the educational environment, nurse educators feel the pressures of tightening resources, increased workload demands, and changes in student characteristics. Adjunct or part-time teachers often are employed as clinical teachers. They may not understand the full scope of the academic nurse educator role and may need guidance to understand the nursing curriculum, requirements, and students. These clinical teachers need to know how a clinical practicum is positioned within the curriculum so they can build upon previous knowledge and position clinical learning appropriately.

Because the context is different for each nursing education program, each curriculum is somewhat unique (DeBoor, 2022). Therefore, the practice of clinical teaching differs somewhat from program to program. It is not possible to recommend a set of clinical teaching strategies that will be equally effective in every nursing education program. Rather, the faculty must make decisions about clinical teaching that are congruent with the planned curriculum and relevant to its context.

THE CURRICULUM PHILOSOPHY

In the sense that it is used most frequently in education, philosophy is a system of enduring shared beliefs and values held by members of an academic or practice discipline that help to guide actions and curriculum implementation. Philosophy as a comprehensive scientific discipline focuses on more than beliefs, but beliefs determine the direction of science and thus form a basis for examining knowledge in any science.

Philosophical statements serve as a guide for examining issues and determining the priorities of a discipline. Although a philosophy does not prescribe specific actions, it gives meaning and direction to practice, and it provides a basis for decision-making and for determining whether one's behavior is consistent with one's beliefs. Without a philosophy to guide choices, a person is overly vulnerable to tradition or fashion.

A curriculum philosophy includes statements of belief about people, society, health, the goals of education, the nature of teaching and learning, and the roles of learners and teachers (DeBoor, 2022). It provides a framework for making curricular and instructional choices and decisions based on a variety of options. The values and beliefs included in a curriculum philosophy provide structure and coherence for a curriculum, but statements of philosophy are meaningless if they are contradicted by actual educational practice or incongruent with the parent institution. In nursing education, a curriculum philosophy directs the curriculum development process by providing a basis for selecting, sequencing, and using content and learning activities while aligning with the mission, vision, and values of the academic institution (Valiga, 2022).

Clinical practica comprise an important part of the overall curriculum, offering opportunities for students to link the curriculum philosophy to their clinical learning and experiences. Clinical practica based on the curriculum philosophy provide a scaffold or structure for the program and direct course sequencing and clinical learning activities. Course configuration must logically build and offer learning opportunities that will enable students to achieve desired outcomes (DeBoor, 2022; Valiga, 2022). Clinical teachers should understand the underlying framework of the curriculum so that they can operationalize the program consistently and align their work with the program mission, philosophy, and organizing framework.

This book provides a framework for planning, guiding, and evaluating the clinical learning activities of nursing students based on the authors' philosophical approach to clinical teaching. That philosophical context for clinical teaching is discussed in the remainder of this chapter.

A PHILOSOPHICAL CONTEXT FOR CLINICAL TEACHING

Every clinical teacher has a philosophical approach to clinical teaching, whether the teacher realizes it or not. That philosophical context determines the teacher's understanding of his or her role, approaches to clinical teaching, selection of teaching and learning activities, use of evaluation processes, and relationships with learners and others in the clinical environment. These beliefs serve as a guide to action, and they profoundly affect how clinical teachers practice, how students learn, and how learning outcomes are evaluated.

Readers may not agree with every element of the philosophical context discussed here, but they should be able to see congruence between what the authors believe about clinical teaching and the recommendations they make to guide effective clinical teaching. Readers are encouraged to articulate their philosophies of nursing education in general and clinical teaching in particular to guide their clinical teaching practice.

A Lexicon of Clinical Teaching

Language has the power to shape thinking, and choice and use of words can affect the way a teacher thinks about and performs the role of clinical teacher. The following terms are defined so that the authors and readers will share a common frame of reference for the essential concepts in this philosophical approach to clinical teaching.

CLINICAL

This word is an adjective, derived from the noun *clinic*. *Clinical* means involving direct observation of the patient. Like any adjective, the word clinical must modify a noun. Nursing faculty members often are heard to say, "My students are in clinical today" or "I am not in clinical this week." Examples of correct use include "clinical practice," "clinical practicum," "clinical instruction," and "clinical evaluation."

CLINICAL TEACHING OR CLINICAL INSTRUCTION

The central activity of the teacher in the clinical setting is clinical instruction or clinical teaching. The teacher does not supervise students. Supervision implies administrative functions such as overseeing, directing, and managing the work of others. Supervision is a function that is more appropriate for professional practice situations, not the learning environment.

The appropriate role of the teacher in the clinical setting is competent guidance. The teacher guides, supports, stimulates, and facilitates learning. The teacher facilitates learning by designing appropriate activities in appropriate settings and allows the student to experience that learning.

CLINICAL EXPERIENCE

Learning is an active, personal process. The student is the one who experiences the learning. Teachers cannot provide the experience; they can provide only the opportunity for the experience. The teacher's role is to plan and provide appropriate activities that will facilitate learning. However, each student will experience activity in a different way. For example, a teacher can provide a guided observation of a surgical procedure for a group of students. Although all students may be present in the operating room at the same time and all are observing the same procedure, each student will experience something slightly different. One of the reasons teachers require students to do written assignments or to participate in clinical conferences is to allow the teacher a glimpse of what students have derived from the learning activities.

ELEMENTS OF A PHILOSOPHICAL CONTEXT FOR CLINICAL TEACHING

The philosophical context of clinical teaching that provides the framework for this book includes beliefs about the nature of the professional practice, essential nurse educator competencies, the importance of clinical teaching, the role of the student as a learner, the need for learning time before evaluation, the climate for learning, the essential versus enrichment curricula, the espoused curriculum versus curriculum-in-use, and the importance of quality over quantity of clinical activities. Each of these elements serves as a guide to action for clinical teachers in nursing.

Clinical Education Should Reflect the Nature of Professional Practice

Nursing is a professional discipline. A professional is an individual who possesses expert knowledge and skill in a specific domain, acquired through formal education in institutions of higher learning and through experience, and who uses that knowledge and skill on behalf of the society by serving specified clients. Professional disciplines are differentiated from academic disciplines by their practice component.

Clinical practice requires critical thinking and problem-solving abilities, specialized psychomotor and technological skills, and a professional value system. Practice in clinical settings exposes students to the realities of professional practice that cannot be conveyed by a textbook or a simulation (Oermann & Gaberson, 2021). Schön (1987) represented professional practice as high, hard ground overlooking a swamp. On the high ground, practice problems can be solved by applying research-based theory and technique. The swampy lowland contains problems that are messy and confusing, and that cannot easily be solved by technical skill. Nursing students must learn to solve both types of problems, but the swampy lowlands problems tend to be those of greatest importance to society. Most professional practice situations are characterized by complexity, instability, uncertainty, uniqueness, and the presence of value conflicts. These are the problems that resist solution by the knowledge and skills of traditional expertise (Schön, 1983).

Professional practice occurs within the context of society, and it must respond to ever-changing social and scientific demands and expectations. The knowledge base and skill repertoire of a professional nurse cannot be static; professional practice requires lifelong learning to prepare for practice in the future. Thus, nursing clinical education must include skills such as identifying knowledge gaps, locating and using new information and technology, developing new and relevant competencies, and initiating or managing change to create systems of care. Because healthcare professionals usually practice as members of interprofessional teams, clinical education of nursing students should also include opportunities for interprofessional education (IPE) (Institute of Medicine, 2011).

A newly released publication of the National Academy of Medicine, *The Future of Nursing 2020–2030: Charting a Path to Achieve Health Equity* (National Academies of Sciences, Engineering, and Medicine [NASEM], 2021), addresses nursing's role in reducing health inequities and improving health and well-being for the U.S. population in the 21st century. Taking into account the COVID-19 global pandemic, including the markedly altered context and rapidly implemented changes in clinical care, nursing education, and nursing leadership, the report anticipates the needs of the population and the nursing profession for the next decade. It includes a set of recommended actions that can make a meaningful impact on deploying the profession more robustly so that nurses will be both prepared for disasters in the future and equipped to engage in the complex but essential work of advancing health equity, addressing social determinants of health, and meeting social needs of individuals and families (NASEM, 2021).

Nursing faculties should not only design curricula to meet predicted needs for current and future nursing practice, but also be prepared to anticipate and quickly respond to emerging needs. Planned clinical learning activities can be modified to allow students to engage in rapidly developing new realities of nursing practice, such as those encountered during the COVID-19 pandemic, or to substitute virtual clinical learning when exposure to actual clinical settings is not possible.

Thus, if clinical learning activities are to prepare nursing students for professional practice, they should reflect the realities of that practice. Students must be exposed to the demands and issues confronting nursing and healthcare. Clinical education should allow students to encounter real practice problems in the swampy lowland. Rather than focus exclusively on teacher-defined, well-structured problems for which answers are easily found in theory and research, clinical educators should expose students to ill-structured problems for which there are insufficient or conflicting data or multiple solutions (Oermann & Gaberson, 2021).

Clinical Teaching Is More Important Than Classroom Teaching

Because nursing is a professional practice discipline, what nurses and nursing students do in clinical practice is more important than what they can demonstrate in a classroom or learning laboratory. Clinical learning activities provide real-life opportunities for the transfer of knowledge to practical situations (Oermann & Gaberson, 2021). Some learners who perform well in the classroom have difficulty applying their knowledge successfully in the clinical area.

If clinical instruction is so important, why doesn't all nursing education take place in the clinical area? Clinical teaching is the most expensive element of any nursing curriculum. Lower student-to-teacher ratios in clinical settings usually require a larger number of clinical teachers than classroom teachers. Students and teachers spend numerous hours in clinical settings; those contact hours typically exceed the number of credit hours for which students pay tuition. Even if the tuition structure compensates for that intensive use of resources, clinical instruction remains an expensive enterprise. Therefore, classroom instruction is used to prepare students for their clinical activities. Students learn prerequisite knowledge in the classroom and through independent learning activities that they later apply and test, first in the simulation laboratory and then in clinical practice.

As we have learned during the recent global COVID-19 pandemic, actual clinical settings may not always be available to nursing students for learning activities. The substitution of simulation activities for clinical practice has increased significantly over the last 2 decades as nursing education programs have encountered barriers to the placement of students in clinical settings, such as increased competition from other programs. The National Council of State Boards of Nursing's (NCSBN) study of the use of simulation as a substitute for traditional clinical practice found that high-quality simulation activities could replace up to 50% of traditional clinical learning activities in prelicensure curricula without significant differences in knowledge acquisition and clinical performance. Specifically, the substitution of up to 50% simulation for actual clinical learning activities produces outcomes similar to those of traditional clinical practice as long as sufficient numbers of faculty members are adequately trained, there is a dedicated simulation lab with appropriate resources, simulation scenarios are realistic and well designed, and debriefing is based on a standardized model (Alexander et al., 2015).

During the recent pandemic, many prelicensure programs found it necessary to substitute an even larger percentage of simulation activities for actual clinical learning activities, with many state boards of nursing relaxing restrictions on the use of simulation in programs where such regulations already existed. Graduate advanced practice nursing' programs also were challenged to find clinical placements for students due to rapid changes in the context of clinical care such as cancelled elective surgeries and office appointments, a scarcity of available preceptors due to lay-offs, and extensive closure of clinical sites to students at all levels. Many graduate programs successfully substituted telehealth and online simulations for a portion of students' clinical practice.

While we have not yet had time to evaluate the effect of these changes on nursing student outcomes, the NCSBN simulation study results suggest that "the quality of the experience, not the number of hours, is crucial. If students would be placed in clinical settings with inadequate opportunity for hands-on experience, employment of simulation by capable faculty with meaningful debriefing may offer a better alternative" (Alexander et al., 2015, p. 41).

The Nursing Student in the Clinical Setting Is a Learner, Not a Nurse

In preparation for professional practice, the clinical setting is the place where the student comes in contact with the patient for testing theories and learning skills. In nursing education, clinical learning activities have historically been confused with caring for patients. In a classic study on the use of the clinical laboratory in nursing education, Infante (1985) observed that the typical activities of nursing students focus on patient care. Learning is assumed to take place while caring for patients. However, the central focus in clinical education should be on learning, not doing, as the student's role. Thus, the role of the student in nursing education should be primarily that of learner, not nurse. For this reason, the term *nursing student* rather than *student nurse* is preferred, because in the former term, the noun *student* describes the role better. Likewise, the term *learning assignment* should be used in place of *patient assignment* to emphasize that students are in the clinical setting to learn how to care for patients, not to provide patient care.

Sufficient Learning Time Should Be Provided Before Performance Is Evaluated

If students enter the clinical area to learn, then it follows that students need to engage in activities that promote learning and to practice the skills that they are learning before their performance is evaluated to determine a grade. Many nursing students perceive that the main role of the clinical teacher is to evaluate, and many nursing faculty members perceive that they spend more time on evaluation activities than on teaching activities. Nursing faculty members seem to expect students to perform skills competently the first time they attempt them, and they often keep detailed records of students' failures and shortcomings, which are later consulted when determining grades. However, skill acquisition is a complex process that involves making mistakes and learning how to correct and then prevent those mistakes. Because the clinical setting is a place where students can test theory and apply it to practice, some of those tests will be more successful than others. Faculty members should expect students to make mistakes and not hold perfection as the standard. Therefore, faculty members should allow plentiful learning time with ample opportunity for feedback before evaluating student performance summatively.

Clinical Teaching Is Supported by a Climate of Mutual Trust and Respect

Another element of this philosophy of clinical teaching is the importance of creating and maintaining a climate of mutual trust and respect that supports learning and student growth. Faculty members must respect students as learners and trust their motivation and commitment to the profession they seek to enter. Students must respect the faculty's commitment to both nursing education and society and trust that faculty members will treat them with fairness and, to the extent that it is possible, not allow students to make mistakes that would harm patients.

The responsibilities for maintaining this climate are mutual, but teachers have the ultimate responsibility to establish these expectations in the nursing program. In most cases, students enter a nursing education program with 12 or more years of school experiences in which teachers may have been viewed as enemies, "out to get students," and eager to see students fail. Nurse educators need to state clearly, early, and often that they see nursing education as a shared enterprise, that they sincerely desire student success, and that they will be partners with students in achieving success. Before expecting students to trust them, teachers need to demonstrate their respect for students; faculty must first trust students and invite students to enter into a trusting relationship with the faculty. This takes time and energy, and sometimes faculty members will be disappointed when trust is betrayed. However, in the long run, clinical teaching is more effective when it takes place in a climate of mutual trust and respect, so it is worth the time and effort.

Clinical Teaching and Learning Should Focus on Essential Knowledge, Skills, and Attitudes

Most nurse educators believe that each nursing education program has a single curriculum. In fact, every nursing curriculum comprises knowledge, skills, and attitudes that are deemed to be essential for safe, competent practice and those that would be nice to have but are not critical. In other words, there is an essential curriculum and an enrichment curriculum. No nursing education program has the luxury of unlimited time for clinical teaching. Therefore, teaching and learning time is used to maximum advantage by focusing most of the time and effort on the most common practice problems that nurses are likely to encounter.

As healthcare and nursing knowledge grow, nursing curricula tend to change additively. That is, new content and skills are added to nursing curricula frequently, but faculty members are reluctant to delete anything. Neither students nor teachers are well served by this approach. Teachers may feel like they are drowning in content and unable to fit everything in; students resort to memorization and superficial, temporary learning, unable to discriminate between critical information and less important material. Faculty members must determine what content is critical and necessary and what information is nice to know but may not be necessary to include. Nurse educators in prelicensure programs should focus on knowledge needed for entry of the novice nurse into professional practice, development of basic competencies to ensure the provision of safe patient care, and formation of a professional value system while making the tough decisions about what content and clinical activities should remain and which can be removed. The faculty of a graduate nursing program should be guided by regulatory requirements and accreditation standards to focus the curriculum on knowledge, competencies, and values needed by advanced practice nurses entering one of the four APRN roles with a specific identified population focus.

The traditionally designed prelicensure curriculum, using blocks of content structured around clinical specialties (e.g., pediatrics, medical–surgical, community health), is one curriculum approach used in nursing education. However, many programs are shifting to a concept-based curriculum that uses core nursing concepts to enhance the development of critical thinking skills (DeBoor, 2022). Concepts frequently used include oxygenation, stress and adaptation, quality and safety, social determinants of health, and collaboration as well as other broad concepts. Clinical activities in a nursing education program using a concept-based curriculum align with concepts discussed in the classroom, facilitating students' understanding and application of the concepts to actual clinical problems and issues.

Every nurse educator should be able to take a list of 10 clinical competencies or learning outcomes and reduce it to five essential competencies or learning outcomes by focusing on what is needed to produce safe, competent practitioners. If faculty members of a nursing education program wanted to design an accelerated program, they would have to decide what content to retain and what could be omitted without affecting the ability of their graduates to pass the licensure or certification examination and practice safely.

Making decisions like these is difficult, but what is often more difficult is getting a group of nurse educators to agree on the distinction between essential and enrichment content. Not surprisingly, these decisions are often made according to the clinical specialty backgrounds of the faculty; the specialties that are represented by the largest number of faculty members are usually deemed to hold the most essential content. These beliefs may explain why a group of nursing faculty members who teach medical–surgical or adult health nursing would suggest that a behavioral health clinical practice session should be cancelled so that all students may hear a guest speaker's presentation on arterial blood gases, or why many nursing faculty members advise students to practice for a year or two after graduation in a medical–surgical setting before transferring to the clinical setting in which students initially express interest, such as behavioral health, community health, or ambulatory settings.

This is not to suggest that the curriculum should consist solely of essential content. The enrichment curriculum is used to enhance learning, individualize activities, and motivate students. Students who meet essential clinical outcomes can select additional learning activities from the enrichment curriculum to satisfy needs for more depth and greater variety. Learners need to spend most of their time in the essential curriculum, but all students should have opportunities to participate in the enrichment curriculum as well.

The Espoused Curriculum Should Be the Curriculum-in-Use

In a landmark guide to the reform of professional education, Argyris and Schön (1974) proposed that human behavior is guided by operational theories of action that operate at two levels. The first level, espoused theory (the paper, official, or legitimate theory), is what professionals say that they believe and do. Espoused theory is used to explain and justify action. The other level, theory-in-use (the practice or operational theory), guides what professionals actually do in spontaneous behavior with others. Professionals often are unable to describe their theories-in-use, but, when they reflect on their behavior, they often discover that it is incongruent with their espoused theory of action. Incongruity between espoused theory and theory-in-use can result in ineffective individual practice as well as discord within a faculty group.

Similarly, a nursing curriculum often operates on two levels. The espoused curriculum is the one that is described in the self-study for accreditation or state approval and in course syllabi and clinical evaluation tools. This is the curriculum that is the subject of endless debate at faculty meetings. However, the curriculum-in-use is what happens. A faculty can agree to include or exclude certain learning activities, goals, or evaluation methods in the curriculum, but when clinical teachers are in their own clinical settings, they often do what seems right to them at the time, in the context of changing circumstances and resources. In fact, one of the competencies included on the National League for Nursing (NLN) Certified Nurse Educator (CNE®) Examination Detailed Test Blueprint is "Respond effectively to unexpected events that affect instruction" (NLN, 2021a). In other words, every teacher must interpret the espoused curriculum in view of circumstances and resources in the specific clinical setting and the individual needs of students and patients at the time. In reality, a faculty cannot prescribe to the last detail what teachers will teach (and when and how) and what learners will learn (and when and how) in clinical settings. Consequently, every student experiences the curriculum differently; hence the distinction between learning *activity* and learning *experience*.

When implementing a concept-based curriculum, both novice and experienced teachers may lose focus on the desired learning outcomes and how they relate to the underlying curriculum concepts. Instead, they adjust their teaching and planned learning activities to their own personal interests and expertise (DeBoor, 2022). Because a curriculum philosophy is designed to provide clear direction to the faculty for making decisions about teaching and learning, the integrity of the program of study may be compromised if the practice of an individual clinical teacher diverges widely from the collective values, beliefs, and ideals of the faculty. While academic freedom is valued in nursing education, faculty need to teach consistently with the philosophy adopted by the faculty as their framework. Thus, the exploration of incongruities between espoused curriculum and curriculum-in-use should engage the whole faculty on an ongoing basis while allowing enough freedom for individual faculty members to operationalize the curriculum in their own clinical teaching settings.

Quality Is More Important Than Quantity

Early on, Infante (1985) wrote, "The amount of time that students should spend in the clinical laboratory has been the subject of much debate among nurse educators" (p. 43). More than 40 years later, this statement still holds true for clinical teaching. Infante proposed that when teachers schedule a certain amount of time (e.g., 8 or 12 hours) for clinical learning activities, it will be insufficient for some students and unnecessarily long for others to achieve a particular learning outcome. The length of time spent in clinical activities is no guarantee of the amount or quality of learning that results. Both the activity and the amount of time need to be individualized.

Most nursing faculty members worry far too much about how many hours students spend in the clinical setting and too little about the quality of the learning that is taking place. A 2-hour activity that results in critical skill learning is far more valuable than an 8-hour activity that merely promotes repetition of skills and habit formation. Nurse educators often worry that there is not enough time to teach everything that should be taught, but a rapidly increasing knowledge base ensures that there will never be enough time. As the NCSBN 2014 simulation study results suggested, the quality of the student's clinical experience, not the number of hours spent in the clinical setting, is most important (Alexander et al., 2015). There is no better reason to identify the critical outcomes of clinical teaching and focus most of the available teaching time on guiding student learning to achieve those outcomes.

USING A PHILOSOPHY OF CLINICAL TEACHING TO IMPROVE CLINICAL EDUCATION

In the following chapters, the philosophical context for clinical teaching articulated here will be applied to discussions of the role of the clinical teacher and the process of clinical teaching. Differences in philosophical approaches can profoundly affect how individuals enact the role of clinical teacher. Every decision about teaching strategy, setting, outcome, and role behavior should be grounded in the teacher's philosophical perspective.

The core values inherent in an educator's philosophy of clinical teaching can serve as the basis for useful discussions with colleagues and testing of new teaching strategies. Reflection on one's philosophy of clinical teaching may uncover the source of incongruities between an individual's espoused theory of clinical teaching and the theory-in-use. When the outcomes of such reflection are shared with other clinical teachers, they provide a basis for the continual improvement of clinical teaching.

Nurse educators are encouraged to continue to develop their philosophies of clinical teaching by reflecting on how they view the goals of clinical education and how they carry out teaching activities to meet those goals. A philosophical approach to clinical education will thus serve as a guide to more effective practice and a means of ongoing professional development.

SUMMARY

The context in which clinical teaching occurs is a major determinant of its effectiveness. The context of the curriculum comprises internal and external influences, expectations, and demands that ground the curriculum and make it unique. The internal contextual factors include the faculty's shared beliefs about the goals of education, the nature of teaching and learning, and the roles of learners and teachers—the philosophical context of the curriculum.

A philosophical context for clinical teaching influences one's understanding of the role of the clinical teacher and the process of teaching in clinical settings. This philosophy includes fundamental beliefs about the value of clinical education, roles and relationships of teachers and learners, and how to achieve desired outcomes.

Terms related to clinical teaching were defined to serve as a common frame of reference. The adjective *clinical* means involving direct observation of the patient; its proper use is to modify nouns such as *practicum, instruction, practice,* or *evaluation.* The teacher's central activity is *clinical instruction* or *clinical teaching* rather than supervision, which implies administrative activities such as overseeing, directing, and managing the work of others. Because learning is an active, personal process, the student is the one who experiences the learning. Therefore, teachers cannot provide *clinical experiences*, but they can offer opportunities and activities that will facilitate learning. Each student will experience a learning activity in a different way.

The philosophy of clinical teaching described in this chapter comprises the authors' shared beliefs about clinical teaching and learning and the roles of teachers and students. Subsequent chapters operationalize this philosophical approach to clinical teaching.

Clinical education should reflect the nature of the professional practice. Practice in clinical settings exposes students to realities of professional practice that cannot be conveyed by a textbook or a simulation. Most professional practice situations are complex, unstable, and unique. Therefore, clinical learning activities should expose students to problems that cannot be solved easily with existing knowledge and technical skills. Whenever actual clinical learning activities cannot be provided, substitution with high-quality simulation opportunities may be preferable.

Another element of the philosophy of clinical teaching concerns the importance of clinical teaching. Because nursing is a professional practice discipline, the clinical practice of nurses and nursing students is more important than what they can demonstrate in a classroom. Clinical education provides opportunities for real-life experiences and the transfer of knowledge to practical situations.

In the clinical setting, nursing students encounter patients for the purpose of applying knowledge, testing theories, and learning skills. Although typical activities of nursing students focus on patient care, learning does not necessarily take place during caregiving. The central high-quality activity of the student in clinical education should be learning, not doing.

Sufficient learning time should be provided before performance is evaluated. Students need to engage in learning activities and practice skills before their performance is evaluated summatively. Skill acquisition is a complex process that involves making errors and learning how to correct and then prevent them. Teachers should allow plentiful learning time with ample opportunity for feedback before evaluating performance.

Another element of this philosophy of clinical teaching is the importance of a climate of mutual trust and respect that supports learning and student growth. Teachers and learners share the responsibility for maintaining this climate, but teachers are ultimately accountable for establishing expectations that faculty and students will be partners in achieving success.

Clinical teaching and learning should focus on essential knowledge, skills, and attitudes. Because every nursing education program has limited time for clinical teaching, this time is used to maximum advantage by focusing on the most common practice problems that learners are likely to encounter. Educators need to identify the knowledge, skills, and attitudes that are most essential for students to learn. Learners need to spend most of their time on this *essential curriculum*, but all students should have opportunities to participate in the *enrichment curriculum* as well.

In clinical settings, the *espoused curriculum* should be the *curriculum-in-use*. Although most faculty members would argue that there is one curriculum for a nursing education program, in reality the espoused curriculum is sometimes interpreted somewhat differently by each clinical teacher. Consequently, every student experiences this curriculum-in-use differently. A faculty cannot prescribe every detail of what teachers will teach and what learners will learn in clinical settings. Instead, it is usually more effective to specify broader outcomes and allow teachers and learners to meet them in a variety of ways. Individual faculty members are cautioned not to take individualizing the curriculum as a license to ignore the shared philosophy that guides curriculum development and implementation.

Finally, the distinction between quality and quantity of clinical learning is important. The quality of a learner's experience is more important than the amount of time spent in clinical activities. Both the activity and the amount of time should be individualized.

CERTIFIED NURSE EDUCATOR (CNE®) EXAMINATION TEST BLUEPRINT COMPETENCIES

1. **Facilitate Learning**
   A. Implement a variety of teaching strategies appropriate to:
      1. content,
      2. setting,
      3. learner needs,
      4. learning style, and
      5. desired learner outcomes
   B. Use teaching strategies based on:
      1. educational theory
   I. Create a positive learning environment that fosters a free exchange of ideas
   L. Respond effectively to unexpected events that affect instruction
2. **Facilitate Learner Development and Socialization**
   D. Create learning environments that facilitate learners' self-reflection, personal goal setting, and socialization to the role of the nurse
4. **Participate in Curriculum Design and Evaluation of Program Outcomes**
   B. Actively participate in the design of the curriculum to reflect:
      1. institutional philosophy and mission,
      2. current nursing and healthcare trends,
      3. community and societal needs,
      4. nursing principles, standards, theory, and research,
      5. educational principles, theory, and research, and
6. **Engage in scholarship, service, and leadership**
   C. Function effectively within the organizational environment and the academic community
      1. Identify how social, economic, political, and institutional forces influence nursing and higher education
      3. Integrate the values of respect, collegiality, professionalism, and caring to build an organizational climate that fosters the development of learners and colleagues
      4. Consider the goals of the nursing program and the mission of the parent institution when proposing change or managing issues

Note: The Certified Nurse Educator (CNE®) Competencies in this and subsequent chapters identify selected competencies that relate to the content in each chapter. The lettering and numbering of competencies correspond to the structure of the CNE Examination Detailed Test Blueprint. The CNE® Handbook with the full list of competencies is available at http://www.nln.org/Certification-for-Nurse-Educators/cne/handbook

Source: National League for Nursing (2021a). Copyright by National League for Nursing. Reprinted with permission.

CERTIFIED ACADEMIC CLINICAL NURSE EDUCATOR® (CNE®cl) EXAMINATION TEST BLUEPRINT COMPETENCIES

1. **Function within the Education and Health Care Environments**
   A. Function in the clinical educator role
      1. Bridge the gap between theory and practice by helping learners to apply classroom learning to the clinical setting
   B. Operationalize the curriculum
      2. Plan meaningful and relevant clinical learning assignments and activities
      3. Structure learner experiences within the learning environment to promote optimal learning
   C. Abide by legal requirements, ethical guidelines, agency policies, and guiding framework
      4. Facilitate learning activities that support the mission, goals, and values of the academic institution and the clinical agency
2. **Facilitate Learning in the Health Care Environment**
   A. Implement a variety of clinical teaching strategies appropriate to learner needs, desired learner outcomes, content, and context
   B. Ground teaching strategies in educational theory and evidence-based teaching practices
   C. Create a positive and caring learning environment
3. **Facilitate Learner Development and Socialization**
   A. Create learning environments that are focused on socialization to the role of the nurse

Note: The Certified Academic Clinical Nurse Educator (CNE®cl) Competencies in this and subsequent chapters identify selected competencies that relate to the content in each chapter. The lettering and numbering of competencies correspond to the structure of the CNE®cl Examination Detailed Test Blueprint. The CNE®cl Handbook with the full list of competencies is available at http://www.nln.org/Certification-for-Nurse-Educators/cnecl/cne-cl-handbook

Source: National League for Nursing. (2021b). Copyright by National League for Nursing. Reprinted with permission.

REFERENCES

Alexander, M., Durham, C. F, Hooper, J. I., Jeffries, P. R., Goldman, N., Kardong-Edgren, S., Kesten, K. S., Spector, N., Tagliareni, E., Radtke, B., & Tillman, C. (2015). NCSBN simulation guidelines for prelicensure nursing programs. *Journal of Nursing Regulation,* *3(6),* 39–42.
Argyris, C., & Schön, D. A. (1974). *Theory in practice: Increasing professional effectiveness.* Jossey-Bass.
DeBoor, S. S. (2022). Curriculum development in nursing. In M. H. Oermann, J. C. De Gagne, & B. C. Phillips (Eds.), *Teaching in nursing and role of the educator: The complete guide to best practice in teaching, evaluation, and curriculum development* (3rd ed., pp. 321–342). Springer Publishing Company.
Infante, M. S. (1985). *The clinical laboratory in nursing education* (2nd ed.) Wiley.
Institute of Medicine. (2011). *The future of nursing: Leading change, advancing health.* National Academies Press.
National Academies of Sciences, Engineering, and Medicine. (2021). *The future of nursing 2020–2030: Charting a path to achieve health equity.* The National Academies Press. https://doi.org/10.17226/25982.
National League for Nursing. (2021a). *Certified nurse educator (CNE®) 2021 candidate handbook.* http://www.nln.org/docs/default-source/default-document-library/cne-handbook-2021.pdf?sfvrsn=2

National League for Nursing. (2021b). *Certified nurse educator (CNEcl®) 2021 candidate handbook.* http://www.nln.org/docs/default-source/default-document-library/cnecl-handbook-2021.pdf?sfvrsn=2

Oermann, M. H., & Gaberson, K. B. (2021). *Evaluation and testing in nursing education* (6th ed.). Springer Publishing Company.

Schön, D. A. (1983). *The reflective practitioner: How professionals think in action.* Basic Books.

Schön, D. A. (1987). *Educating the reflective practitioner.* Jossey-Bass.

Valiga, T. M. (2022). Curriculum models and course development. In M. H. Oermann, J. C. De Gagne, & B. C. Phillips (Eds.), *Teaching in nursing and role of the educator: The complete guide to best practice in teaching, evaluation, and curriculum development* (3rd ed., pp. 343–355). Springer Publishing Company.

A robust set of instructor resources designed to supplement this text is located at http://connect.springerpub.com/content/book/978-0-8261-6705-7. Qualifying instructors may request access by emailing textbook@springerpub.com.

Outcomes of Clinical Teaching

To justify the enormous expenditure of resources on clinical education in nursing, teachers must have clear, realistic expectations of the desired outcomes of clinical learning. What knowledge, skills, and values can be learned only in clinical practice and not in the classroom or through independent learning activities?

Nurse educators have traditionally focused on the *process* of clinical teaching. Many hours of discussion in faculty meetings have been devoted to how and where clinical learning takes place, which clinical activities should be required, and how many hours should be spent in the clinical area. However, current accreditation criteria for higher education in general and nursing in particular focus on evidence that the educational program is producing important intended outcomes of learning. Therefore, the effectiveness of clinical teaching should be judged on the extent to which it produces such outcomes.

This chapter discusses broad outcomes of nursing education programs that can be achieved through clinical teaching and learning. These outcomes may be operationally defined and stated as competencies to be useful in guiding teaching and evaluation. Competencies for clinical teaching are discussed in Chapter 5.

INTENDED OUTCOMES

Since the 1980s, accrediting bodies in higher education have placed greater emphasis on measuring the performance of students and graduates, holding faculty and institutions accountable for the outcomes of their educational programs. Outcomes are the products of educational efforts—the behaviors, characteristics, qualities, or attributes that learners display at the end of an educational program. Teachers are responsible for specifying outcomes of nursing education programs that are congruent with the current and future needs of society. Changes in healthcare delivery systems, demographic trends, technological advances, and developments in higher education influence the competencies needed for professional nursing practice. A nursing faculty must take these influences into account when designing a context-relevant, evidence-informed curriculum (Iwasiw et al., 2020).

In the curriculum development process, after the faculty agrees on the philosophical context for the nursing education program, it formulates curriculum outcome statements (Iwasiw et al., 2020). The desired outcomes for clinical teaching contribute to the achievement of the overall curriculum outcomes and therefore should be congruent with them.

In nursing education, several different terms are used to refer to professional abilities that learners are expected to demonstrate at program completion. *Outcomes* can be used to indicate the actual abilities demonstrated by program graduates or the intended or expected results of the education program. The latter connotation is more accurately referred to as *outcome statements*. Other terms used to denote such outcomes are *terminal objectives* (usually associated with a behaviorist philosophical approach) and *goals* (more broadly stated). Expectations of performance at the end of a curriculum level or course are often termed *competencies*. In this book, we use the term *outcomes* to refer to the intended or expected results of clinical teaching.

The curriculum reform movement of the 1980s focused on the importance of outcomes rather than processes in improving the quality of teaching and learning in nursing education. This approach suggests that an orderly curriculum design does not take into account each learner's individual needs, abilities, and learning style and that learners can reach the same goal using different paths. Development of an outcome-driven curriculum begins with specifying the desired ends and then selecting content and teaching strategies that will bring about those ends.

Thus, planning for clinical teaching should begin with identifying learning outcomes that are necessary for safe, competent nursing practice. These outcome statements are derived from the philosophical approach chosen to guide curriculum development and are related to the three domains of learning: cognitive (knowledge and intellectual skills), psychomotor (skills and technological abilities), and affective (professional attitudes, values, and beliefs) (Oermann & Gaberson, 2021). They also include outcomes that incorporate more than one of these domains.

Cognitive Domain Outcomes

Clinical learning activities enable students to transfer knowledge learned in the classroom and through other learning activities to real-life situations. In clinical practice, theory and scientific evidence are translated into practice. By participating in clinical activities, students extend the knowledge that they acquired in the classroom, simulation lab, and self-directed learning. To use resources effectively and efficiently, clinical learning activities should focus on the development of knowledge that cannot be obtained in the classroom or other settings.

As discussed in Chapter 1, new content is added to nursing curricula frequently, reflecting the growth of new knowledge in nursing and healthcare. If the faculty is not willing to delete content that is no longer current or essential, the potential exists for creating a congested, content-saturated curriculum in which both students and teachers lose focus on the essential knowledge outcomes. Nurse educators thus need to develop evidence-based teaching skills that will help them to critically evaluate the evidence for content additions and deletions and decide what knowledge is essential for students to acquire. For nursing education programs that prepare candidates for licensure or certification, consulting the licensure or certification examination test plans will help the faculty to focus attention on essential program content. The National Council of State Boards of Nursing (NCSBN®) test plans for the National Council Licensing Examinations (NCLEX®) registered nurses (NCSBN, 2018) and practical nurses (NCSBN, 2019), and the American Association of Colleges of Nursing (AACN) publication *The Essentials: Core Competencies for Professional Nursing Education* (AACN, 2021) are helpful resources for selecting and organizing essential content in undergraduate and graduate programs in nursing.

Knowing how to practice nursing involves higher-level cognitive abilities such as problem solving, critical thinking, decision making, clinical reasoning, and clinical judgment. Traditional pedagogies that emphasize memorizing content and applying it in clinical practice are not sufficient for teaching the higher-level thinking abilities necessary to ensure high-quality nursing care and patient safety in the complex environments of the contemporary healthcare system. Newer approaches such as narrative pedagogy promote teaching the process of thinking instead of content. Shifting emphasis away from covering content to engaging students in understanding the evolving context for nursing practice promotes the development of thinking from multiple perspectives. When faculty members intend to teach higher-level thinking, they should use approaches that engage students as participants in questioning, interpreting, and thinking about significant issues from multiple perspectives.

Multiple terms are used to refer to how nurses use higher-level cognitive skills in practice (Griffits et al., 2017; Tyo & McCurry, 2019). Although they are often used interchangeably, *problem solving, critical thinking, clinical reasoning, clinical decision-making*, and *clinical judgment* skills have important differences that affect how they are taught and evaluated.

PROBLEM SOLVING

Clinical learning activities provide rich sources of realistic practice problems to be solved. Some problems are related to patients and their health needs; some arise from the clinical environment. As discussed in Chapter 1, most clinical problems tend to be complex, unique, and ambiguous. The ability to solve clinical problems is thus an important outcome of clinical teaching and learning, and the nursing process itself is a problem-solving approach. Most nurses and nursing students have some experience in problem solving, but complex problems of clinical practice often require new methods of reasoning and problem-solving strategies. Nursing students may not be functioning on a cognitive level that permits them to solve clinical problems effectively. To achieve this important outcome, clinical activities should expose the learner to realistic clinical problems of increasing complexity.

Many nurse educators and nursing students believe that problem solving is synonymous with critical thinking. However, the ability to solve clinical problems, while necessary, is insufficient for professional nursing practice, because it focuses on the solution or outcome instead of a more complete understanding of a situation in context. Problem solving involves identifying and defining the problem, collecting relevant data, proposing and implementing solutions, and evaluating their effectiveness. Students cannot solve problems for which they lack understanding and a relevant knowledge base. Only when students have a deep understanding of the problem in its context can they apply their knowledge and previous experience with similar patients as a framework for solving it (Oermann & Gaberson, 2021).

CRITICAL THINKING

Critical thinking is an important outcome of nursing education. Early emphasis on developing critical thinking skills was stimulated by previous criteria for the accreditation of prelicensure nursing education programs, but it is no longer an accreditation standard. However, current standards, competencies, and recommendations from the Institute of Medicine (IOM, 2011), Quality and Safety Education for Nurses (QSEN) Institute (QSEN, 2014a, 2014b), and AACN (2021) address the importance of nurses who can think critically to promote patient safety and achieve cost-efficient, quality patient outcomes. The complexity of patient needs, the ever-expanding amount of healthcare information that nurses need to process in clinical settings, and multiple ethical issues faced by nurses require the ability to think critically to arrive at sound judgments about patient care (Oermann & Gaberson, 2021).

Because critical thinking is integral to the ability to practice professional nursing, most employers of new nursing graduates expect them to demonstrate this competency. Nurse educators face the challenge of developing critical thinkers who are able to practice in the ever-changing healthcare environment of the future. This challenge suggests that clinical learning activities must focus intently on developing students' critical thinking skills and dispositions throughout the nursing education program.

Many definitions of critical thinking exist, and the faculty must agree on a definition that is appropriate for a given program to provide direction for teaching and assessing this outcome as well as communicating the construct effectively to students. Critical thinking is an intellectual process that involves analysis, logic, seeking information, discriminating between relevant and irrelevant data, applying standards, predicting outcomes, and drawing valid conclusions. It is purposeful, outcome-directed, and evidence-based (Alfaro-LeFevre, 2020; Griffits et al., 2017). Students who think critically:

- Ask questions and are curious and willing to search for answers.
- Consider alternate perspectives and explanations.
- Question current practices.
- Are open-minded (Oermann & Gaberson, 2021).

Although most educators would classify critical thinking as a cognitive domain outcome, some definitions of critical thinking characterize it as a composite of attitudes, knowledge, and skills. It involves the ability to seek and analyze truth systematically and with an open mind as well as attitudinal dimensions of self-confidence, perseverance, flexibility, creativity, open-mindedness, intellectual integrity, and inquisitiveness (Griffits et al., 2017). Critical thinking is not restricted only to clinical situations. Professionals in every discipline use critical thinking, and this often results in uncertainty about how to measure and evaluate this important outcome. However, clinical learning activities help learners to develop discipline-specific critical thinking skills as they observe, participate in, and evaluate nursing care in an increasingly complex and uncertain healthcare environment.

CLINICAL REASONING

Clinical reasoning is an essential feature of nursing competence that is often demonstrated by experienced nurses. Clinical reasoning is discipline-specific and applied in clinical settings. In nursing, clinical reasoning involves the process of evaluating the quantity, quality, and reliability of available evidence; analyzing and evaluating patient information; and making professional judgments about patient management. The result of clinical reasoning is *clinical judgment*, the inference or conclusion arrived at through clinical reasoning (Alfaro-LeFevre, 2020).

Effective clinical reasoning, like the more general process of critical thinking, is dependent on a deep understanding of the context of a particular patient. It is the ability to reason as clinical situations change, grasping the nature of patients' needs as they change over time. Clinical experience of appropriate duration, diversity, and quality is crucial for developing nursing students' clinical reasoning.

CLINICAL DECISION MAKING

Professional nursing practice requires nurses to make decisions about patient care involving problems, possible solutions, and the best approach to use in a particular situation. Other decisions involve managing the clinical environment, care delivery, and other activities (Oermann & Gaberson, 2021). The decision-making process involves gathering, analyzing, weighing, and valuing information in order to choose the best course of action from among several alternatives. However, nurses rarely know all possible alternatives, benefits, and risks; thus, clinical decision making usually involves some degree of uncertainty.

Clinical decision making should be guided by national standards of nursing practice such as the American Nurses Association (ANA), *Scope and Standards of Practice* (2021), specialty organization standards, and evidence-based practice (EBP) guidelines such as the American Society of PeriAnesthesia Nurses *Perianesthesia Nursing Standards, Practice Recommendations, and Interpretive Statements* (2020), and healthcare organization standards of care, policies and procedures, and critical paths (Alfaro-LeFevre, 2020). However, an essential element of decision making is recognizing when such standards and guidelines are not relevant to the particular clinical context (Alfaro-LeFevre, 2020). Decisions are also influenced by an individual's values and biases and by cultural norms, which affect the way the individual perceives and analyzes the situation. In nursing, clinical decision making is mutual and participatory with patients and staff members so that the decisions are more likely to be accepted. Clinical learning activities should involve learners in many realistic decision-making opportunities to produce this outcome.

CLINICAL JUDGMENT

According to the results of a 2013–2014 NCSBN Practice Analysis, newly licensed nurses are responsible for many complex decisions made in healthcare. If these decisions are based on sound clinical judgment, adverse healthcare events may be preventable. Based on these findings and those of additional research studies, the NCSBN developed a comprehensive clinical judgment model that depicts the process of clinical nursing judgment to serve as a model for measuring competence in using that process on the nursing licensure examination (Dickison et al., 2019).

Clinical judgment is the outcome of critical thinking and decision making. It is an iterative process that uses nursing knowledge to recognize cues about a clinical situation, generate and evaluate hypotheses, take evidence-based action, and evaluate outcomes in order to produce satisfactory clinical outcomes. The NCSBN Clinical Judgment Model (CJM) includes the following cognitive operations of nursing clinical judgment: cue recognition, hypotheses generation, hypotheses evaluation, taking action, and evaluating the outcomes. Because clinical judgments must be made within the unique context of each clinical encounter, the CJM includes contextual conditions or factors that contribute to the quality of clinical nursing judgment. These *conditioning factors* are classified as internal or individual (e.g., knowledge, skills, personal characteristics, level of prior experience) and external or environmental (e.g., task complexity, time pressures, resources, health record data, consequences, risks) to the nurse (Dickison et al., 2019).

There is ample evidence in the literature that newly licensed nurses have difficulty entering the workforce because they lack clinical judgment ability, and that this lack of preparedness is partially attributed to insufficient development of this ability in realistic clinical practice settings in their academic programs. However, there is less evidence of the effectiveness of specific pedagogies to support clinical judgment formation (Monagle et al., 2018). One clinical teaching strategy that may promote the development of clinical judgment is the use of structured reflection activities such as reflective journaling and debriefing of difficult clinical situations in group discussion (Monagle et al., 2018). The NCSBN CJM also may be used as a task model or education tool to teach the process of clinical judgment to nursing students based on a specific clinical scenario or unfolding case study. Task models define the cognitive operations of the CJM, the contextual factors or conditions that "set the stage" for the scenario, and the expected nursing actions that students need to perform (Dickison et al., 2019).

Evaluation of clinical judgment may be limited by the scarcity of discipline-specific measurement tools. The Lasater Clinical Judgment Rubric (Lasater, 2007) may be used for formative evaluation of nursing students' development of clinical judgment abilities (Lasater, 2011). Based on four aspects of clinical judgment identified by Tanner (Tanner, 2006), this rubric uses 11 dimensions that describe a trajectory of clinical judgment development in prelicensure students. The rubric may be useful in guiding student reflection on their clinical experiences during debriefing, clinical conferences, or journaling activities, and as a basis for giving students' feedback on their thinking as expressed in these activities. For summative evaluation, the NCSBN CJM may be used to guide faculty members' design of tests and clinical evaluation tools for assessing clinical judgment by targeting specific cognitive operations involved in that skill (Dickison et al., 2019).

Psychomotor Domain Outcomes

Skills are another important outcome of clinical learning. Nurses must possess adequate psychomotor, communication, technological, and organizational skills to practice effectively in an increasingly complex healthcare environment. Skills often have cognitive and attitudinal dimensions, but the skill outcomes that must be produced by clinical teaching typically focus on the performance component.

PSYCHOMOTOR SKILLS

Psychomotor skills are integral to nursing practice, and any deficiency in these skills among new graduates often leads to criticism of nursing education programs. Psychomotor skills enable nurses to perform effectively in action situations that require neuromuscular coordination. These skills are purposeful, complex, movement-oriented activities that involve an overt physical response. The term *skill* refers to the ability to carry out physical movements efficiently and effectively, with speed and accuracy. Therefore, psychomotor skill is more than the capability to perform; it includes the ability to perform proficiently, smoothly, and consistently under varying conditions and within appropriate time limits. Psychomotor skill learning requires practice with feedback in order to refine performance until the desired outcome is achieved. Thus, clinical learning activities should include plentiful opportunities for the practice of psychomotor skills with knowledge of results to facilitate the skill-learning process.

However, psychomotor skill development involves more than technical proficiency. While performing technical skills, nursing students and staff members must also perform caring behaviors, critical thinking, clinical reasoning, problem solving, and clinical decision making. However, the ability to integrate all of these competencies at once is not usually achieved until the technical skill component is so well developed that it no longer requires the nurse's or nursing student's conscious attention for successful performance. It is only at this point that the learner sees the whole picture and is able to focus on the patient as well as the technical skill performance.

INTERPERSONAL SKILLS

Interpersonal skills are used throughout the nursing process to assess patient and family needs, plan and implement care, evaluate the outcomes of care, and record and disseminate information. These skills include communication abilities, therapeutic use of self, and using the teaching process. Interpersonal skills involve knowledge of human behavior and social systems, but there is also a motor component largely comprising verbal behavior, such as speaking and writing, and nonverbal behavior, such as facial expression, body posture and movement, and touch. To encourage the development of these outcomes, clinical learning activities should provide opportunities for students to form therapeutic relationships with patients; to develop collaborative relationships with other health professionals; to document patient information, plans of care, care given, and evaluation results; and to teach patients, family members, and staff members individually and in groups.

Results of a study of a national sample of hospital nurse leaders' perceptions of the professional behaviors that new nurses need revealed communication and conflict-management skills to be among the most important of those behaviors (Sortedahl et al., 2020). In addition to communicating with patients, the most highly ranked skill, important communication behaviors also included listening to and communicating with families, prescribers, nursing assistants, managers, nurse colleagues, and other healthcare team members. Important conflict-related skills included using conflict management techniques, identifying signs of aggressive behavior in patient and family members, delivering feedback about improving performance, and addressing incivility in nurse colleagues. While Sortedahl et al. (2020) recommended that nursing faculty members emphasize the development of these essential competencies in the classroom, authentic clinical learning activities in real clinical settings would provide opportunities for students to apply knowledge to practice, receive guidance in reflecting on their experiences, and obtain feedback to guide improvement.

ORGANIZATIONAL SKILLS

Nurses need organization and time management skills to practice competently in a complex environment. In clinical practice, students learn how to set priorities, manage conflicting expectations, and sequence their work to perform efficiently. Sortedahl et al. (2020) found that hospital nurse leaders identified prioritization skills to be among the most important expectations of new nurses. It seems reasonable to expect that nurse leaders in other healthcare settings would have similar expectations.

One organizational skill that has become an important job expectation for professional nurses is delegation. In most healthcare settings, patient care is provided by a mix of licensed and assistive personnel, and professional nurses must know how to delegate various aspects of patient care to others. "When certain nursing care needs to be delegated, it is imperative that the delegation process and the jurisdiction [nurse practice act] be clearly understood so that it is safely, ethically and effectively carried out" (NCSBN and ANA, 2019, p. 1). Nurses need to know both the theory and skill of delegation—what to delegate, to whom, and under what circumstances—and to understand the legal aspects of empowering another person to carry out delegated tasks. However, students will not learn these skills unless they are given opportunities to practice them with faculty guidance. They need to learn to communicate clearly what is to be done; why, when, and how it should be done; and expectations for response or report back to the delegator. As discussed in Chapter 7, if clinical learning assignments focus exclusively on total patient care activities, students will not gain enough experience in carrying out this delegation responsibility to perform it competently as graduates.

Nursing faculty members, clinical teachers, administrators, and staff members in clinical facilities should provide opportunities for nursing students to understand delegation as a skill set that must be practiced in order to be performed competently. These skills may be initially developed in simulation activities. Debriefing after the simulation should focus not only on students' performance of delegation skills but also on the clinical judgment process that resulted in the decision to delegate the work to others during the simulation and the effect that the simulated delegation would have had on clinical outcomes.

Depending on the level of the learner (graduate or undergraduate student), clinical activities also provide opportunities to develop leadership and management skills. These skills include the ability to manage the care of a group of patients, to evaluate the performance of self and others, to allocate and coordinate resources, to work as part of a healthcare team, to ensure patient safety and quality of care, and to manage one's own career development. Among a national sample of hospital nurse leaders, Sortedahl et al. (2020) found that the leadership abilities in new nurses, such as proposing solutions to problems, self-confidence, taking appropriate risks, and empowering others, were rated moderately to very important.

Clinical teachers may model these skills to students as well as encourage staff members and preceptors in the clinical setting to do so. Examples of modeling opportunities include serving on a unit or institution-wide practice committee, demonstrating how to deal with a safety concern or healthcare error, and how to delegate effectively, as previously described. Because such activities are not always visible to nursing students in clinical settings, clinical teachers, preceptors, and staff members should discuss the rationale for their decisions and actions with students, intentionally making the thinking process more apparent.

Affective Domain Outcomes

Clinical learning also produces important affective outcomes—beliefs, values, attitudes, and dispositions that are essential elements of professional nursing practice (Oermann & Gaberson, 2021). Affective outcomes represent the humanistic and ethical dimensions of nursing. Professional nurses are expected to hold and act on certain values about patient care, such as respect for the patient's uniqueness, supporting patient autonomy and right to choose, and the confidentiality of patient information. The values of professional nursing are expressed in the American Nurses Association *Code of Ethics for Nurses* (2015), and the nursing faculty should introduce the code early in any nursing education program and reinforce its values by planning clinical learning activities that help students to develop these values.

Additionally, professional nurses must be able to use the processes of moral reasoning, values clarification, and values inquiry. In an era of rapid knowledge and technology growth, nursing education programs must also produce graduates who are lifelong learners, committed to their own continued professional development.

Students form the role of professional nurse in the clinical setting, where accountability is demanded and the consequences of choices and actions are readily apparent. The clinical setting provides opportunities for students to develop, practice, and test these affective outcomes. Clinical education should expose students to strong role models, including nursing faculty members and practicing nurses who demonstrate a commitment to professional values, and it should provide value development opportunities that serve to support role formation.

Integrated Domain Outcomes

Although in the previous discussion we attempted to classify outcomes according to cognitive, psychomotor, or affective domain, some intended outcomes of clinical learning include elements of all three domains. Two examples are cultural competence and healthcare quality and patient safety competence.

CULTURAL COMPETENCE

The U.S. population is becoming more racially and ethnically diverse. Based on the U.S. Census Bureau's 2017 National Population Projections, by the year 2060, the percentage of non-Hispanic White American residents will fall from 61% to 44%. The percentage of Black or African American residents is expected to increase from 13% to 15%, and the percentage of American residents of Asian origin will increase from 6% to 9%. The population of American residents of Hispanic origin is projected to increase from 18% to 28%, and the percentage of American residents who identify as being of two or more races will likely double, from 3% to 6% (Vespa et al., 2020). To respond competently to these demographic changes, nursing students must be prepared to deal with diversity in all of its forms. The AACN publications *Cultural Competency in Baccalaureate Nursing Education* (2008) and *Establishing a Culturally Competent Master's and Doctorally Prepared Nursing Workforce* (2009) address the need to integrate cultural competence in baccalaureate and graduate nursing education to support the development of patient-centered care that identifies, respects, and addresses differences in patients' values, preferences, and expressed needs. This rationale includes a focus on eliminating health disparities, achieving social justice for vulnerable populations, and functioning in a global environment and in partnership with other healthcare disciplines. Promoting culturally competent care is a priority in nursing and nursing education. Clinical teachers should plan learning activities that will challenge learners to explore cultural differences and to develop culturally appropriate responses to patient needs.

Cultural competence has no specific endpoint; it is an ongoing developmental process by which nurses understand, appreciate, and incorporate cultural expressions and worldviews into the care of patients and interactions with other healthcare providers. The development of cultural competence begins with awareness of cultural diversity and specific knowledge about cultural values, beliefs, rules, and traditions of the nurse's own culture. A concept related to cultural awareness is that of cultural humility, the belief that one's own culture is not the only or best one. These concepts cannot be learned only in the classroom; they require experience with culturally diverse patients over time and reflection on those experiences.

HEALTHCARE QUALITY AND PATIENT SAFETY COMPETENCIES

An important set of outcomes of clinical teaching is an evidence-based interprofessional practice within a quality improvement (QI) and patient safety framework. Competencies in quality and safety science are an important part of curricula to prepare all healthcare professionals. In nursing, the QSEN project was initiated in 2005 to transform healthcare by "addressing the challenge of preparing future nurses with the knowledge, skills, and attitudes necessary to continuously improve the quality and safety of the healthcare systems in which they work" (QSEN, 2014c). The knowledge, skills, and attitudes (KSAs) necessary to deliver safe quality care are related to six QSEN competencies: patient-centered care, teamwork and collaboration, EBP, QI, safety, and informatics (QSEN, 2014c). These competencies have been integrated into prelicensure and graduate nursing education programs as well as nurse residency programs.

The patient-centered care competency is defined as "Recogniz[ing] the patient or designee as the source of control and full partner in providing compassionate and coordinated care based on respect for patient's preferences, values, and needs" (QSEN, 2014b). QSEN prelicensure KSAs related to this competency include describing cultural, ethnic, and social backgrounds as sources of patient, family, and community values; providing care with respect for the diversity of human experience; and supporting care for patients whose values differ from one's own (QSEN, 2014b). KSAs for graduate students include integrating knowledge of multiple models of pain and suffering; assessing and treating pain and suffering based on patient values, preferences, and expressed needs; and valuing patients' expertise with their own health (QSEN, 2014a). Development of these KSAs can be facilitated through actual and simulated learning activities that allow learners to reflect on their experiences to identify gaps between current practice and practice that is informed by patient needs, values, and preferences.

Teamwork and collaboration is defined as "Function[ing] effectively within nursing and interprofessional teams, fostering open communication, mutual respect, and shared decision making to achieve quality patient care" (QSEN, 2014b). KSAs related to this competency for prelicensure students include describing scope of practice and roles of healthcare team members, functioning competently within one's own scope of practice as a team member, and respecting the centrality of the patient as a member of the healthcare team (QSEN, 2014b). Graduate student KSAs include identifying system barriers and facilitators of team effectiveness, participating in the creation and implementation of systems that support effective teamwork, and valuing the impact of system solutions on team functioning (QSEN, 2014a). Clinical learning activities in settings that offer natural opportunities to function as members of existing interprofessional teams, such as the operating room, promote acquisition of these KSAs.

The definition of EBP is "Integrat[ing] best current evidence with clinical expertise and patient/family preferences and values for delivery of optimal healthcare" (QSEN, 2014b). For this competency, prelicensure KSAs include describing reliable sources of evidence reports and clinical practice guidelines, consulting with clinical experts before deviating from evidence-based protocols, and valuing the need for continuous practice improvement based on new knowledge (QSEN, 2014b). Graduate student KSAs include determining evidence gaps within specialty practice, using efficient and effective search techniques to answer clinical questions, and valuing the need for ethical performance of research and QI (QSEN, 2014a). Depending on the level of the student, clinical learning activities provide rich opportunities to learn to deliver quality care based on reliable evidence and clinical guidelines for generalist or specialty nursing practice.

QI is defined as "Us[ing] data to monitor the outcomes of care processes and use improvement methods to design and test changes to continuously improve the quality and safety of healthcare systems" (QSEN, 2014b). KSAs related to this competency for prelicensure students include explaining the merit of measurement and variation in assessing quality of care, contributing to a root cause analysis of a sentinel event; and appreciating the impact of unwanted variation on patient care (QSEN, 2014b). For graduate students, KSAs include describing common quality measures in specialty practice, ensuring ethical management of QI projects, and valuing the role of measurement in quality patient care (QSEN, 2014a). Nursing faculty members should create clinical learning opportunities for students to collect data or use existing data to monitor quality of care, and to participate in or conduct QI projects, depending on the level of student.

The safety competency is defined as "Minimiz[ing] risk of harm to patients and providers through both system effectiveness and individual performance" (QSEN, 2014b). Prelicensure KSAs include describing factors that produce a culture of safety, using strategies to reduce reliance on memory, and valuing one's own role in error prevention (QSEN, 2014b). Graduate student KSAs related to this competency include describing best practices for promoting patient and provider safety specialty practice, employing a systems focus rather than individual blame when errors or close calls occur, and valuing the use of organizational error reporting systems (QSEN, 2014a). Nursing faculties should model the safety competency by "appreciat[ing] the cognitive and physical limits of human performance" (QSEN, 2014a), creating a just culture within their nursing education programs, and encouraging students to be forthcoming about and to learn from their errors and close calls. Planning clinical learning opportunities for students to use national patient safety resources in the clinical setting, partner with patients and their families to enhance safe care, and view patient safety through the lens of a total systems approach will facilitate their attainment of the safety KSAs.

The definition of the informatics competency is "Us[ing] information and technology to communicate, manage knowledge, mitigate error, and support decision making" (QSEN, 2014b). The growing use of electronic health records (EHRs) in various clinical settings requires students to have knowledge of this technology and at least a beginning ability to use EHRs to acquire patient information, use it to plan care, and document assessment findings and care given. The IOM's report *The Future of Nursing: Leading Change, Advancing Health* (2011) stated the expectation that nurses "use a variety of technological tools and complex information management systems that require skills in analysis and synthesis to improve the quality and effectiveness of care." This expectation implies that in addition to knowing how to document care electronically, nursing students must understand the concept of meaningful use of health information and value the use of nursing terminologies and classification systems to codify nursing data. Related QSEN KSAs for prelicensure students include giving examples of how technology and information management relate to patient safety and quality of care, using the EHR to document and plan patient care, and appreciating the need to seek lifelong learning of information technology skills (QSEN, 2014b). Graduate student KSAs include critiquing taxonomic and terminology systems used to enhance interoperability of information and knowledge management systems, participating in the creation of clinical decision-making supports and alerts, and appreciating the need for collaboration in developing patient care information systems (QSEN, 2014a). The most effective way to attain these outcomes is to integrate health information technology learning throughout the curriculum instead of offering it in a single course.

UNINTENDED OUTCOMES

Although nurse educators usually have intended outcomes in mind when they design clinical learning activities, those activities may produce positive or negative unintended outcomes as well. Positive unintended outcomes include career choices that students and new graduate nurses make when they have clinical experiences in various settings. Exposure to a wide variety of clinical specialties stimulates learners to evaluate their own desires and competence to practice in those areas and allows them to make realistic career choices. For example, nursing students who do not have clinical learning activities in a postanesthesia care unit are unlikely to choose postanesthesia nursing as a specialty. However, if students participate in clinical activities in a postanesthesia care unit, some will realize that they are well suited to practice nursing in this area, while others will decide that postanesthesia nursing is not for them. In either case, students will have a realistic basis for their career choices.

Clinical learning activities can produce negative unintended outcomes as well. Nurse educators often worry that students will learn bad practice habits from observing other nurses in the clinical environment. Often, students are taught to perform skills, document care, or organize their work based on reliable evidence, practice standards or guidelines, the instructor's preferences, or school or agency policy. However, students may observe staff members in the clinical setting who adapt skills, documentation, and organization of work to fit the unique needs of patients or the environment. Students often imitate the behaviors they observe, such as taking shortcuts and using work-arounds while performing skills, including omitting steps that the teacher may believe are important to produce safe, effective outcomes. The power of role models to influence students' behavior and attitudes should not be underestimated. However, the clinical teacher should be careful not to label the teacher's way as correct and all other ways as incorrect. Instead, the teacher should encourage learners to discuss the differences in practice habits that they have observed, evaluate them in terms of evidence for practice, and identify more positive role models.

Nursing students often report anxiety associated with clinical practice. High levels of anxiety can negatively affect students' mental and physical health, learning abilities, ability to interact effectively with healthcare team members, and ability to provide safe, compassionate patient care (Cornine, 2020). Many research studies have focused on interventions to reduce anxiety; Cornine's integrative review of nonsimulation strategies to reduce undergraduate nursing students' anxiety in clinical settings identified three categories of interventions that had some evidence of decreasing students' anxiety, although the strength of the evidence was generally weak. *Student-led interventions* included strategies such as expressive self-regulatory writing before clinical practice, and use of personal digital devices as reference tools during clinical practice. *Faculty-led behavioral interventions* that reduced anxiety through faculty interactions with students included use of "inviting teaching behaviors" (Cornine, 2020, p. 231) such as conveying respect for students and creating a positive learning environment. *Faculty-led structural interventions* include changes in the context for learning such as pairing students for clinical learning assignments, using a limited number of clinical learning sites by assigning students to a "home clinical site" for as many clinical practica as possible, and "prelab" activities such as receiving a clinical learning assignment, gathering data, and preparing a plan of care in advance of the scheduled clinical learning activities (Cornine, 2020, p. 231). Although many nursing faculty members believe that techniques such as deep breathing, meditation, mindfulness practice, and guided general relaxation exercises are effective in preventing clinical-related anxiety, there is little high-quality evidence that these interventions when used alone are effective. Published studies that identify the causes of or reasons for student anxiety related to clinical practice are scarce, and it is unlikely that one type of intervention would be equally effective in reducing anxiety from all causes; more research on this topic is needed.

Another negative unintended outcome of clinical learning may be academic dishonesty. Academic dishonesty is intentional participation in deceptive practices such as lying, cheating, or false representation regarding one's academic work. While academic dishonesty is typically viewed as classroom-related conduct, nursing students' actions in clinical settings, such as falsely documenting assessment findings, breaking patient confidentiality, and failing to report errors also must be considered (McClung & Gaberson, 2021). Clinical teachers often try to instill the traditional healthcare cultural value that good nurses do not make errors. A standard of perfection is unrealistic for any practitioner, let alone nursing students whose mistakes are an inherent part of learning new knowledge and skills. A teacher's emphasis on perfection in clinical practice may produce the unintended result of student dishonesty to avoid punishment for making mistakes. Punishment for mistakes, in the form of low grades or negative performance evaluations, is not effective in preventing future errors. The unintended result of punishment for mistakes may be that learners conceal errors or lack of knowledge or skill. Students bluffing their way through tasks or failure to report errors can have dangerous consequences for patients in clinical settings, and also creates lost opportunities for learners to learn to correct and then prevent their mistakes.

An ANA position statement recommends a just culture model as an alternative to a punitive system. In the language of the patient safety movement, a just culture "seeks to create an environment that encourages individuals to report mistakes so that the precursors to errors can be better understood in order to fix the system issues" (ANA, 2010, p. 2). If the instructor establishes a learning climate of mutual trust and respect, sets a standard of excellence instead of perfection, acknowledges the possibility of errors, assures students of respectful treatment when they admit their inadequacies, and models exemplary academic and professional integrity, students will be less likely to behave dishonestly (McClung & Gaberson, 2021).

SUMMARY

Outcomes of clinical teaching include abilities in cognitive, psychomotor, and affective domains. Current nursing education program accreditation criteria focus on evidence that meaningful outcomes of learning have been produced. The effectiveness of clinical teaching can be judged on the extent to which it produces intended learning outcomes.

Clinical learning activities should focus on the development of *knowledge* that cannot be acquired in the classroom or other learning settings. Higher-level knowledge outcomes include cognitive skill in problem solving, critical thinking, clinical decision making, clinical reasoning, and clinical judgment. Nurses need *problem solving* ability to find solutions to patient- or healthcare environment-related problems that are typically unique, complex, and ambiguous. *Critical thinking* is a process used to determine a course of action after collecting appropriate data, analyzing the validity and utility of the information, evaluating multiple lines of reasoning, and coming to valid conclusions. Critical thinking is facilitated by attitudinal dimensions of self-confidence, maturity, and inquisitiveness.

Clinical learning activities help learners to develop discipline-specific *clinical reasoning* skills as they observe, participate in, and evaluate nursing care. *Clinical decision making* involves gathering, analyzing, weighing, and valuing information in order to choose the best course of action from among a number of alternatives. Because nurses rarely know all possible alternatives, benefits, and risks, clinical decision making usually involves some degree of uncertainty. Clinical education should involve learners in realistic situations that require them to make decisions about patients, staff members, and the clinical environment in order to produce this outcome. *Clinical judgment* is the outcome of critical thinking and decision making. This process includes the operations of cue recognition, hypotheses generation, and hypotheses evaluation, taking action, and evaluating the outcomes. Clinical teachers facilitate students' development of clinical judgment ability by providing learning opportunities in realistic clinical practice settings, applying a clinical judgment task model to a specific clinical scenario or unfolding case study, and using structured reflection activities such as journaling and debriefing of difficult simulated or real clinical situations.

Psychomotor skills are another important outcome of clinical learning. Many psychomotor skills have important cognitive and attitudinal dimensions. *Interpersonal skills* are used to assess client needs, plan and implement patient care, evaluate the outcomes of care, and record and disseminate information. Important interpersonal skills needed by nurses include communication, therapeutic use of self, teaching patients and others, and using conflict management techniques. Nurses need *organizational skills* in order to set priorities, manage conflicting expectations, sequence their work to perform efficiently, and delegate nursing tasks to others appropriately. Clinical learning activities also provide opportunities for learners to develop leadership and management skills.

Clinical learning also produces important affective outcomes that represent the humanistic and ethical dimensions of nursing. Professional nurses are expected to hold and act on certain values with regard to patient care and to use the processes of moral reasoning, values clarification, and values inquiry. These values are developed and internalized through the process of professional role formation. In an era of rapid knowledge and technological growth, nursing education programs must also produce graduates who are lifelong learners, committed to their own continued professional development.

Some outcomes, such as cultural competence and healthcare quality and patient safety competencies, encompass all three domains. Examples of these competencies were provided.

Clinical learning activities also produce unintended positive and negative outcomes. Exposure to a wide variety of clinical specialties stimulates learners to evaluate their own desires and competence to practice in those areas and allows them to make realistic career choices. However, observing various role models in the clinical environment may result in students' learning bad practice habits. Nursing students often report anxiety associated with clinical practice, which can negatively affect their mental and physical health, learning abilities, ability to interact effectively with healthcare team members, and ability to provide safe, compassionate patient care. Several interventions to reduce anxiety were discussed, although the strength of the evidence to support these interventions is generally weak. The unintended result of a teacher's unrealistic emphasis on perfection in clinical practice may be academically dishonest behavior among students. Suggestions for promoting academic honesty in clinical learning were provided.

CNE® EXAMINATION TEST BLUEPRINT CORE COMPETENCIES

1. **Facilitate Learning**
   A. Implement a variety of teaching strategies appropriate to:
      5. desired learner outcomes
   G. Model reflective thinking practices, including critical thinking
   H. Create opportunities for learners to develop their own critical thinking skills
   I. Create a positive learning environment that fosters a free exchange of ideas
   P. Act as a role model in practice settings
   Q. Foster a safe learning environment
2. **Facilitate Learner Development and Socialization**
   B. Provide resources for diverse learners to meet their individual learning needs
   D. Create learning environments that facilitate learners' self-reflection, personal goal setting, and socialization to the role of the nurse
   E. Foster the development of learners in these areas:
      1. cognitive domain
      2. psychomotor domain
      3. affective domain
   G. Encourage professional development of learners

CNE®cl EXAMINATION TEST BLUEPRINT CORE COMPETENCIES

1. **Function within the Education and Health Care Environments**
   A. Function in the clinical educator role
      5. Act as a role model of professional nursing within the clinical learning environment
   B. Operationalize the curriculum
      3. Identify learners' goals and outcomes
      6. Implement clinical learning activities to help learners develop interprofessional collaboration and teamwork skills
      7. Provide opportunities for learners to develop problem-solving and clinical reasoning skills related to course objectives (e.g., learning outcomes)

2. **Facilitate Learning in the Health Care Environment**
    A. Create opportunities for learners to develop critical thinking and clinical reasoning skills
    B. Promote a culture of safety and quality in the healthcare environment
4. **Apply Clinical Expertise in the Health Care Environment**
    E. Demonstrate sound clinical reasoning
5. **Facilitate Learner Development and Socialization**
    A. Mentor learners in the development of professional nursing behaviors, standards, and codes of ethics
    C. Promote professional integrity and accountability
    E. Encourage ongoing learner professional development via formal and informal venues
    G. Create learning environments that are focused on socialization to the role of the nurse
    J. Encourage various techniques for learners to manage stress (e.g., relaxation, meditation, mindfulness)

REFERENCES

Alfaro-LeFevre, R. (2020). *Critical thinking, clinical reasoning, and clinical judgment: A practical approach* (7th ed.). Elsevier.

American Association of Colleges of Nursing. (2008). *Cultural competency in baccalaureate nursing education.* Retrieved from https://www.aacnnursing.org/Portals/42/AcademicNursing/CurriculumGuidelines/Cultural-Competency-Bacc-Edu.pdf

American Association of Colleges of Nursing. (2009). *Establishing a culturally competent master's and doctorally prepared nursing workforce.* Retrieved from https://www.aacnnursing.org/Portals/42/AcademicNursing/CurriculumGuidelines/Cultural-Competency-Grad-Edu.pdf

American Association of Colleges of Nursing. (2021). *The essentials: Core competencies for professional nursing education.* Author.

American Nurses Association. (2010). *Just culture* [position statement]. Author.

American Nurses Association. (2015). *Code of ethics for nurses with interpretive statements.* http://nursingworld.org/DocumentVault/Ethics-1/Code-of-Ethics-for-Nurses.html

American Nurses Association. (2021). *Nursing: Scope and standards of practice* (4th ed.). Author.

American Society of PeriAnesthesia Nurses. (2020). *2021-2022 Perianesthesia nursing standards, practice recommendations, and interpretive statements.* Author.

Cornine, A. (2020). Reducing student anxiety in the clinical setting: An integrative review. *Nursing Education Perspectives, 41*(4), 229–234. Retrieved from https://doi.org/10.1097/01.NEP.0000000000000633

Dickison, P., Haerling, K. A., & Lasater, K. (2019). Integrating the National Council of State Boards of Nursing Clinical Judgment Model into nursing educational frameworks. *Journal of Nursing Education, 58*(2), 72–78. Retrieved from https://doi.org/10.3928/01484834-20190122-03

Griffits, S., Hines, S., Moloney, C., & Ralph, N. (2017). Characteristics and processes of clinical reasoning in nurses and factors related to its use: A scoping review protocol. *JBI Database of Systematic Reviews and Implementation Reports, 15*(12), 2832–2836. https://doi.org/10.11124/JBISRIR-2016-003273

Institute of Medicine. (2011). *The future of nursing: Leading change, advancing health.* National Academies Press.

Iwasiw, C. L., Andrusyszyn, M.-A., & Goldenberg, D. M. (2020). *Curriculum development in nursing education* (4th ed.). Jones & Bartlett Learning.

Lasater, K. (2007). Clinical judgment development: Using simulation to create an assessment rubric. *Journal of Nursing Education, 46*(11), 496–503. Retrieved from https://doi.org/10.3928/01484834-20071101-04

Lasater, K. (2011). Clinical judgment: The last frontier for evaluation. *Nurse Education in Practice, 11*(2), 86–92. https://doi.org/10.1016/j.nepr.2010.11.013

McClung, E. L., & Gaberson, K. B. (2021). Academic dishonesty among nursing students: A contemporary view. *Nurse Educator, 46*(2), 111–115. https://doi.org/10.1097/NNE.0000000000000863

Monagle, J. L., Lasater, K., Stoyles, S., & Dieckmann, N. (2018). New graduate nurse experiences in clinical judgment: What academic and practice educators need to know. *Nursing Education Perspectives, 39*(4), 201–206. https://doi.org/10.1097/01.NEP.0000000000000336

National Council of State Boards of Nursing. (2018). *Test plan for the National Council Licensure Examination for registered nurses*. https://www.ncsbn.org/2019_RN_TestPlan-English.pdf

National Council of State Boards of Nursing. (2019). *Test plan for the National Council Licensure Examination for practical nurses*. https://www.ncsbn.org/2020_NCLEXPN_TestPlan-English.pdf

National Council of State Boards of Nursing and American Nurses Association. (2019). *National guidelines for nursing delegation*. Retrieved from https://www.ncsbn.org/NGND-PosPaper_06.pdf

Oermann, M. H., & Gaberson, K. B. (2021). *Evaluation and testing in nursing education* (6th ed.). Springer Publishing Company.

Quality and Safety Education for Nurses Institute. (2014a). *Graduate QSEN competencies*. Retrieved from http://qsen.org/competencies/graduate-ksas

Quality and Safety Education for Nurses Institute. (2014b). *Pre-licensure KSAs*. Retrieved from http://qsen.org/competencies/pre-licensure-ksas

Quality and Safety Education for Nurses Institute. (2014c). *Project overview: The evolution of the Quality and Safety Education for Nurses initiative*. Retrieved from http://qsen.org/about-qsen/project-overview

Sortedahl, C., Ellefson, S., Fotsch, D., & Daley, K. (2020). The professional behaviors new nurses need: Findings from a national survey of hospital nurse leaders. *Nursing Education Perspectives, 41*(4), 207–214. https://doi.org/10.1097/01.NEP.0000000000000622

Tanner, C. A. (2006). Thinking like a nurse: A research-based model of clinical judgment in nursing. *Journal of Nursing Education, 45*(6), 204–211. https://doi.org/10.3928/01484834-20060601-04

Tyo, M. B., & McCurry, M. K. (2019). An integrative review of clinical reasoning teaching strategies and outcome evaluation in nursing education. *Nursing Education Perspectives, 40*(1), 11–17. https://doi.org/10.1097/01.NEP.0000000000000375

Vespa, J., Medina, L., & Armstrong, D. M. (2020). *Demographic turning points for the United States: Population projections for 2020 to 2060*. U.S. Census Bureau. Retrieved from https://www.census.gov/content/dam/Census/library/publications/2020/demo/p25-1144.pdf

3

Developing Clinical Learning Sites: Prelicensure Through Advanced Practice

Nursing care occurs in diverse settings where there are patients (individuals, families, groups, and communities) who can benefit from the services of a professional nurse. Professional nurses assume multiple roles as they work with patients of all ages, races, ethnic groups, and cultures. These patients have the full scope of health promotion; health maintenance; and acute, chronic, and rehabilitation care needs.

In an ideal world, all nursing students would have clinical learning activities in all settings, with all patient populations, and in all professional nursing roles, and they would be prepared to adapt to rapid changes with patients, health issues, care locations, and approaches to care. Students would have opportunities to work with people from cultures other than their own and implement care that recognizes the global influences on both health and illness.

Nursing education does not exist in such an ideal world. All students cannot participate in every learning activity nor can every student provide care for all these diverse groups during their nursing education. Faculty must make difficult choices about clinical education with the hope that the breadth and depth of students' clinical learning activities result in the development of the core competencies and skills needed for safe and effective nursing practice. For students who are already licensed nurses and pursuing advanced degrees, their clinical experiences must help them grow as professionals as they move to more advanced levels of practice. Their clinical education should focus on a more autonomous role. They need to develop skilled decision making and use advanced assessment, diagnosis, planning, implementation, and evaluation skills to provide coordinated care.

This chapter explores options for providing clinical learning opportunities for undergraduate and graduate nursing students in a wide variety of clinical sites. Examples are provided of clinical learning opportunities in specialized patient care areas not used regularly for clinical learning, community-based settings such as camps and wellness centers, clinical learning at distant sites, and international settings.

NEED FOR DIVERSE AND VARIED CLINICAL SETTINGS

The traditional approach to prelicensure clinical nursing education involves a faculty member working with a group of students (approximately 6–12, although this can vary from program to program), typically on an acute care unit in a hospital, for a portion of a clinical shift. At the graduate level, the apprenticeship model using a preceptor-student teaching method has been the primary approach used for advanced practice nursing education (American Association of Colleges of Nursing [AACN], 2021a). These approaches, while frequently used in nursing education, may provide an unpredictable, rapidly changing, and haphazard learning environment and may no longer be sustainable given limited preceptor availability and growing competition for clinical sites (AACN, 2021a; Gubrud-Howe, 2020).

Regardless of educational level, factors such as changing patient demographics, variable diagnoses and acuity of patients, diverse care needs, and advances in medical technology impact the learning opportunities during clinical practice. Because of the high patient acuity and complexity, many sites do not permit achievement of the full scope of clinical learning objectives. Collaboration with other disciplines, acting as a change agent, being a patient advocate, and the development of many key assessment and psychomotor skills can be difficult in a setting where all patients are critically ill. Because of the increasingly specialized nature of many acute care units (e.g., cardiovascular, orthopedic, endocrine), it is challenging for students to see a broad scope of patient problems and gain a generalist perspective of care when they have a finite number of clinical hours and a predetermined schedule.

Additionally, due to decreasing length of inpatient stays and economic pressures to provide care in outpatient and community settings, limited (and, in some cases, decreased) numbers of clinical learning activities take place on hospital units that provide care for children, individuals with psychiatric illnesses, and women and families during pregnancy and childbirth. Even with these challenges, faculty teaching prelicensure students may still believe that traditional rotations through medical–surgical specialty areas with specific numbers of clinical hours in those areas are important. However, these clinical hours may also include observation and simulation experiences and use of a wide variety of alternative settings without clinical teachers directly present to oversee patient care.

Even when traditional acute care placements are appropriate, implementing clinical learning activities in such settings can be challenging. High demand for clinical placements from nursing education programs (often with rapidly increasing enrollments) and other healthcare professions programs have overwhelmed many acute care agencies. Both staff members and patients can be asked to interact with students 24 hours a day, 7 days a week. As a result, acute care agencies often place limitations on the numbers of students per unit or the days and times that students can be present. In some cases, the mandated clinical group size is so limited that some students in a clinical group must be scheduled for other clinical learning activities elsewhere so that fewer students are present on the clinical unit. In other cases, the group size must be kept very small, a remedy that is usually neither economically feasible nor ideal for learning and meeting the educational goals of the course and the program. Engaging in these alternate clinical activities may decrease students' opportunity to actively participate in learning the professional nursing role and may also consume the time and resources of staff in these other areas. Faculty members must evaluate the appropriateness of observation activities, address concerns about student guidance in the absence of a clinical instructor, and support staff members as they encounter different students arriving for observation activities each day.

The rapidly rising cost of healthcare in acute care settings and the demand for safe, quality care led to the examination of healthcare delivery at a national level. The Institute of Medicine's (IOM, 2011) report, *The Future of Nursing: Leading Change, Advancing Health*, encouraged the transformation of the healthcare system from acute care to community settings. Nursing has made progress in meeting these recommendations, but further work remains to advance nursing education and address scope of practice issues (National Academies of Sciences, Engineering, and Medicine [NASEM], 2016). Past education approaches that have been used in clinical education may no longer prepare nurses for future practice roles.

Faculty have re-examined clinical nursing education and explored alternative approaches. They have shifted emphasis from acute care to primary care and increased the variety of clinical settings used for teaching to allow for a broader scope of experience for students. Additionally, national and international leaders have advocated for nursing education to provide enhanced education that integrates social determinants of health, as these issues shape health and health concerns (National League for Nursing [NLN], 2019). Unfortunately, the social determinants of health are not adequately incorporated into nursing education (Tilden et al., 2018). Yet, addressing how social, economic, environmental, cultural, and political forces impact health provides for unique emerging clinical learning opportunities, many of which will take place outside of acute care settings.

Another driving force for the use of diverse settings for clinical learning is a call to increase the global and cultural competencies of graduates of nursing education programs. Nursing has issued guidelines and suggested competencies for nursing students and programs to develop needed knowledge and development of culturally competent practice (NLN, 2016). Clinical learning experiences need to support the development of graduates who can provide culturally responsive care and practice from a global perspective. Examples of these experiences include:

▪ Participation in a cultural immersion experience.
▪ Participation in community projects involving community members—for example, health fairs, community forums, and the like—to understand concerns, values, and beliefs about healthcare.
▪ Development of partnerships with community organizations such as churches, businesses, schools, or community groups serving vulnerable populations.
▪ Service-learning opportunities working with populations such as immigrants, migrants, underserved or indigenous groups.

REIMAGINING CLINICAL LEARNING SETTINGS

Nursing care can be learned wherever students have contact with patients. Learning objectives do not prescribe a specific setting where the learning activities must take place. The core components of a clinical learning activity can be present in settings other than acute care hospital units and might include patient contact; opportunities for students to have an active role in assessment, goal setting, and then planning, implementing, and evaluating care; clinical reasoning and problem-solving opportunities; competent guidance (from the clinical teacher or someone designated to take on the teaching role in that site); and skill development (intellectual as well as psychomotor).

Benefits

Reimagining and transforming clinical placements for nursing students have multiple benefits. These include preparing students to be a part of a healthcare team and system in which the acute care hospital is but one part. Not only will students learn about the varied settings in which healthcare is provided, but they will also have opportunities to develop skills that these settings are best able to provide. For example, development of a psychomotor skill such as initiation of IV therapy, including the clinical assessment and decision-making skills that go with this routine procedure, might be best learned in a perioperative setting. Development of therapeutic communication competencies might be best achieved in rehabilitation settings where it is possible to have sustained patient contact. The best opportunities to learn care planning, evaluation, and revision might be available in a home health setting where multidisciplinary care planning is fully integrated into patient services. Or, for advanced practice nursing students, development of care coordination skills may be best achieved through a preceptorship in a nursing clinic.

Clinical learning activities in community-based settings allow nursing students to work with patients where they live and work. Students see the challenges that patients face as they implement self-care for health promotion and maintenance, as well as see the impact on family members. Collaboration with other members of the healthcare team is a natural, necessary, and active part of care delivery in community-based settings.

Nursing students can participate in creatively designed, rigorous, high-quality clinical learning activities almost anywhere. This chapter discusses clinical learning opportunities in alternative patient care sites, community-based sites, distant sites, and international settings. It also reviews various practical aspects of implementing clinical learning activities in these settings by addressing common agency, faculty, and student problems and suggesting solutions for such problems.

EXAMPLES OF ALTERNATIVE CLINICAL LEARNING SETTINGS

Clinical learning activities in alternative settings include opportunities for students to meet specific learning objectives while caring for patients. Four categories will be used as examples of such activities. The first consists of specialized patient care areas that are not used regularly as clinical learning sites. Some of these patient care sites (e.g., the operating room [OR]) have been virtually eliminated as clinical learning sites by prelicensure nursing education programs, while others (e.g., outpatient clinics, nursing homes) are underused, despite the rich learning opportunities provided for students in these settings. The second category includes community-based sites where provision of healthcare may not be the prime focus of the site or agency but provide learning opportunities for clinical nursing students. Examples are schools, camps, or community agencies. An example of a learning activity in a community-based site is service learning. With the growth of technology and online nursing education, distance sites provide a third category of alternative clinical learning opportunities. The fourth category is the use of international clinical learning activities. Although these learning opportunities may be brief (often 1 week), students gain valuable experiences in diverse international settings while serving as part of a team providing health services.

There are other clinical learning activities not included in this discussion. One is an observation in which students' objectives are best achieved while they maintain a nonparticipant role in the clinical setting. Another is a special event held as part of a clinical rotation (such as a trip to an art gallery or attending a play), designed to help students increase a specific skill, competency, or self-awareness. Also, clinical observations and interactions that are part of a didactic course are not included. Although potentially valuable as learning activities, riding in an ambulance with emergency medical service providers or visiting a hospital, clinic, or patient group as part of a course is not a clinical learning activity if there is no patient care in which the student participates.

CLINICAL LEARNING IN SPECIALIZED PATIENT CARE SITES

With the diversity of clinical practice sites, there are many examples of clinical learning activities in specialized patient care sites that are often underutilized in clinical education. Several examples will be used to illustrate how such sites can be optimized.

Outpatient Clinics

Outpatient settings such as primary care practices, specialty clinics, and rehabilitation programs are often difficult to use effectively for prelicensure clinical learning sites because of the lack of sufficient RN role models and the difficulty placing large numbers of students at one site, which can make clinical teaching by the faculty difficult. This can be addressed through placement of students in a single large clinical facility. Major medical centers may have multiple specialty clinics and centers that allow students to participate in a multidisciplinary approach to patient care focused on specific problems. For example, clinics that focus on pain management, wounds, gastroenterology, women's health, behavioral and mental health, diabetes, rehabilitation and sport medicine, and others may be appropriate for student learning. Depending upon geographic location and availability, faculty can also consider outpatient oncology centers, dialysis centers, rural clinics, or Indian health services as possible clinical learning sites. Students will have opportunities to engage in assessment, teaching, and delivery of focused care while interacting with a wide range of healthcare providers in these settings. Nursing staff members provide mentoring of the students while clinical teachers are available and provide regular supervisory visits. Student–teacher conferencing activities allow for an assessment of student learning as well as an opportunity for students to ask questions. Group conferencing with several clinical nursing students can be used to share experiences with other students and enable them to make comparisons and contrasts between the learning settings, the care provided, and the patients seen.

Clinics also provide excellent clinical learning opportunities for graduate nursing students. Working with staff in these settings allows for students to engage in the practice environment while expanding their care responsibilities and role. The students gain specialized competencies needed for advanced practice roles. Graduate students can refine skills of advanced assessment, develop differential diagnostic abilities, engage in decision making, and demonstrate their clinical judgment and decision making in these settings.

Operating Room (OR) and Other Perioperative Settings

Most nursing education programs eliminated an OR clinical rotation from their undergraduate curricula many years ago, but in doing so, nursing faculty have overlooked rich clinical learning opportunities. Many hospitalized patients for whom acute care nurses provide care pass through the OR at some time during their hospitalization. Knowledge about patients' surgical experiences can greatly enhance the knowledge and skills of the nurse caring for the patients both before and after surgery. Perioperative environments are ideal settings for learning application of the nursing process, and perioperative clinical learning activities can contribute to the achievement of a wide variety of program outcomes. In addition to developing expected skills like aseptic technique, students see the use of the latest technology both in the surgical procedures and in the overall care of surgical patients. Students learn about safety, effective communication, and work with an interdisciplinary team.

Nursing students can develop a wide array of psychomotor skills in perioperative settings, such as catheter care, maintenance of IV lines, pain management, skin and wound care, positioning, and care of unconscious patients. Additionally, inclusion of perioperative learning activities in undergraduate nursing curricula will increase nurses' knowledge of patients' surgical experiences. It may also increase the number of nursing students who choose the perioperative specialty after graduation, possibly helping to minimize the predicted shortage of nurses in the perioperative setting.

One way to include more perioperative clinical learning activities is with a practicum or capstone experience with preceptor guidance (Fleming et al., 2019). Such capstone courses allow students to apply knowledge and nursing principles learned from various courses throughout the program while being guided by an expert OR clinician. Another approach used by nursing programs to provide these learning experiences is through elective clinical courses. These elective courses offer students clinical learning experiences in perioperative, intraoperative, and postanesthesia care units, thus allowing students to experience the continuum of care while simultaneously developing specialized skills (Maneval et al., 2020).

Nursing Homes and Extended Care Facilities

Competency in the care of older adults, including frail elderly individuals, is a desired outcome of all nursing curricula. Given the growing aging population in the United States, almost all graduates will be caring for elderly patients, regardless of their future work setting or level of education. An underused clinical learning setting for gaining knowledge and competencies about care for the elderly is the nursing home or extended care facility.

Nursing homes provide an opportunity for students to practice multiple psychomotor skills while addressing the complex care needs of the elderly population. With a rich variety of patients, learning needs can be matched with clinical learning assignments as students provide holistic care while developing their health assessment, communication, leadership, and delegation skills with a wide range of residents. Additionally, students learn about the complex health issues of this population as they address multiple health problems, polypharmacy concerns, cognitive impairments, and changes in functional health status of this population. Nursing homes provide many opportunities for students to practice implementing care that has a long-term impact.

Another benefit of student clinical learning in nursing homes is the opportunity to learn about the nursing role in improvement of care for the residents of the facility. Clinical teachers can serve as clinical experts and role models, and students have the time needed to implement and support programs that help patients achieve objectives that are hard to meet in today's rapidly changing acute healthcare environment. These settings also provide rich opportunities to learn and practice delegating nursing tasks to other licensed and unlicensed members of the care team.

There are some barriers to high-quality clinical learning experiences in nursing homes. One barrier is the negative attitude some students have toward elderly people, either a pre-existing attitude or because of a previous nursing home experience. Providing opportunities for positive experiences and designing activities to engage in attitude exploration can help students build effective relationships and attitudes toward this growing population (Parker et al., 2021; Watson et al., 2020).

Faculty members need to carefully consider the agency selected for this clinical learning experience. Because there can be wide variability in quality of care provided to residents from facility to facility, it is critical for the faculty to assess indicators of quality in nursing homes and select appropriately. One measure that may provide insight into quality of care is the adequacy of staffing and appropriate role models. To provide information about other measures of nursing home quality, the Medicare website on nursing homes (www.medicare.gov/nursinghomecompare/search.html) presents reports about nursing home performance on indicators such as quality measures, staffing, and health inspections. This website supplies regular updates and overall ratings for over 15,000 Medicare- and Medicaid-certified nursing homes nationwide.

Once the quality of the nursing home is assessed, the teacher assigned to this clinical site should work on developing a partner relationship with the nursing home staff. This reciprocal relationship will help to build alliances and enable all staff members, teachers, and students to work collaboratively in delivering care, addressing patients' healthcare needs while providing relevant learning opportunities. While at the clinical site, faculty need to actively support student learning as they confront care challenges and deal with a variety of social and emotional issues (Watson et al., 2020). Students can use this experience to improve collaboration skills as they work with a wide variety of staff members, including nursing assistants, licensed practical or vocational nurses, RNs, physical therapists, occupational therapists, dieticians, social workers, and administrators. Lastly, clinical teachers should plan structured orientation programs that provide needed information to adequately prepare students, particularly for the social and clinical aspects they will encounter.

Hospice and Palliative Care

Competency in delivering end-of-life care is an expected student outcome of nursing education, yet many students may not have opportunities to develop the skills needed in caring for these patients. It can be difficult to achieve these competencies in traditional cure-focused clinical settings where students have limited exposure and opportunity to interact with dying patients and their families. Clinical learning in hospice settings is an excellent way to expose students to the issues related to end-of-life care and to provide opportunities to develop many skills needed in all nursing roles and settings. Clinical teachers in community or mental health courses can work with hospice and palliative care providers to arrange for students to partner with nurses and provide care to families receiving hospice or palliative care services. Clinical teachers at both the undergraduate and graduate levels can use the recommended end-of-life education consortium resources to guide these clinical educational experiences (AACN, 2021b). Given the sensitive issues that arise during end-of-life care, it is important for clinical teachers to consider the emotional needs of students during these experiences and provide opportunities to discuss feelings. This can be accomplished through written reflective journals and structured clinical conference activities that encourage reflection and debriefing about the experiences.

CLINICAL LEARNING IN COMMUNITY-BASED CLINICAL SITES

Almost all patients cared for by nurses in the acute care setting come from and return to the community. In addition, many issues, particularly those related to health promotion and maintenance and management of chronic disease, are best addressed in community settings. Community settings also offer many learning opportunities for development of key skills and competencies that are hard to meet in the acute care environment. For these reasons, inclusion of community-based clinical learning activities in nursing curricula is important. Community-based learning activities are often implemented under the umbrella of service learning. In service learning, students work collaboratively with community partners to meet both course and community objectives. Reflection on the experience and development of a sense of civic engagement are essential components.

Community-based experiences can occur in a wide variety of settings. Traditionally, these include health departments, schools, home health agencies, camps, shelters, day care centers for children or senior citizens, prisons, and wellness centers where students complete a wide variety of nursing interventions. Given the shift from acute to community care, nursing programs have formed partnerships and identified unique community-based experiences. For example, the use of a therapeutic riding/equestrian assisted program can provide an innovative clinical learning site that focuses on physical and mental health for individuals in the community (Hamilton et al., 2018; Obarzanek & Pieper, 2020). Other nursing programs have also developed novel clinical learning opportunities. For example, student pairs visit client homes identified through an interdisciplinary partnership with a fire department (Yoder & Pesch, 2020). Food pantries as well as home delivered meal services for seniors provide a clinical learning experience allowing students to understand population health concerns (Campbell & Berg, 2018; Shaffer et al., 2018). Another example of a community-based learning experience involves a home visitation program for first-time low-income mothers and infants through the nurse family partnership program (Knight et al., 2020; Yorga, 2020).

Service Learning

In service learning, students participate in an organized service activity that meets identified community needs and through this experience gain a deeper understanding of the nurse's role in society. Service learning combines teaching, reflection, and community-based projects. Through these projects students can learn about the health disparities in their community and become more aware of social determinants of health (Tillman et al., 2020).

Benefits of service learning to students include developing skills in communication, critical thinking, and collaboration; a community perspective and commitment to health promotion and health equity in the community; a deeper awareness of diversity and cultural influences on health; and leadership abilities (Gresh et al., 2020; McGahee et al., 2018; Taylor & Leffers, 2016). Benefits to the community include having control of the service provided and recipients of service becoming better able to serve themselves and be served by their own actions.

As nursing education programs include more community-based learning activities, opportunities to incorporate service learning increase. Meaningful community-based service learning opportunities are based on relationships between the academic unit and the community to be served. For such partnerships to work effectively, there must be a good fit between the academic unit's mission and goals and the needs of the community. A key element of service learning is the community partner's identification of need (Taylor & Leffers, 2016).

Similar to other clinical learning activities, planning for a service-learning activity begins with the teacher's decision that these learning activities would help students to achieve one or more course outcomes. The success of service learning depends on the embedding of this pedagogy in an existing academic course with clearly defined outcomes (Taylor & Leffers, 2016). The teacher should determine how much time to allot to this activity, keeping in mind that the time spent in service learning would replace and not add to the total time available for other clinical activities for that course.

Schools

Decreased inpatient pediatric census and improved preventive care have led to the reduction of clinical learning opportunities for nursing students, particularly in smaller community hospitals. Nontraditional community-based clinical learning sites such as schools are popular. School-based clinical learning activities provide excellent alternative opportunities for development of pediatric health assessment and promotion skills. This learning is enhanced if it takes place in the context of an ongoing program that demonstrates the principles of family-centered care and public health nursing rather than being a one-time event when the students drop into a school to provide sporadic care such as taking height and weight measurements or teaching about healthy lifestyles. Nursing students need to develop skills related to health promotion and well childcare, disease prevention, safety, nutrition, and growth and development. Schools provide ideal opportunities for nursing student development in these areas. Additionally, partnering with a school district for clinical experiences allows students to have learning opportunities involving assessment, teaching, as well as care for children with an array of acute and chronic health conditions. When working with a school, nursing students can also administer medications, practice developmentally appropriate communication, and collaborate with a variety of professionals within the school (Pohl et al., 2017).

Camps

Another community-based site that can meet many clinical learning objectives, particularly those related to the care of children with acute and chronic illnesses, is a camp. Clinical learning activities in summer camps for children provide a rich learning opportunity for nursing students to learn about growth and development, use physical assessment skills, and manage illnesses and emergencies while also gaining insight about primary care. Camps that focus on specific health problems or chronic illnesses, such as diabetes, asthma, cancer, or developmental delays, allow nursing students to learn about these health problems during this immersion experience at the camp. Students develop communication skills, deliver clinical care, engage in interpersonal relationship building, demonstrate social problem-solving, and promote health (Hendrickx et al., 2020). For students to be adequately prepared for the experiences, they may need appropriate clinical clearances (as discussed later in this chapter) and they should also be familiar with the camper's typical health problems and common medications administered. Since camp nurse responsibilities occur around the clock, students need to be prepared to deliver nursing care at all hours of the day and night, and ultimately deal with the camp living conditions and fatigue that may occur. Clinical teachers who guide these learning activities need to provide opportunities for student reflection on their experiences and appropriate mentoring during the experience.

Wellness Centers

Wellness centers or interprofessional clinics offer a creative alternative to traditional clinical learning sites. These centers allow nurses, alone or in collaboration with other healthcare providers, to manage health services that focus on health promotion, disease prevention, health education, and wellness. Typically, these wellness centers or clinics are located in the community in places such as public housing, community or recreation centers, homeless shelters, senior centers, storefronts, or churches where they serve vulnerable and underserved populations. Sometimes, clinical teachers or preceptors serve as clinicians for the site and teach nursing students there as well (Shaffer et al., 2018). Educators in this dual role as clinical teachers and care providers serve as powerful nursing role models for students, and their first-hand knowledge of the community enriches the students' learning experiences as well as allows them to advocate for the populations served. However, when this clinical model is used, nursing programs face the challenge of providing services during school breaks and holidays and need to carefully plan programs and activities that are not disrupted by an interruption of services.

At these wellness centers and clinics, students have opportunities to address critical public health problems such as food insecurity, mental health concerns, addiction recovery, and other health issues. Students gain valuable experience assessing critical community and neighborhood concerns and providing needed health services while establishing interprofessional relationships and advocating for those in underserved communities. They can design programs and provide holistic care to vulnerable individuals across the life span.

CLINICAL LEARNING AT DISTANT SITES

Distance education has become a respected and effective method of providing higher education in the United States. The U.S. Department of Education National Center for Education Statistics (2020) reported that 6.9 million students are learning online, with enrollments in online education continuing to grow. The COVID-19 pandemic accelerated the use of distance education as nursing programs needed to quickly modify their educational delivery approaches because of the pandemic health concerns.

Students choose distance education programs for a variety of reasons, including issues related to distance from, and therefore access to, on-campus programs as well as the convenience of anytime, anyplace learning opportunities. Many distance learning programs operate asynchronously, allowing students to choose what time of the day or week they will participate. This makes distance learning programs especially attractive to adult learners who may be working or raising families or both while furthering their education.

But what about clinical education? Students enrolled in post-licensure undergraduate programs (RN-to-BSN) and graduate-level education may pursue distance education. The content in these programs depends heavily on acquiring not only the didactic knowledge base but also a set of necessary clinical skills. Ultimately, students must be able to demonstrate that they can apply clinical judgment and function as safe, competent practitioners in a clinical environment. This is the segment of their education that cannot be completely taught or learned using computer technologies.

Faculty members in distance education programs need to carefully consider how students will acquire the necessary clinical skills and how these students will be evaluated. Available clinical sites and knowledgeable, skilled preceptors are needed. Typically, those preceptors working with online students are physically located in or near students' own communities, which may be hundreds of miles or more away from the nursing program. Although nurse educators have been able to provide didactic education to students who live almost anywhere using internet technologies, schools traditionally have had affiliations only with clinical sites located geographically close to their campuses, thus requiring development of new clinical sites for distance learners. The process of securing an appropriate clinical placement for students at distant locations involves a series of checks and balances to ensure that students receive the education they need. The specific steps involved in selecting, preparing, evaluating, and rewarding preceptors are discussed in more detail in Chapter 11.

Evaluating students in the clinical setting is an ongoing challenge for preceptors and nursing faculty but can be particularly challenging with distance education. Goals of evaluation include identification of student strengths and problem areas as well as documentation of student progress. Faculty members must carefully screen and orient preceptors while developing and maintaining trusting work relationships with clinical preceptors who are at a distance. Contact between the nursing education program faculty member and the preceptor during a student's clinical experience needs to be timely and consistent. Preceptors need to know how to reach the designated faculty member with questions and concerns. At the same time, teaching and completing student evaluations can be time-consuming for the preceptor, and the nursing education program needs to avoid imposing unnecessary reporting burdens. When working at a distance, electronic communication using email, or other synchronized audiovisual communication, such as Zoom, can be helpful to busy preceptors and faculty members alike.

Various tools have been developed by faculty members to assist in the evaluation process. Student self-evaluation is essential and includes regular written evaluations, reflections on clinical experiences, and plans for improvement. Involvement of the preceptor in written assessments provides documentation of the preceptor's observations of student performance that are necessary evidence for the faculty member's decision making. Self-identification of areas needing improvement can be stressful for students but is the basis for a mature practitioner's growth and should be fostered by the nursing education program.

Evaluation of clinical competence is more challenging when students are located in a distant setting. Some programs may require students to visit a campus for evaluation sessions and demonstration of essential clinical skills. Sometimes objective structured clinical examinations (OSCEs) are used for this evaluation, particularly with nurse practitioner students. Online nurse practitioner programs are creatively using video enhanced OSCEs to assess performance using an online teleconferencing platform (Day et al., 2018). Regardless of in-person or remote, these exams assess student clinical competency with standardized patients portraying typical clinical problems. Students rotate through various stations and demonstrate skills such as history taking, assessments, or clinical procedures while a faculty evaluator uses a checklist or other rating tool to evaluate performance. However, this type of evaluation may cause stress and anxiety among participants (Goh et al., 2019). To ensure valid and reliable assessments of student performance, clinical teachers need to carefully select and train standardized patients and use appropriately designed data collection tools that are linked to clinical competencies and critical performance elements. Other emerging possibilities include telehealth applications, virtual communities, and virtual interactive video conferencing. Regardless of the method used, faculty need to plan for clinical learning at distance sites and carefully consider student guidance and evaluation. Chapter 13 is on teaching and evaluating students in distance-based programs and expands this discussion.

CLINICAL LEARNING IN INTERNATIONAL SITES

Clinical placements in international sites can be rich opportunities to expand students' comfort and competence in the care of diverse patient populations, beyond that which can be gained in coursework focusing on such content. International learning experiences may increase cultural awareness and sensitivity while developing a better understanding of global issues (Gosse & Katic-Duffy, 2020). On a personal level, students may explore values, develop confidence, and learn or refine other skills. Nursing students whose clinical activities take place within other cultures, in both developed and developing countries, are challenged intellectually and emotionally to become more culturally aware.

Clinical experiences at international sites present unique challenges and require adequate preparation for both the student and the faculty member. Various factors must be considered as part of the planning process. The source institution for the nursing education program may have an international placement office that can assist with arrangements, offer travel suggestions, and facilitate the selection of appropriate sites. Establishing relationships with key personnel at the host location may enhance collaboration and facilitate planning. Once a site has been selected, preliminary and early travel arrangements should be completed because some preparation and planning time may be required. Students and faculty members must ensure that they are protected from developing health problems when traveling abroad. Participants will need to have updated immunizations and maintain current health and travel insurance. Depending upon the location of travel, they may also need to take preventive medications such as antimalarial drugs or get additional vaccinations. Most immunization series must be started well in advance of the planned trip. Students will need passports with an expiration date well beyond the end of the planned learning activity. Completion of necessary paperwork usually includes a waiver of responsibility of the source educational institution and a separate application for the international activity.

Another important part of preparation involves understanding the practice environment, healthcare system, and nursing regulations at the destination site. Determine what students can legally do at the clinical site. Are there practice boundaries and restrictions on the nursing care that they can provide? Students need to be prepared and understand that nursing practice, as well as the settings for that care, will be different. Make sure that students stay within regulated boundaries. Depending on the host location and type of site, verification of licensure of graduate nursing students and accompanying clinical teachers, and protocols to cover any nursing care to be delivered by students may be needed.

An understanding of the overall culture, customs, politics, economics, traditions, communication patterns, and values of the community and country in which they will be placed is also essential. This knowledge will be helpful and will ensure that students demonstrate respect and appreciation for the culture and challenges that the patients face.

Emergency planning is also essential. Make sure that students know what to do if they become separated from the group. Have a frank discussion of what students and clinical teachers should do in case of a natural disaster or public health concern. Where should they go? When? Whom should they contact and how can that contact be completed? Monitor the U.S. Department of State website (www.travel.state.gov) for travel warnings for U.S. citizens and follow cautions and warnings.

Opportunities for reflection and sharing of experiences are critical because students may encounter emotional issues that need to be addressed. Even with adequate pretrip planning, students may not be prepared for the health disparities and complex health and cultural issues they encounter, the limited resources available, the stereotypes they may experience, and their ethnocentric thinking (Gosse & Katic-Duffy, 2020). Journaling (traditional or electronic format), development of a photo-log, and sharing their experiences with classmates who did not participate provide opportunities for students to explore their feelings and reflect on their learning.

PRACTICAL ASPECTS OF CLINICAL PLACEMENTS IN DIVERSE SITES

When considering practical aspects of clinical placements in diverse sites, there are two major areas of concern. The first reflects the regulatory and accreditation requirements for clinical learning activities; the second involves preparation of the agency, clinical teachers, and students. All clinical learning activities must meet the requirements of state law and regulations (often set by the board of nursing) as well as the policies and requirements of accreditation agencies, the nursing education program (or its parent institution), and the site at which the clinical activities are to take place. Each nursing education program also has procedures in place that describe how contracts and similar formal communication with an agency are to be handled. While often clear from the school's perspective, this is not always the case from the agency's side. This is an important point for agencies that usually do not negotiate such contracts and for which there is no clearly identified contact person. Some agencies that appear to be freestanding may be part of larger agencies. When the agency is part of a larger entity (e.g., a hospital system, local government program, state health department, school district, or federal agency such as the Department of Veterans Affairs), it can be both difficult and time-consuming to get the contract signed by all relevant parties. These agreements can dictate student and faculty requirements needed prior to entering the clinical agency for learning. These agreements are especially important when dealing with smaller agencies that may not have procedures in place related to orientation or placement of students in their facilities.

Adhering to the agency guidelines is important to avoid conflicts, especially when multiple programs (nursing and other health professionals) are seeking placements for the same time period. Even if students are at one of the clinical entity's sites, the policy for the overall entity must be followed. Often, smaller and nontraditional sites (e.g., day care settings, church programs, food kitchens) and even some formal agencies that do not have large numbers of staff (e.g., day treatment programs for substance abusers, assisted living facilities) do not require or have a formal orientation program. The clinical teacher should work with the staff to determine what preparation the students need to optimize their learning as well as to protect and provide the best care for the patients they will encounter. A larger institution (e.g., a major hospital system) may be the parent organization of smaller community-based programs, and students may need to complete the full agency orientation to be placed in even a small, peripheral program. If these requirements become too onerous, expensive, or time-consuming, the value of clinical learning activities at these sites may be questioned by the nursing education program faculty and administration. Legal aspects of clinical learning experiences are more fully explored in Chapter 6, and a few aspects highly relevant to the use of diverse sites are presented in Exhibit 3.1.

EXHIBIT 3.1 Areas of Consideration When Placing Students in Diverse Clinical Sites

LEGAL AND REGULATORY ISSUES

Does the placement meet requirements of relevant state laws and accompanying regulations related to approval, contract, faculty ratios, nature of faculty guidance, and student scope of practice?
Must the clinical teacher be present for clinical learning activities for students to practice direct patient care?
Can preceptors be used in the setting and in the manner planned?
Can the clinical teacher delegate guidance and evaluation of students' learning to an RN on staff at the agency, if the clinical teacher is not present but in the building?
How and where are students documenting care?

NURSING EDUCATION PROGRAM ISSUES

Is a contract or legal agreement required?
Is travel reimbursement available?

(continued)

EXHIBIT 3.1 Areas of Consideration When Placing Students in
Diverse Clinical Sites (*continued*)

If the planned clinical learning activity will take place over more than the usual hours and day
of a traditional clinical activity (e.g., on parts of most days of the week, during school breaks,
on weekends), is this reflected in the clinical teacher's workload and compensation?
Are there specific requirements of the education program's accreditation body that affect the
planned clinical learning activity?

AGENCY ISSUES

What are the agency's rules and policies related to nursing student clinical activities? Can the
student deliver care or are they primarily observing care?
Does the agency require a contract with the nursing education program? If so, who handles
contracts with education programs?
How are requests for clinical placements from multiple nursing education and other programs
handled?
What are the agency rules for student clearance (e.g., criminal background, child or elder abuse
records, drug screening)?
If screenings or background checks beyond the requirements of the nursing education program
are required, who pays for them?
Does the nursing education program need to document that students have demonstrated CPR or
other competencies?
What are the health requirements, such as tuberculosis testing or immunizations?
Are there specific Health Insurance Portability and Accountability Act or patient privacy
statements that must be completed?
Does the agency need to keep a record of students for legal or regulatory purposes, or to obtain
future funding based on the value of student service to the organization? If yes, what is needed
from the nursing education program?

STUDENT ISSUES

What modes of transportation are available? Is there parking?
What measures will help to ensure safety of students?
What is the required orientation?

Agency Preparation

As competition for clinical sites continues, clinical teachers seek creative ways to
effectively and efficiently secure appropriate student learning opportunities. Clinical
agency administrators and educators are also ready to embrace creative approaches
that will decrease nursing program competition and rivalry in securing clinical
sites. They should also work collaboratively to provide an equitable approach that
will meet agency, nursing program, and student needs. Educational programs and
healthcare providers must work together to meet common goals. One approach is
the formation of a clinical placement consortium. In this model, school representatives, service agency liaisons, and clinical agency representatives meet to find
appropriate learning opportunities for all. The use of web-based programs or course
management systems is one way to manage and display clinical placement requests
and facilitate open communication and negotiation among consortium members.

Another approach to secure student clinical placements involves development of partnerships between healthcare organizations and nursing education programs. Academic service partnerships, also known as academic–practice partnerships, are formal collaborative relationships between agencies that allow for sharing of knowledge, resources, clinical expertise, and opportunities with the intent of promoting both better patient care and nursing education. Formal partnerships generally allow for better access to clinical placements because the partners have clearly articulated a shared vision and mutually agreed upon goals and have re-envisioned the roles of teacher and staff members. Partners work together to facilitate quality care, enhance student skill acquisition, and promote transition to practice (Shephard Battle, 2018).

Regardless of the type of relationship with the clinical agency or location of the clinical site, there are some basic considerations that will help to ensure a collegial work relationship with agency leaders and nursing staff. Details of the clinical learning activity (when will students be there, what are their learning goals, what are they expected to do, and how can they participate) must be communicated with the staff. Settings that rarely host nursing students, as well as those that often do, can have problems getting this information to the staff members who will have the most contact with the students. Explore if there are methods to electronically share information with staff, such as through email, so that it is disseminated in a convenient and efficient way. Misunderstandings about student activities and objectives do occur and can jeopardize the learning experience. Often course syllabi, clinical objectives, and guides to the clinical learning activity are provided to administrative staff of a clinical agency but may not be shared with the staff members who are directly working with the students and could benefit from access to this information. A meeting with the staff members who will work directly with the students, along with providing multiple copies of these written materials, will facilitate communication and ensure that the right people have the right information.

Including nursing staff in planning clinical learning activities can also prevent potential problems. Seeking input from staff nurses and understanding their workload demands can help clinical teachers plan effectively for student learning activities. Realizing the existing demands on staff members, such as precepting new nurses or supervising other staff members, will help clinical teachers form realistic expectations of the time available to assist students.

Clinical Teacher Preparation

Clinical teachers may need additional education, mentoring, and support as they implement clinical learning activities in new and diverse settings. A highly skilled clinical teacher who is at ease while teaching students to care for acutely ill patients in a critical care unit may not have the knowledge and skills needed to care for those patients in their homes a week after discharge. Like their students, clinical teachers may find that the fine points of adapting care to the home setting while respecting the family in their home and dealing with the virtual loss of the multiple support systems of the acute care setting will be new to them.

The organization and structure of clinical teaching outside of acute care settings will often be new to a faculty member. Some logistical issues will need to be addressed. If the students are not all in the same setting, how will faculty members conduct their clinical teaching activities at multiple sites? How will students and teachers communicate with each other? How will clinical conferences occur? What written assignments will be submitted to the teacher and how and when will it be returned to students? Electronic technology can provide solutions for some of these issues. Course management platforms can be used to create forums for posting clinical updates and news, submission of course assignments, or asynchronous discussion boards. Other electronic communication methods can be used to remain in touch with students during clinical practice. These methods include cell phones, although they are not always permitted at clinical sites. Text messaging can be used to provide support and instant access between clinical teachers and students during clinical learning experience activities. Use of this service is inexpensive and easy to use, and it allows for instant connectivity. Some computer applications such as Remind (www.remind.com) are available and can help teachers to schedule automatic announcements. They can also be used to share messages without revealing the clinical teacher's phone number.

Clinical teachers with nursing students in diverse sites, perhaps at different sites at the same time, have complex teaching obligations. Some sites, particularly those that are community based or international, have work hours that extend beyond the days, times, or even weeks when traditional clinical learning activities occur. In those situations, teachers may need to maintain partnerships that enable a collaborative approach to meet student and program needs.

Student Preparation

When students have clinical learning activities in unfamiliar sites or where the learning opportunities are not immediately clear to them, students may feel confused, insecure, isolated, and unprepared for the experience. Provision of specific objectives, learning activities, preparation expectations, activity guides, and written expectations will greatly facilitate learning and make the expectations clear. This is especially true if the faculty member will not be present at the site at all times. Exhibit 3.2 is an example of specific preparation, objectives, activities, and written expectations for a community-based experience. Orientation for the clinical experience is based on agency, site, and student needs. Regardless of the clinical setting, an overall orientation to the course expectations with a review of frequently used skills can be helpful. A discussion about preconceptions and expectations also will provide students with essential preparation that will enable them to feel confident and prepared for the experience.

EXHIBIT 3.2 Example of Instructions to Students for Community Clinical Sites

PREPARATION FOR ALL COMMUNITY CLINICAL LEARNING ACTIVITIES

Review objectives and activities as listed for each assignment and do assign reading before arriving at the site.

Review key facts or existing guides (e.g., immunization schedules or classification of hypertension in adults) appropriate for the clinical area.

Be at the site at the time indicated by your instructor.

Wear your clean uniform (including identification) and follow the dress code. Dress appropriately for the weather.

(continued)

EXHIBIT 3.2 Example of Instructions to Students for Community Clinical Sites (*continued*)

Bring a black pen, watch with a second hand, stethoscope, notebook, electronic references, and pocket reference books, as appropriate, for the clinical learning activity.
Check on transportation and directions to the site.
Have contact information for your instructor (cell phone number, etc.) with you at all times.
Share your schedule (where and when you are going) with your class partner.
Bring a charged cell phone.
Have the phone number and name of the site contact person.

SPECIFIC PREPARATION BEFORE THE CLINICAL LEARNING ACTIVITY STARTS

Read assigned chapters in the course text.
Complete and submit the clinical preparation worksheet to your instructor.

GENERAL CLINICAL ACTIVITY GUIDELINES

Work with the staff for an optimal learning experience.
Your instructor will visit the site each day and be available by cell phone or text messaging.
You should complete assessments, documentation, and teaching as described in the Clinical Activities. You may only administer medications under the direct observation of the RN identified by your instructor.
Review any unfamiliar medical diagnoses, medications, and care needed for patients you are seeing.
Ask for help if something is unclear.

CLINICAL ACTIVITIES

During this clinical learning activity, students will work with staff members to:

Follow agency policy for client intake for the visit, including completion of initial assessments and placement of clients and charts with the appropriate provider.
Review patients' health records for history, diagnoses, medications, and lab test results.
Follow patients through the physical exam to the end of the visit, if provider and patient agree.
Implement health teaching after review by the instructor.
Complete the required clinical report.

Student safety during the clinical learning experience will also need to be addressed. This is an issue in all clinical activities, but it is especially important in situations where students may be in an unfamiliar area, making home visits, or going alone or in small groups to clinical sites at various times during the day or evening. Teachers must provide explicit guidelines for student safety during learning activities and document them in the course syllabus. Safety guidelines should address proper methods of communication with faculty, agency, and patients. Students should have the following information prior to the start of the clinical experience: clinical teacher and emergency contact information, clear travel directions, a reliable vehicle with adequate fuel, availability of a charged cell phone, and guidelines for appropriate dress and behavior while in a patient's home or at an agency or facility without an instructor present. The students must also be prepared for appropriate actions they may need to take if they find themselves in a dangerous situation, be it at an agency, out in the community, or at a patient's home. The faculty member should provide education for how students can prevent and avoid situations that involve harassment or potential violence. It is important to promote a culture of safety and also teach students what to do if they experience an adverse event during the clinical time (García-Gámez et al., 2019).

Regular brief visits by the clinical teacher to each clinical site will help prevent problems and address issues that may arise from staff and students during the experience. Individual and group conferences with students will allow for sharing of experiences and provide additional time to assess learning and growth.

SUMMARY

Nursing care occurs anywhere clients need the services of a professional nurse, and nursing students can learn to provide care wherever they have contact with clients. Traditionally, much of clinical nursing education has occurred in acute care settings because of long-held assumptions about how nurses must be prepared to practice. However, decreasing length of inpatient stays, high patient acuity, economic pressures to provide care in outpatient and community settings, and increasing competition with other educational programs for the same clinical sites have limited clinical learning opportunities located in traditional acute care settings. Using diverse sites for clinical learning activities can prepare nursing students for the challenges of contemporary nursing practice as clients, health needs, care locations, and approaches to care change over time.

This chapter discussed options for planning and providing clinical learning opportunities for undergraduate and graduate nursing students in a wide variety of clinical sites. Examples of clinical learning opportunities in four categories were presented. The first category included clinical learning in specialized patient care areas that are not used regularly as clinical learning sites (e.g., outpatient clinics, the OR, nursing homes and extended care facilities, and hospice and palliative care settings). These sites offer rich learning opportunities for students. The second category included community-based settings such as camps and wellness centers and clinics. The third category is clinical learning at distant sites. The final category is the growing use of international clinical learning opportunities.

Practical aspects of clinical placements in diverse sites were also discussed. Two main areas of concern are the need to meet regulatory and accreditation requirements and the need for adequate preparation of agency staff members, clinical teachers, and students. Examples of methods and tools used for the preparation of agency staff members, clinical teachers making the transition from traditional acute care sites, and nursing students were provided.

CNE® EXAMINATION TEST BLUEPRINT CORE COMPETENCIES

1. **Facilitate Learning**
   A. Implement a variety of teaching strategies appropriate to:
      2. Setting
      3. Learner needs
      5. Desired learner outcomes

    C. Modify teaching strategies and learning experiences based on consideration of learners':
       1. Cultural background
       2. Past clinical experiences
    H. Create opportunities for learners to develop their own critical thinking skills
    M. Develop collegial working relationships with clinical agency personnel to promote positive learning environments
    O. Demonstrate the ability to teach clinical skills
    P. Act as a role model in practice settings
    Q. Foster a safe learning environment

2. **Facilitate Learner Development and Socialization**
    D. Create learning environments that facilitate learners' self-reflection, personal goal setting, and socialization to the role of the nurse
    E. Foster the development of learners in these areas
       1. Cognitive domain
       2. Psychomotor domain
       3. Affective domain
    F. Assist learners to engage in thoughtful and constructive self and peer evaluation

4. **Participate in Curriculum Design and Evaluation of Program Outcomes**
    A. Demonstrate knowledge of curriculum development including:
       1. Selecting appropriate clinical experiences
    H. Collaborate with community and clinical partners to support educational goals

6. **Engage in Scholarship, Service, and Leadership**
    A. Function as a change agent and leader:
       1. Function as a change agent and leader
         ■ Model cultural sensitivity when advocating for change
       4. Implement strategies for change within the:
         ■ Nursing program
         ■ Local community
       6. Adapt to changes created by external forces

CNE®cl EXAMINATION TEST BLUEPRINT CORE COMPETENCIES

1. **Function within the Education and Health Care Environments**
    B. Operationalize the Curriculum
       1. Assess the congruence of the clinical agency to curriculum, course goals, and learner needs when evaluating clinical sites
       4. Prepare learners for clinical experiences (e.g., facility, clinical expectations, equipment, and technology-based resources)
    C. Abide by Legal Requirements, Ethical Guidelines, Agency Policies, and Guiding Framework
       1. Apply ethical and legal principles to create a safe clinical learning environment
       4. Inform others of program and clinical agency policies, procedures, and practices
       5. Adhere to program and clinical agency policies, procedures, and practices when implementing clinical experiences
       6. Promote learner compliance with regulations and standards of practice

2. **Facilitate Learning in the Health Care Environment**

   A. Implement a variety of clinical teaching strategies appropriate to learner needs, learner outcomes, content, and context

   D. Create opportunities for learners to develop critical thinking and clinical reasoning skills

3. **Demonstrate Effective Interpersonal Communication and Collaborative Interprofessional Relationships**

   B. Foster a shared learning community and cooperate with other members of the healthcare team

   C. Create multiple opportunities to collaborate and cooperate with other members of the healthcare team

   F. Use clear and effective communication in all interactions (e.g., written, electronic, verbal, non-verbal)

   N. Communicate performance expectations to learners and agency staff

5. **Facilitate Learner Development and Socialization**

   G. Create learning environments that are focused on socialization to the role of the nurse

6. **Implement Effective Clinical Assessment Evaluation Strategies**

   K. Evaluate the quality of the clinical learning experiences and environment

REFERENCES

American Association of Colleges of Nursing. (2021a). *APRN clinical training task force report brief.* https://www.aacnnursing.org/News-Information/APRN-Clinical-Training-Task-Force-Report-Brief

American Association of Colleges of Nursing. (2021b). *End-of-life nursing education consortium (ELNEC) fact sheet.* https://www.aacnnursing.org/Portals/42/ELNEC/PDF/ELNEC-Fact-Sheet.pdf

Campbell, S., & Berg, J. M. (2018). Nursing student collaborative with Meals on Wheels: Home visits for at-risk senior adults. *Nursing Education Perspectives, 39*(3), 190–191. https://doi.org/10.1097/01.NEP.0000000000000230

Day, C., Barker, C., Bell, E., Sefcik, E., & Flournoy, D. (2018). Flipping the objective structured clinical examination: A teaching innovation in graduate nursing education. *Nurse Educator, 43*(2), 83–86. https://doi.org/10.1097/NNE.0000000000000421

Fleming, L., Lorenzen, R., Stanek, J., Williams, M., & Mendel, H. (2019). Transition in care model for a senior-level clinical immersion experiences. *Nurse Educator, 45*(1), 39–42. https://doi.org/10.1097/NNE.0000000000000657

García-Gámez, M., Morales-Asencio, J. M., García-Mayor, S., Kaknani-Uttumchandani, S., Marti-Garcia, C., Lopez-Leiva, I., León-Campos, A., Fernandez-Ordoñnez, E., García-Guirrero, A., & Iglesias-Parra, M. R. (2019). A scoping review of safety management during clinical placements of undergraduate nursing students. *Nursing Outlook, 67*(2019), 765–775. https://doi.org/10.1016/j.outlook.2019.06.003

Goh, H. S., Zhang, H., Lee, C. N., Wu, X. V., & Wang, W. (2019). Value of nursing objective structured clinical examinations: A scoping review. *Nurse Educator, 44*(5), E1–E6. https://doi.org/10.1097/NNE.0000000000000620

Gosse, N. L., & Katic-Duffy, A. (2020). Nursing student and faculty perceptions of reciprocity during international clinical learning experiences: A qualitative descriptive study. *Nurse Education Today, 84*(2020), 1–6. https://doi.org/10.1016/j.nedt.2019.104242

Gresh, A., LaFave, S., Thamilselvan, V., Batchelder, A., Mermer, J., Jacques, K., Greensfelder, A., Buckley, M., Cohen, Z., Coy, A., & Warren, N. (2020). Service learning in public health nursing education: How COVID-19 accelerated community-academic partnership. *Public Health Nursing, 38*, 248–257. https://doi.org/10.1111/phn.12796

Gubrud-Howe, P. (2020). Teaching in the clinical setting. In D. M. Billings & J. A. Halstead (Eds.), *Teaching in nursing: A guide for faculty* (6th ed., pp. 328–352). Elsevier.

Hamilton, M. R., Delaney, E., & Hall, K. (2018). We're not just horsing around: Creating innovative community clinical experiences utilizing diverse opportunities. *Nursing Education Perspectives, 39*(2), 123–125. https://doi.org/10.1097/01.NEP.0000000000000164

Hendrickx, L., Pelzel, H., Burdette, L., & Hartung, N. (2020). Pediatric clinical for nursing students in rural areas: The camp nursing experiences. *Online Journal of Rural Nursing and Health Care, 20*(1), 142–155. https://doi.org/10.14574/ojrnhc.v20i1.603

Institute of Medicine. (2011). *The future of nursing: Leading change, advancing health.* National Academies Press.

Knight, C. C., Selleck, C. S., Wakefield, R., Horton, J. E., Wilson, M. E., & Harper, D. C. (2020). Development of an academic practice partnership to improve maternal child health. *Journal of Professional Nursing, 36*(2020), 116–122. https://doi.org/10.1016/j.profnurs.2019.10.003

Maneval, R., Hepburn, M., Brooks, C., Tamburi, M., Chin, S. D. N., Prado-Inzerillo, M. Haghenbeck-Nunnink, K. T., & Flaum, S. J. (2020). Enhancing the undergraduate nursing education experience with clinical elective courses. *Journal of Professional Nursing, 37*(2), 366–372. https://doi.org/10.1016/j.profnurs.2020.04.014

McGahee, T., Bravo, M., Simmons, L., & Reid, T. (2018). Nursing students and service learning: Research from a symbiotic community partnership with local schools and Special Olympics. *Nurse Educator, 43*(4), 215–218. https://doi.org/10.1097/NNE.0000000000000445

National Academies of Sciences, Engineering, and Medicine. (2016). *Assessing progress on the Institute of Medicine report The Future of Nursing.* The National Academies Press. https://doi.org/10.17226/21838

National League for Nursing. (2016). *Achieving diversity and meaningful inclusion in nursing education.* http://www.nln.org/docs/default-source/about/vision-statement-achieving-diversity.pdf?sfvrsn=2

National League for Nursing. (2019). *A vision for integration of social determinants of health in nursing education curricula.* http://www.nln.org/docs/default-source/default-document-library/social-determinants-of-health.pdf?sfvrsn=2

Obarzanek, L., & Pieper, B. (2020). The use of equine-assisted programs for nontraditional undergraduate clinical pediatric experiences. *Teaching and Learning in Nursing, 15*(2), 145–151. https://doi.org/10.1016/j.teln.2020.01.002

Parker, C. N., Harvey, T., Johnston, S., & MacAndrew, M. (2021). An exploration of knowledge of students and staff at residential aged care facilities and implications for nursing education. *Nurse Education Today, 96*(2021), 104639. https://doi.org/10.1016/j.nedt.2020.104639

Pohl, C., Jarvill, M., Akman, O., & Clark, S. (2017). Adapting pediatric clinical experiences to a changing healthcare environment. *Nurse Educator, 42*(2), 105–108. https://doi.org/10.1097/NNE.0000000000000315

Shaffer, K., Swan, B. A., & Bouchaud, M. (2018). Designing a new model for clinical education: An innovative approach. *Nurse Educator, 43*(3), 145–148. https://doi.org/10.1097/NNE.0000000000000468

Shephard Battle, L. H. (2018). Academic-practice partnerships and patient outcomes. *Nursing Management, 49*(1), 34–40. https://doi.org/10.1097/01.NUMA.0000527717.13135.f4

Taylor, S. L., & Leffers, J. M. (2016). Integrative review of service-learning assessment in nursing education. *Nursing Education Perspectives, 37*, 194–200.

Tilden, V. P., Cox, K. S., Moore, J. E., & Naylor, M. D. (2018). Strategic partnerships to address adverse social determinants of health: Redefining healthcare. *Nursing Outlook, 66*(3), 233–236. https://doi.org/10.1016/j.outlook.2018.03.002

Tillman, P., Thomas, M., & Buelow, J. R. (2020). Impact of service learning on student attitudes toward the poor and underserved. *Nurse Educator, 45*(6), 316–320. https://doi.org/10.1097/NNE.0000000000000807

United States Department of Education National Center for Education Statistics. (2020). *Fast facts: Distance learning*. https://nces.ed.gov/fastfacts/display.asp?id=80

Watson, J., Horseman, Z., Fawcett, T., Hockley, J., & Rhynas, S. (2020). Care home nursing: Co-creating curricular content with student nurses. *Nurse Education Today, 84*(2020), 104233. https://doi.org/10.1016/j.nedt.2019.104233

Yoder, C. M., & Pesch, M. S. (2020). An academic-fire department partnership to address social determinants of health. *Journal of Nursing Education, 59*(1), 34–37. https://doi.org/10.3928/01484834-20191223-08

Yorga, K. W. (2020). Looking beyond the walls for clinical experiences. *Journal of Nursing Education, 59*(8), 423–424. https://doi.org/10.3928/01484834-20200723-01

A robust set of instructor resources designed to supplement this text is located at http://connect.springerpub.com/content/book/978-0-8261-6705-7. Qualifying instructors may request access by emailing textbook@springerpub.com.

Preparing for Clinical Learning Activities

Nurse educators should consider several factors in preparing for clinical learning activities. Equipping students to enter the clinical setting must be balanced with preparing staff members for the presence of learners in a service setting while also respecting the needs of patients. This chapter describes the roles and responsibilities of faculty members, staff members, and others involved in clinical teaching and suggests methods of preparing students and staff members for clinical learning activities. Strategies for crafting clinical learning activities are discussed in Chapter 7.

UNDERSTANDING THE CONTEXT FOR CLINICAL LEARNING ACTIVITIES

To begin preparations for clinical teaching and learning, nurse educators should reflect on the context in which these activities take place. Teachers and learners use an established healthcare or community setting for a learning environment, thus becoming guests within that setting. What are the implications for clinical teaching and learning effectiveness under these conditions?

Over the last century, basic preparation for professional nursing has moved from service-based training and apprenticeships to academic educational programs in institutions of higher learning. As a result of this service-education separation, the clinical teacher and students who enter a clinical setting for learning activities are often regarded as guests of the healthcare agency or community site. They participate in the activities of the established system and attempt to follow the norms of its culture, but they are not a constant presence. They must rely on relationships they develop within the agency to facilitate their sense of belonging to support student learning (Dahlke & Hannesson, 2016; Oosterbroek et al., 2019).

Traditionally, clinical teachers and students in an academic nursing education program comprise a temporary system within the permanent culture of the clinical setting. A temporary system is a set of individuals who work together on a complex task over a limited period of time. Although clinical teachers are professional colleagues to nursing staff members and are viewed as nurses by patients, their primary role is that of educator. Even if they are employed by the agency as a staff member on a casual or part-time basis in addition to their academic positions, faculty members enact a different role in that agency when they are guiding the clinical learning activities of students, and role confusion is often inevitable.

Being a good guest involves knowing and adhering to the established routines, policies, and practices of the clinical setting. Clinical teachers negotiate with staff members for access to learning opportunities and resources while simultaneously protecting students from criticism and preventing errors. Often, students point out discrepancies between nursing staff practice and the standards or procedures that the students were taught. The teacher needs to explain such differences in terms of choice of approach to solving a clinical problem, when appropriate, rather than offering a value judgment. When possible, the clinical teacher should point out staff members who are positive role models of clinical excellence and professionalism. The clinical teacher juggles the complex responsibilities of supporting student learning, developing trusting relationships with staff, and ensuring the delivery of safe quality care.

At times, a clinical teacher's desire for positive relationships with staff members, reluctance to delay or slow patient care, and concern for patient and student safety result in minimizing students' risk taking in an effort to prevent errors. For example, teachers may select assignments for students that allow them to demonstrate previously developed competencies rather than choose learning activities that will challenge students to deepen their understanding and develop higher skill levels. If the teacher expects that a student will not be able to complete patient care activities in a timely manner, the instructor may forego a rich opportunity for the student to learn to prioritize, organize, and complete a complex set of tasks for the patient and to work collaboratively and efficiently with other healthcare team members efficiently. Excessive gatekeeping actions of this kind do not allow students to exhibit clinical problem solving, organize care activities, and learn to take appropriate, calculated risks.

Although clinical teachers and nursing students are seen as guests in the healthcare environment, they are also a vital resource to a healthcare agency. Students represent potential future employees. The learning environment encountered during the clinical experience can impact the recruitment and job seeking of graduates (Steele-Moses et al., 2018). Exposure to and immersion in clinical specialty areas influence nursing student decisions about practice upon graduation. Positive clinical learning experiences may encourage nursing students to consider future employment in that agency, and nursing staff members who nurture the development of students can have a powerful influence on such a choice (Kapaale, 2020).

Many staff members, however, are unaware of or misinterpret these teaching expectations; they expect nursing students to participate fully in all unit activities assume responsibility for patient care, and take the same kinds of patient assignments and complete the same patient care tasks as staff members. They may recall their own clinical education as being more rigorous than the contemporary clinical activities that they witness; communicating those perceptions to nursing students can produce self-doubt, discouragement, and dissatisfaction among the novices. The teacher as culture broker must allow students to experience the real world of clinical nursing and, at the same time, communicate to staff members that trends and current issues in nursing education mean that "it's not your mother's nursing school." Keeping clinical agency staff members, managers, and administrators informed about the nature of contemporary nursing education and keeping students updated on current challenges and priorities in the healthcare environment will help to integrate students more effectively into the real world of clinical nursing.

SELECTING CLINICAL SETTINGS

Clinical teachers may have sole responsibility for selecting the settings in which clinical learning activities occur, or their input may be sought by those who make these decisions. In either case, selection of clinical sites should be based on important criteria such as compatibility of school and agency philosophy, availability of opportunities to meet learning objectives, geographical location, agency licensure or accreditation, availability of positive role models, the complexity of patients, level of student, purpose, and type of course, and physical resources (Fressola & Patterson, 2017). In some areas, selection of appropriate clinical settings may be difficult because of competition among several nursing programs, and nursing programs must typically contract with a variety of agencies to provide adequate learning opportunities for students. Additionally, as nursing programs increase enrollments, they face the challenge of securing adequate clinical placements, particularly in specialty areas such as pediatrics. Programs may be forced to use numerous clinical sites, which increases the time and energy required for teachers to develop relationships with staff, to obtain necessary information about agencies, and to develop and maintain competence to practice in diverse settings. It also creates an administrative burden to manage clinical agency approval, track student health requirement compliance, and coordinate clinical activities.

Selection Criteria

Nurse educators should conduct a careful assessment of potential clinical sites before selecting those that will be used. Faculty members who are also employed in clinical agencies may provide some of the necessary information, and teachers who have instructed students in an agency can provide ongoing input into its continued suitability as a practice site. State boards of nursing may have specific reporting requirements or forms that need to be completed as part of the selection and approval process for clinical sites. Nursing education programs may need to provide additional information for board of nursing review. For an example of an agency data form see www.dos.pa.gov/ProfessionalLicensing/BoardsCommissions/Nursing/Documents/Applications%20and%20Forms/agency_data_form.pdf.

Assessment of potential clinical agencies should address the following criteria:

- *Opportunity to achieve learning outcomes:* Are sufficient opportunities available to allow learners to achieve learning objectives? For example, if planning, implementing, and evaluating preoperative teaching is an important course objective, the average preoperative patient census must be sufficient to permit learners to practice these skills. If the objectives require learners to practice direct patient care, does the agency allow this, or will learners only be permitted to observe? Will learners from other educational programs be present in the clinical environment at the same time? If so, how much competition for the same learning opportunities is anticipated? Will there be an adequate patient census to ensure that appropriate learning opportunities are available?
- *Level of the learner:* If the learners are undergraduate students at the beginning level of the curriculum, the agency must provide ample opportunity to practice basic skills. Graduate students need learning activities that will allow them to develop advanced practice skills. Does the clinical agency permit graduate students to practice independently or under the guidance of a preceptor, without an

on-site instructor? Are undergraduate students in a capstone course permitted to participate in clinical learning activities under the guidance of an appropriate staff member as preceptor, without the physical presence of a faculty member?

■ *Degree of control by faculty:* Does the agency staff recognize the authority of the clinical teacher to plan appropriate learning activities for students, or do agency policies limit or prescribe the kinds and timing of student activities? Do staff members restrict the types of learning activities available? Do agency personnel view learners as additions to the staff and expect them to provide service to patients, or do they acknowledge the role of students as learners?

■ *Availability of role models for students:* As previously discussed, students often imitate the behaviors they observe in nursing staff members. Are the agency staff members positive role models for students and new staff nurses? If learners are graduate students who are learning advanced practice roles, are strong, positive role models available to serve as preceptors and mentors? Do they have the educational and experiential qualifications to guide students appropriately? Is staffing adequate to permit staff members to interact with students and participate in their learning, or are they overburdened? Are staff dismissive, exclusionary, and rude, or are they cooperative, inclusive, supportive, and welcoming of students?

■ *Geographical location:* Although the geographical location of the clinical agency is not usually the most important selection criterion, it can be a crucial factor when a large number of clinical agencies must be used. Travel time between the campus and clinical settings for faculty and students must be considered, especially if learning activities are scheduled in both settings on the same day. Is travel to the agency via public transportation possible and safe, especially if faculty and students must travel in the evening or at night? Are public transportation schedules convenient; do they allow students and faculty to arrive at the agency in time for the scheduled start of activities, and do they permit a return trip to campus or home without excessive wait times? Does the value of available learning opportunities at the agency outweigh the disadvantages of travel time and cost?

■ *Physical facilities:* Are physical facilities such as conference space, locker rooms, cafeteria or other dining facility, library, and parking available for use by clinical teachers and students?

■ *Staff relationships with teachers and learners:* Do staff members respond positively to the presence of students, engage in effective communications with faculty and students, and welcome appropriate questions from them? Will the staff members cooperate with teachers in selecting appropriate learning activities, participate in orientation activities for faculty and students, and provide useful guidance and feedback about student performance?

■ *Orientation needs:* Some clinical agencies require faculty members to attend scheduled orientation sessions before they take students into the clinical setting. The time required for such orientation must be considered when selecting clinical agencies. If faculty members are also employed in the agency as casual or per diem staff, this orientation requirement may be waived. Can any parts of the orientation be completed without being present in the agency, such as online or via self-study? Is the clinical teacher who is new to a clinical setting permitted to work in the staff nurse role for several days prior to bringing students to the agency, to become familiar with the routines and to begin to form collaborative relationships with staff members? Are technology initiatives occurring that require faculty and student orientation, password clearances, and access to computer systems? If so, are there mechanisms in place for training and to allow clinical teachers and students to use these systems as part of the clinical learning activities?

■ *Opportunity for interdisciplinary activities:* As interprofessional skill development emerges as a critical component of nursing education, consider if there are opportunities for learners to practice as members of an interdisciplinary healthcare team. Will learners have contact with other healthcare practitioners, such as physical therapists, pharmacists, nutritionists, respiratory therapists, social workers, infection control personnel, and physicians?

■ *Agency requirements:* Unless the educational program and the clinical facility are parts of the same organization, a legal contract or agreement usually must be negotiated to permit students and faculty to use the agency as a clinical teaching site. Such contracts or agreements typically specify requirements such as school and individual liability insurance; competence in cardiopulmonary resuscitation; professional licensure for clinical teachers, graduate students, and RN-to-BSN students; immunization and other health requirements; dress code; use of name tags or identification badges; requirements for student drug testing; and requirements for criminal background checks for students and clinical teachers.

■ *Agency licensure and accreditation:* Accreditation requirements for educational programs may specify that clinical learning activities take place in accredited healthcare organizations. If the agency must be licensed to provide certain health services, it is appropriate to verify current licensure before selecting that agency as a clinical site.

■ *Costs:* In addition to travel expenses, there may be other costs associated with use of an agency for clinical learning activities. Any fees charged to schools for use of the agency or other anticipated expenses to the educational program and to individual clinical teachers and students should be assessed.

■ *Regulatory board approvals:* State boards of nursing often require review and approval of clinical sites before a new site can be used for clinical nursing education. Faculty members or administrators may need to provide information about the healthcare institution, including bed capacity and average daily patient census, a list of other nursing education programs using the facility, number of students who will use the facility, and specific scheduling information.

Healthcare agencies are mandating these requirements to ensure patient safety and comply with various regulations. Currently, the Centers for Disease Control and Prevention (CDC, 2019) and the Advisory Committee on Immunization Practices (ACIP) of the CDC recommend that health profession students receive measles, mumps, rubella, hepatitis B, varicella, influenza, tetanus, diphtheria, and pertussis vaccines. Given the changing nature of vaccines, particularly regarding COVID-19, recommendations are regularly updated. Therefore, teachers need to periodically check these guidelines for new information and consult with healthcare agencies to align with their requirements. Students may need to demonstrate compliance by showing evidence of immunizations or immunity, or they may require booster immunizations. Many healthcare facilities may have additional or site-specific clinical requirements such as mandatory drug testing. Institutions may require testing for a specific panel of drugs or drug classifications. Typically, students have a narrow window of time for completion of the drug testing at the start of a clinical practicum and must follow a specific protocol for this testing. Depending upon state regulations, students may also need to complete a variety of background checks to screen for offenses and criminal arrest records. These background checks may include child abuse, elder abuse, and criminal history checks. Some agencies require that students meet the same requirements that their staff members must meet, which may include financial background checks. All of these requirements should be communicated to students in print and, for ease of retrieval, in an online electronic format. Early and clear communication with students about these requirements will help to ensure that students understand them and have sufficient time to gather evidence of completion by the specified deadlines.

The list of clinical requirements may be quite lengthy and may require significant time and financial investment for students to comply; however, they must be completed before a student can begin clinical activities at a clinical site and risk violating the nursing education program's contract with the agency and jeopardize future access to that clinical site. Another concern for the educational institution involves managing these records. When gathering personal information about students, nursing education program personnel need to protect student privacy and prevent inappropriate disclosure of personal information obtained for clinical requirements. Some programs contract with agencies that serve as a repository for the various student health requirements and background checks. These companies review the materials submitted by students and provide reports to the nursing program that can guide decisions about completion of the requirements. Student consent is essential when releasing personally identifiable information to such outside agencies to ensure compliance with the Family Education Rights and Privacy Act (FERPA) (20 U. S. C. § 1232g; 34 CFR Part 99). Thus, nursing education programs should have guidelines for disclosure and a method of keeping this private information separate from students' academic records.

Sufficient time must be allowed before the anticipated start of clinical activities to negotiate a contractual agreement that specifies rights and responsibilities. Legal counsel may be involved in negotiating these legally binding documents that specify roles and responsibilities (Fressola & Patterson, 2017). Clinical teachers must usually have current unencumbered professional nursing licenses for each state in which they instruct in the clinical area, unless the clinical agencies are located in states that have adopted the Nurse Licensure Compact (NLC; National Council of State Boards of Nursing, n.d.). Over 30 states allow nurses to practice in NLC states as long as they live in a NLC state and hold and meet license requirements in their home state. Other states have nurse licensure compact legislation pending.

PREPARATION OF FACULTY MEMBERS

When selection of the clinical site or sites is complete, the nurse educator must prepare for the teaching and learning activities that will take place there. Areas of preparation that must be addressed include clinical competence, familiarity with the clinical environment, and orientation to the agency or setting.

Clinical Competence

Clinical competence has been documented as an essential characteristic of effective clinical teachers. Clinical competence includes theoretical knowledge, expert clinical skills, and judgment in the practice area in which teaching occurs (Oermann & Gaberson, 2021).

Standards for accreditation and state approval of nursing education programs may require nurse faculty members to have advanced clinical preparation in graduate nursing programs in the clinical specialty area in which they are assigned to teach. In addition, faculty members should have sufficient clinical experience in the specialty area in which they teach. This is particularly important for faculty members who will provide direct, on-site guidance of students in the clinical area; the combination of academic preparation and professional work experience supports the teacher's credibility and confidence. Students often identify the ability to demonstrate nursing care in the clinical setting as an essential skill of an effective clinical instructor (Gubrud-Howe, 2020).

Clinical teachers should maintain current clinical knowledge through participation in continuing education and practice experience. Nurse educators who have a concurrent faculty practice or joint appointment in a clinical agency, or who work part time in a clinical role in addition to their academic assignment, are able to maintain their clinical competence by this means, especially if they practice in the same specialty area and clinical agency in which they teach.

Familiarity With the Clinical Environment

If the clinical teacher is entering a new clinical area, they may ask to work with the staff for a few days prior to returning to the site with students. This enables the teacher to practice using equipment and technology that may be unfamiliar and to become familiar with the agency environment, policies, and procedures. If this is not possible, the teacher should at least observe activities or shadow a nursing staff member in the clinical area to discern the characteristics of the patient population, the usual schedule and pace of activities, the types of learning opportunities available to develop desired outcomes, the diversity of healthcare professionals in the agency, and the presence of other learners (Jaroneski & Przymusinski, 2019).

As previously mentioned, a clinical agency may require faculty members whose students use the facility to attend an orientation program. Orientation sessions vary in length, from several hours to a day or more, and typically include introductions to administrators, managers, and staff development instructors; clarification of policies such as whether students may administer IV medications; review of documentation procedures; and safety procedures. Faculty members may be asked to demonstrate competent operation of equipment, such as infusion pumps, that their students will be using or to submit evidence that they have met the same competency standards that are required of nursing staff members. They may also need computer training so they can access electronic health records.

ADJUNCT AND PART-TIME TEACHERS

As nursing programs face increasing enrollments, combined with faculty retirements, fiscal constraints, and changing program needs, adjunct or part-time teachers are often hired for clinical teaching responsibilities. Practicing nurses with their extensive clinical knowledge and expertise in the practice setting may fill the needed teacher vacancies. Drawing upon their knowledge of the clinical setting, they can effectively help students learn nursing care practices; however, these skilled clinicians may lack the necessary educational preparation needed to successfully carry out the clinical teacher role (Summers, 2017). Specifically, these clinical teachers may need to understand student policies, curriculum, and evaluation practices that are necessary to help students make the connection between theory and practice and provide safe patient care. It is important that all clinical teachers, particularly those newly hired, be oriented to their role, responsibilities, and expectations. Providing opportunities for support and connection with other teachers, integration into the program, and faculty development opportunities aimed at addressing clinical teaching and learning needs will enhance retention and success in the clinical teacher role.

PREPARATION OF CLINICAL AGENCY STAFF

Preparation of the clinical agency staff usually begins with the nursing education program's initial contact with the agency when negotiating an agreement or contract between the program and the agency. Establishing an effective working relationship with the nursing staff is an important responsibility of the clinical teacher. Ideally, nursing staff members would be eager to work with the faculty member to help students meet their learning goals. Indeed, in academic health centers and other teaching institutions, participation in education of learners from many healthcare disciplines is a normal job expectation. Serving as a preceptor or working with students may be used for recertification or rewards through a clinical ladder program (Ulrich, 2019). Regardless of the reasons for working with students, some staff members will enjoy working with students more than others. Because teachers cannot usually choose which staff members will be involved with students, it is important for the teacher to communicate the following information to all staff members.

Clarification of Roles

Staff members often expect the instructor to be responsible for the care of patients with whom students are assigned to work. Many clinical teachers remark that if they have 10 students and each student is assigned two patients, the instructor is responsible for 30 individuals. These role expectations are both unrealistic and unfair to all involved parties.

Although the clinical teacher is ultimately responsible for student learning, students have much to gain from close working relationships with staff members. Staff members can serve as useful role models of nursing practice in the real world; students can observe how staff members must adapt their practice to fit the demands of a complex, ever-changing clinical environment. At the same time, staff members are often stimulated and motivated by students' questions and the current information that they can share. The presence of students in the clinical environment often reinforces staff members' competence and expertise, and many nurses enjoy sharing their knowledge and skill with novices. Clinical teachers should therefore encourage staff members to participate in the instruction of learners within guidelines that teachers and staff members develop jointly. Students should be encouraged to use selected staff members as resources for their learning, especially when they have questions that relate to specific patients for whom the staff members are responsible.

An important point of role clarification is that the responsibility for patient care remains with staff members of the clinical agency, as mentioned earlier. If a student is assigned learning activities related to care of a specific patient, a staff member, often called the primary nurse, is assigned the overall responsibility for that patient's care. Students are accountable for their own actions, but the primary nurse and student should collaborate to ensure that patient needs are met. Staff members may give reports about patient status and needs to students who are assigned to work with those patients. Students should be encouraged to ask questions of staff members about specific patient care requirements; to share ideas about patient care; and to report changes in patient condition, problems, and tasks that they will not be able to complete, and the need for assistance with tasks (Kan & Stabler-Haas, 2018).

Role expectation guidelines such as these should be discussed with staff members and managers. When mutual understanding is achieved, the guidelines may be written and posted or distributed to relevant personnel and students.

Level of Learners

Staff members can have reasonable expectations of learner performance if they are informed of the students' levels of education and experience. Beginning students and novice staff members will need more guidance; staff members working with these learners should expect frequent questions and requests for assistance. More experienced learners may need less assistance with tasks but more guidance on problem solving and clinical decision making. Sharing this information with staff members allows them to plan their time accordingly and to anticipate student needs.

It is especially important for faculty members to tell agency personnel what specific tasks or activities learners are permitted and not permitted to do. This decision may be guided by educational program or agency policy, the curriculum sequence, or by the specific focus of the learning activities on any given day. For example, during one scheduled clinical session, an instructor may want students to practice communication and active listening skills during health history data collection without relying on physical care tasks. The instructor should share this information with the staff and ask them to avoid involving students in physical care on that day.

Learning Outcomes

The overall purpose and desired outcomes of the clinical learning activities should be communicated to staff members. As demonstrated in the previous example, knowledge of the specific objectives for a clinical session permits staff members to collaborate with the teacher in facilitating learning. If students have the specific learning objective of administering intramuscular injections, staff members can be asked to notify the teacher if any patient needs an injection that day so that the student can take advantage of that learning opportunity.

Knowledge of the learning objectives allows staff members to suggest appropriate learning activities, even if the teacher is unable to anticipate the need. For example, an elderly patient who is confused may be admitted to the nursing unit; the staff nurse who is aware that students are focusing on nursing interventions to achieve patient safety might suggest that a student be assigned to work with this patient.

Need for Positive Role Modeling

The need for staff members to be positive role models for learners is a sensitive but important issue. As previously discussed, teachers often worry that students will learn bad practice habits from experienced nurses who may take shortcuts when giving care. When discussing this issue with staff members, instructors should avoid implying that the only right way to perform skills is the teacher's way. Instead, the teacher might ask staff members to point out when they are omitting steps from procedures and to discuss with learners the rationale for those actions. In this way, staff nurses can model how to think like a nurse, a valuable learning opportunity for nursing students.

Asking staff nurses to be aware of the behaviors that they model for students and seeking their collaboration in fostering students' professional role development is an important aspect of preparing agency staff to work with learners. To accomplish this goal, instructors need to establish mutually respectful, trusting relationships with staff members and to sustain dialogue about role modeling over a period of time.

The Role of Staff Members in Evaluation

Agency staff members have important roles in evaluating learner performance. The clinical performance of learners must be evaluated formatively and summatively. Formative evaluation takes the form of feedback to the student during the learning process; its purpose is to provide information to be used by the learner to improve performance. Summative evaluation occurs at the end of the learning process; its outcome is a judgment about the worth or value of the learning outcomes (Oermann & Gaberson, 2021). Summative evaluations usually result in academic grades or personnel decisions such as promotions or merit pay increases.

Teachers should explain carefully their expectations about the desired involvement of staff members in evaluating student performance. Agency personnel have an important role in formative evaluation by communicating with teachers and learners about student performance. Because staff members are often in close contact with students during clinical activities, their observations of student performance are valuable, but the teacher should keep in mind that staff members may have different expectations for student performance than the instructor does. Staff members should be encouraged to report to the teacher any concerns that they may have about student performance as well as observations of exemplary performance; clinical instructors should accept this input and then validate the report by their own observations. Staff members should also feel free to praise students, point out any errors they may have made, or make suggestions for improving performance. Immediate, descriptive feedback is necessary for learners to improve their performance, and often staff members are better able than teachers to provide this information to students.

However, it is the teacher's responsibility to make summative evaluation decisions. Staff members should know that they are an important source of data on student performance and that their input is valued, but that it is the clinical teacher who ultimately certifies competence or assigns a grade.

PREPARING THE LEARNERS

Students need cognitive, psychomotor, and affective preparation for clinical learning activities. It is the clinical teacher's responsibility to assist students with such preparation as well as to assess its adequacy before students enter the clinical area.

Cognitive Preparation

General prerequisite knowledge for clinical learning includes information about the learning outcomes; the clinical agency; and the roles of teacher, student, and staff member. Students may be expected to prepare ahead of time for each clinical learning session (Gubrud-Howe, 2020). This preparation may include one or more of the following tasks: gathering information from patient records; interviewing patients and family members; assessing patient needs; performing physical assessments; reviewing relevant pathophysiology, nursing, nutrition, and pharmacology textbooks; and completing written assignments such as a patient assessment, plan of care, concept map, or instructor-designed preparation sheet. In some programs, students complete these types of learning activities during and following their clinical learning activities.

Teachers should ensure that the expected cognitive preparations for clinical learning do not carry more importance than the clinical learning activities themselves. That is, learning should be expected to occur during the clinical learning activities as well as during preclinical preparation. If students receive their learning assignments in advance of the scheduled clinical activity, they can be reasonably expected to review relevant textbook information and to anticipate potential patient problems and needs. If circumstances permit a planning visit to the clinical agency, the student may meet and interview the patient and review the patient's health record. However, requiring extensive written assignments to be completed before the actual clinical activity implies that learning takes place only before the student enters the clinical area. Students cannot be expected to formulate a realistic plan of care before assessing the patient's physical, psychosocial, and cultural needs; this assessment may begin before the actual clinical activity, but it usually comprises a major part of the student's activity in the clinical setting. Thus, preclinical planning should focus on preparations for the learning that will take place in clinical practice. For example, the teacher may require students to formulate a tentative nursing diagnosis from available patient information, formulate a plan for collecting additional data to support or refute this diagnosis, and plan tentative nursing interventions based on the diagnosis. A more extensive written assignment submitted after the clinical activity may require students to evaluate the appropriateness of the diagnosis and the effectiveness of the nursing interventions.

Additionally, because students often copy information from textbooks (or, regrettably, from other students) to complete such requirements, written assignments submitted before the clinical learning activity may not show evidence of clinical reasoning and problem solving, let alone comprehension and retention of the information. For example, some teachers require students to prepare for medication administration during the clinical experience. Students often copy published pharmacologic information without attempting to retain this information and to think critically about why the medication was prescribed or how a particular patient might respond to it. A better approach is to ask students to reflect on the pharmacologic actions of prescribed drugs and to be prepared to discuss relevant nursing care implications, either individually with the instructor or in a group conference. If it is not possible for students to determine in advance which drugs are being used to treat patients whose care they will be participating in, the clinical instructor may ask students to study particular drug classifications and their prototype drugs and to be prepared to seek and use appropriate information resources when the student obtains the drug list. For example, if students are studying nursing care of patients who are at risk of a cerebral vascular accident, they should be familiar with several classifications of antihypertensive drugs and understand the common desired, side, and adverse effects. Students can then formulate a tentative plan of care for these patients and then modify and individualize the plan when they are able to assess specific patients.

Nursing students should learn to use a variety of reference materials both to prepare for clinical practice and as resources during clinical learning activities. Electronic mobile devices are popular resources that can be used to access reference materials and save time in the clinical setting. Students can use smartphones, tablets, computer applications, and ebooks to support clinical learning. Faculty members should consider the cost, connectivity issues, training needs, technology support, access, privacy and confidentiality concerns, available software, and student comfort with use if requiring these devices. Teachers may need to plan technology training sessions, collaborate with campus and clinical site technology support personnel, and develop policies and guidelines for appropriate use during clinical learning. Additional information about teaching with technology can be found in Chapter 10.

We recommend that students be expected to complete some cognitive preparation before clinical practice, but extensive, detailed written preparation assignments are unrealistic and often shift focus away from learning *during* clinical activities. Encouraging students' identification and use of appropriate, available information resources during clinical practice facilitates development of clinical reasoning and problem-solving abilities.

Meeting with students during a preclinical conference, either in a group or individually, also allows for assessment of student preparation as well as offers anticipatory guidance. Clinical teachers can use questioning techniques to determine if students have adequate knowledge to care for patients. It also provides an opportunity for clarification about anticipated nursing care and allows for correction of students' misconceptions before patient care is provided. Clinical teachers can assess student preparation and feel assured that students have an appropriate plan for care. Exhibit 4.1 provides sample questions that clinical teachers might use for preclinical conferences with students.

EXHIBIT 4.1 Sample Preclinical Conference Questioning

What are your priority nursing assessments?
What is your plan of care for the day? What nursing care will you provide first?
What lab or diagnostic tests were performed recently? What are the results? What are your nursing actions based upon these results?
What medications are prescribed for your patient that will need to be administered? Why is the patient taking each medication? What are the actions, side effects, and nursing implications of these medications?

Psychomotor Preparation

Skill learning is an important outcome of clinical teaching. As students develop into competent care providers, they need to have adequate time to learn psychomotor skills in a practice setting and be given appropriate and informative feedback to enhance performance. When learning complex skills, it is more efficient for students to practice the parts first in an environment such as a simulation center or skills laboratory, free from the demands of the actual practice setting (Durham & Baker, 2018). In such a setting, students can investigate and discover alternative ways of performing skills, and they can make errors and learn to correct them without fear of harming patients. Thus, students should have ample skill practice time before they enter the clinical area so that they are not expected to perform a skill for the first time in a fast-paced, demanding environment.

It is the clinical teacher's responsibility to ensure that students have developed the desired level of skill before entering the clinical setting. The use of clinical simulation and technology in a nursing skills lab provides students with realistic learning opportunities to develop psychomotor skills in a controlled environment. Use of clinical simulation activities allows students to practice and refine psychomotor skills and incorporates cognitive and affective learning as well. Exhibit 4.2 provides additional suggestions for teachers to use for psychomotor skill teaching and learning. Chapter 9 presents a comprehensive discussion of the use of clinical simulation.

EXHIBIT 4.2 Strategies for Enhancing Psychomotor Skill Learning

Focus on commonly used psychomotor skills.
Use technology and a variety of teaching–learning methods (visual, auditory, tactile).
Include demonstration and succinct explanations when teaching skills.
Offer a realistic environment for skill learning.
Physically guide students during early psychomotor skill learning.
Allow students opportunities to test different ways of performing skills but ensure critical.
elements of the psychomotor skills are performed correctly.
Provide focused practice opportunities over time, not just a single practice session.
Cluster steps of a psychomotor skill to facilitate memory.
Practice psychomotor skills to become proficient, coordinated, and efficient.
Intersperse psychomotor skill practice with other learning activities.
Design learning activities that allow students to observe skill performance of others.
Alternate psychomotor skill practice and observation of others' skills practice.
Use simulation for psychomotor skill practice and follow this with debriefing.
Provide prompt, positive feedback and coaching about psychomotor skill performance.
Incorporate prompts or cues to allow students to problem solve during psychomotor skill learning.
Provide formative feedback to correct psychomotor performance errors.
Use summative evaluation to verify skill learning.
Incorporate practice to refresh performance if a psychomotor skill is not used frequently.

Source: Adapted from Aldridge, M. D., & Hummel, F. (2019). Nursing students' perceptions of skills learning: A phenomenological study. *Nurse Educator, 44*(3), 170-174. doi:10.10197/NNE.0000000000000569; Oermann, M. H., Muckler, V. C., & Morgan, B. (2016). Framework for teaching psychomotor and procedural skills in nursing. *The Journal of Continuing Education in Nursing, 47*(6), 278-282. doi:10.3928/00220124-20160518-10

Affective Preparation

Affective preparation of students includes strategies for managing their anxiety and for fostering confidence and positive attitudes about learning. Most students have some anxiety about clinical learning activities (Gubrud-Howe, 2020). Students report that their initial clinical experience on a unit and being observed by the clinical teacher are among the most commonly identified anxiety-producing situations for them (Wang et al., 2019). The teacher plays a critical role in mediating that anxiety and stress and may employ strategies to identify students' fears and reduce their anxiety to a manageable level. A preclinical conference session might assess learners' specific concerns and assure students of the teacher's confidence in them, desire for their success, and availability for consultation and guidance during the clinical activities.

For example, during a preclinical conference on the first day of clinical practice in a course, the instructor may state that it is common for students to feel anxious before a clinical activity but that anxiety usually decreases during the experience. The teacher may encourage students to identify and name the specific source and nature of their anxieties; once these are identified, the teacher can help students to use a problem-solving approach to identify helpful responses. For instance, if students express concern that something may happen that they will not know how to handle, the teacher may help students to list all the potential adverse events and then brainstorm possible responses to them. Throughout such a discussion, teachers should reassure students of their availability to answer questions and assist them with clinical reasoning and problem solving during the clinical learning activities. Other strategies, such as orientation, can be used to ensure students are adequately prepared.

Orientation to the Clinical Agency

Like clinical teachers, students also need a thorough orientation to the clinical agency in which learning activities will take place. This orientation may take place before or on the first day of clinical activities. Staff members often assist the teacher in orienting students to the agency and helping them to feel welcome and comfortable in the new environment.

Orientation should include:

- The geographical location of the agency
- The physical setup of the specific unit where students will be placed
- Names, titles, and roles of personnel
- Location of areas such as rest rooms, dining facilities, conference rooms, and locker rooms
- Information about transportation and parking
- Agency and unit policies
- Daily schedules and routines
- Emergency protocols (e.g., fire drills, rapid response codes, cardiac arrest procedures, and equipment)
- Patient information documentation systems, including establishment of passwords and acquiring computer access to electronic health records and bedside medication administration systems

In addition, students need to have a telephone number at the clinical setting where they can be contacted in case of family emergency, know what procedures to follow in case of illness or other reason for absence on a clinical day, understand the uniform or dress requirements, and know what equipment to bring (e.g., stethoscope) and what to leave at home (e.g., personal valuables).

Given the growth of informatics in healthcare settings, faculty need to consider this for student orientation needs. Gone are the days of showing students hard-copy charts and explaining medication administration records and then moving quickly to delivering care. Instead, students need access codes for technology used at the clinical site. They will also need training for computer use, such as bar-coded bedside medication systems and electronic health records before they can fully deliver care. Preparing students for use of the electronic health record may require a special training session for students. Staff development practitioners or information technology staff may need to schedule designated electronic health record training and arrange access for students. Clinical teachers need to coordinate this technology training with nurse educators and healthcare information technology personnel. Of course, clinical teachers also need to ensure that they are up to date on this training so that they are prepared to guide student learning in the clinical setting. Unfortunately, some clinical agencies are restricting student access to the electronic health record by only allowing read-only access, limited documentation, and restricted diagnostic results creating variability in skill development for these students. Educators are encouraged to dialogue with clinical agencies to ensure appropriate access and training. If unsuccessful, they may want to adopt an academic electronic health record system that students can use and practice in a simulated laboratory setting (Hansbrough et al., 2020).

Not all of this orientation information needs to be presented on site; some creative clinical teachers have developed electronic resources that provide a virtual tour of the facility. If the agency uses computer software to document patient information, the instructor may be able to acquire a copy of the software application and make it available in the school's computer facility. Or the nursing program may purchase bar code scanning equipment that can be used to simulate medication administration in clinical practice labs. Learners can be expected to review these resources before coming to the clinical site. Self-directed electronic learning modules can be used to orient and prepare students for the clinical experience ensuring an efficient, flexible, and cost-effective delivery method for training. Mandatory education required by healthcare facilities, such as fire safety, Health Insurance Portability and Accountability Act (HIPAA) training, infection control, or other topics can be delivered electronically. Clinical teachers and students can review needed training and complete appropriate evaluation materials. Spreadsheets or online systems can efficiently track compliance and completion of learning. Electronic delivery of clinical information can also be used throughout the year to share ongoing updates with clinical teachers and students in an efficient manner.

The First Day

Students almost always perceive the first day of clinical learning activities in a new setting as stressful; this is especially true of learners in their initial clinical nursing course. Students' first exposure to the clinical environment can either promote their independence as learners or foster dependence on the instructor due to fear. Clinical teachers should plan specific activities for the first day that will allow learners to become familiar with and comfortable in the clinical environment and at the same time alleviate their anxiety. These activities may include tours, conferences, games, and special assignments. Another creative option involves having experienced nursing students serve as peer mentors. These experienced students may help reduce situation-specific anxiety felt by beginning students during their first clinical experience (Kachaturoff et al., 2020).

Even if learners have attended an agency orientation, it is helpful to take them on a tour of the specific areas they will use for learning activities, pointing out locations such as rest rooms, drinking fountains, fire alarms and extinguishers, emergency equipment, elevators, stairwells, and emergency exits. The instructor should introduce learners to staff members by name and title. If students need agency-specific identification badges, parking permits, or passwords for use of the computer system, the teacher may make the necessary arrangements ahead of time or accompany students to the appropriate locations where these items can be acquired. If an empty patient room is available, the instructor may demonstrate the use of equipment such as bed controls, call bells, oxygen delivery systems, and lighting controls.

Special assignments may include review and discussion of patient records, practice of computer documentation, and a scavenger hunt to help learners locate typical items needed for patient care. Exhibit 4.3 is an example of a scavenger hunt activity used in orienting students to a medical–surgical unit of a hospital. Learners may be asked to observe patient care for a specified period of time, interview a patient or family member, shadow a nurse, or complete a short written assignment focused on documenting an observation.

EXHIBIT 4.3 A Scavenger Hunt Strategy

ANYWHERE GENERAL HOSPITAL, UNIT 2C

Work in pairs to search for the location of the items or areas listed in the following. Check them off as you find them.

Locker room
Restrooms
Oxygen tank
Fire alarms
Fire extinguishers
Emergency exits
Patient teaching materials
Nurse manager's office
Medication dispensing systems
Linen carts
Kitchen
Utility room
Biohazardous waste containers
Waterless hand sanitizer dispensers
Reference materials
Conference room
Medical supply carts (IV bags, dressing change materials, gloves)
Computer workstations
Pulse oximeter
Wheelchairs

These activities may be followed by a short group conference, during which students are encouraged to discuss their impressions, experiences, and feelings. The teacher should review the roles of students, teacher, and staff members and should emphasize lines of communication. For example, students need to know who to ask for help and under what circumstances—that is, when to ask questions of staff members and when to seek assistance from the teacher. Handouts summarizing these expectations and requirements are useful because students can review them later when their anxiety is lower. If a dining facility is available in the clinical setting, pre- or postclinical conferences may take place in that location to allow students to relax with refreshments away from patient care areas. The conference may conclude by making plans for the next day of clinical practice, including selecting assignments and discussing how learners should prepare for their learning activities. Selection of clinical assignments is discussed in detail in Chapter 7.

SUMMARY

This chapter described the roles and responsibilities of faculty, staff members, and others involved in clinical teaching and suggested strategies for preparing students and staff members for clinical learning. The teacher and learners comprise a temporary system within the permanent culture of the clinical setting. Negative consequences of this relationship can be avoided by establishing and maintaining regular communication between the instructor and staff members. Clinical teachers function as culture brokers and border spanners to help integrate students more fully into the real world of nursing practice.

Settings for clinical learning should be selected carefully, based on important criteria such as compatibility of school and agency philosophy, licensure and accreditation, availability of opportunities to meet learning objectives, geographical location, availability of positive role models, and physical resources. Selection of appropriate clinical settings may be complicated by competition among several nursing programs for a limited number of agencies. Specific criteria for assessing the suitability of potential clinical settings were discussed.

When clinical sites have been selected, educators must prepare for teaching and learning activities. Areas of preparation include clinical competence, familiarity with the clinical environment, and orientation to the agency. Clinical competence has been documented as an essential characteristic of effective clinical teachers and includes knowledge and expert skill and judgment in the clinical practice area in which teaching occurs. Teachers may maintain clinical competence through faculty practice, joint appointment in clinical agencies, part-time clinical employment, and continuing nursing education activities. The teacher may become familiar with a new clinical setting by working with or observing the staff for a few days prior to returning to the site with students. The clinical agency may require faculty members to attend an orientation program that includes introductions to agency staff, clarification of policies concerning student activities, and review of skills and procedures. Adjunct and part-time clinical teachers need to ensure they are familiar with the curriculum, course, policies, and procedures.

Preparation of the clinical agency staff usually begins with the teacher's initial contact with the agency. Roles of teachers, students, and staff members should be clarified so that staff members have guidelines for their participation in the instruction of learners. An important point of role clarification is that, although students are accountable for their own actions, the responsibility for patient care remains with staff members of the clinical agency. Staff members also need to be aware of specific learning objectives, the level of the learner, the need for positive role modeling, and expectations concerning their role in evaluating student performance. Although staff members' feedback is valuable in formative evaluation, the teacher is always responsible for summative evaluation of learner performance.

Students need cognitive, psychomotor, and affective preparation for clinical learning activities. Cognitive preparation includes information about the learning objectives; the clinical agency; and the roles of teacher, student, and staff member. Students may be expected to prepare for each clinical learning session through readings, interviewing patients, and completing written assignments. However, requirements for extensive written assignments to be completed before the actual clinical activity may imply that learning takes place only before the student enters the clinical area.

The instructor has a responsibility to assess that students have the desired level of skill development before entering the clinical setting. When learning complex skills, it is more efficient for students to practice the parts first in a simulated setting such as a skills laboratory, free from the demands of the actual practice setting. Students should have ample skill practice time before they enter the clinical area so that they are not expected to perform a skill for the first time in a fast-paced, demanding environment.

Affective preparation of students includes strategies for managing their anxiety and for fostering confidence and positive attitudes about learning. Most students have some anxiety about clinical learning activities. Mild or moderate anxiety often serves to motivate students to learn, but excessive anxiety hinders concentration and interferes with learning. In preparation for clinical learning activities, teachers may employ strategies such as a structured preclinical conference to identify students' fears and reduce their anxiety to a manageable level.

Students also need a thorough orientation to the clinical agency in which learning activities will take place. This orientation should include information about the location and physical setup of the agency, relevant agency personnel, agency policies, daily schedules and routines, and procedures for responding to emergencies and for documenting patient information.

Students almost always perceive the first day of clinical learning activities in a new setting as stressful. Clinical teachers should plan specific activities for the first day that will allow learners to become familiar with and comfortable in the clinical environment and at the same time alleviate their anxiety. These activities include tours, conferences, games, and special assignments.

CNE® EXAMINATION TEST BLUEPRINT CORE COMPETENCIES

1. **Facilitate Learning**
   D. Use information technologies to support the teaching–learning process
   H. Create opportunities for learners to develop their own critical thinking skills
   I. Create a positive learning environment that fosters a free exchange of ideas
   K. Demonstrate personal attributes that facilitate learning (e.g., caring, confidence, patience, integrity, respect, and flexibility)
   M. Develop collegial working relationships with clinical agency personnel to promote positive learning environments

O. Demonstrate ability to teach clinical skills
P. Act as a role model in practice settings
Q. Foster a safe learning environment

2. **Facilitate Learner Development and Socialization**
   D. Create learning environments that facilitate learners' self-reflection, personal goal setting, and socialization to the role of the nurse
   E. Foster the development of learners in these areas
      1. cognitive domain
      2. psychomotor domain
      3. affective domain

4. **Participate in Curriculum Design and Evaluation of Program Outcomes**
   A. Demonstrate knowledge of curriculum development including:
      4. selecting appropriate learning activities
      5. selecting appropriate clinical experiences
   H. Collaborate with community and clinical partnerships that support the educational goals

5. **Pursue Systematic Self-Evaluation and Improvement in the Academic Nurse Educator Role**
   A. Engage in activities that promote one's socialization to the role
   E. Participate in professional development opportunities that increase one's effectiveness in the role

6. **Engage in Scholarship, Service, and Leadership**
   C. Function effectively within the organizational environment and the academic community
      3. Integrate the values of respect, collegiality, professionalism, and caring to build an organizational climate that fosters the development of learners and colleagues

CNE®cl EXAMINATION TEST BLUEPRINT CORE COMPETENCIES

1. **Function within the Education and Health Care Environments**
   A. Function in the Clinical Educator Role
      1. Bridge the gap between theory and practice by helping learners to apply classroom learning to the clinical setting
      2. Foster professional growth of learners (e.g., coaching, reflection, and debriefing)
      4. Value the contributions of others in the achievement of learner outcomes (e.g., health team, families, and social networks)
   B. Operationalize the Curriculum
      1. Assess the congruence of the clinical agency to curriculum, course goals, and learner needs when evaluating clinical sites
      2. Plan meaningful and relevant clinical learning assignments and activities.
      4. Prepare learners for clinical experiences (e.g., facility, clinical expectations, equipment, and technology-based resources)
      5. Structure learner experiences within the learning environment to promote optimal learning
      7. Provide opportunities for learners to develop problem-solving and clinical reasoning skills related to course objectives (e.g., learning outcomes)

    C. Abide by Legal Requirements, Ethical Guidelines, Agency Policies, and Guiding Framework
       1. Apply ethical and legal principles to create a safe clinical learning environment
       4. Inform others of program and clinical agency policies, procedures, and practices
       5. Adhere to program and clinical agency policies, procedures and practices when implementing clinical experiences
       6. Promote learner compliance with regulations and standards of practice

2. **Facilitate Learning in the Health Care Environment**
    A. Implement a variety of clinical teaching strategies appropriate to learner needs, learner outcomes, content, and context
    D. Create opportunities for learns to develop critical thinking and clinical reasoning skills
    G. Develop collegial working relationships with learners, faculty colleagues, and clinical agency personnel

3. **Demonstrate Effective Interpersonal Communication and Collaborative Interprofessional Relationships**
    B. Foster a shared learning community and cooperate with other members of the healthcare team
    C. Create multiple opportunities to collaborate and cooperate with other members of the healthcare team
    E. Act as a role model showing respect for all members of the healthcare team, professional colleagues, clients, family members, as well as learners
    F. Use clear and effective communication in all interactions (e.g., written, electronic, verbal, non-verbal)
    K. Maintain an approachable, nonjudgmental, and readily accessible demeanor
    M. Demonstrate effective communication in clinical learning environments with diverse colleagues, clients, cultures, healthcare professionals, and learners
    N. Communicate performance expectations to learners and agency staff

5. **Facilitate Learner Development and Socialization**
    G. Create learning environments that are focused on socialization to the role of the nurse

6. **Implement Effective Clinical and Assessment Evaluation Strategies**
    B. Implement both formative and summative evaluation that is appropriate to the learner and learning outcomes
    E. Provide timely, objective, constructive, and fair feedback to learners
    H. Assess and evaluate learner achievement of clinical performance expectations
    I. Use performance standards to determine learner strengths and weaknesses in the clinical learning environment
    K. Evaluate the quality of the clinical learning experiences and environment

REFERENCES

Aldridge, M. D., & Hummel, F. (2018). Nursing students' perceptions of skills learning: A phenomenological study. *Nurse Educator, 44*(3), 170–174. https://doi.org/10.1097/NNE.0000000000000569

Centers for Disease Control and Prevention. (2019). *Advisory Committee on Immunization Practices (ACIP) vaccine recommendations and guidelines.* https://www.cdc.gov/vaccines/hcp/acip-recs/index.html

Dahlke, S., & Hannesson, T. (2016). Clinical faculty management of the challenges of being a guest in clinical settings: An exploratory study. *Journal of Nursing Education*, 55(2), 91–95. https://doi.org/10.3928/01484834-20160114-06

Durham, C. F., & Baker, D. E. (2018). Learning laboratories as a foundation for nursing excellence. In M. H. Oermann, J. C. De Gagne, & B. Phillips (Eds.), *Teaching in nursing and role of the educator* (2nd ed., pp. 155–177). Springer Publishing Company.

Fressola, M. C., & Patterson, G. E. (2017). *Transition from clinician to educator: A practical approach.* Jones & Bartlett.

Gubrud-Howe, P. (2020). Teaching in the clinical setting. In D. M. Billings & J. A. Halstead (Eds.), *Teaching in nursing: A guide for faculty* (6th ed., pp. 328–352). Elsevier.

Hansbrough, W., Dunker, K. S., Ross, J. G., & Ostendorf, M. (2020). Restrictions on nursing students' electronic health information access. *Nurse Educator*, 45(5), 243–247. https://doi.org/10.1097/NNE.0000000000000786

Jaroneski, L. A., & Przymusinski, L. A. (2019). *So you want to teach clinical? A guide for new nursing clinical instructors.* Routledge.

Kachaturoff, M., Caboral-Stevens, M., Gee, M., & Lan, V. M. (2020). Effects of peer-mentoring on stress and anxiety levels of undergraduate nursing students: An integrative review. *Journal of Professional Nursing*, 36(2020), 223–228. https://doi.org/10.1016/j.profnurs.2019.12.007

Kan, E. Z., & Stabler-Haas, S. (2018). *Fast facts for the clinical nursing instructor* (3rd ed.). Springer Publishing Company.

Kapaale, C. C. (2020). Validating factors that influence student nurse intention regarding perioperative nursing. *Journal of Nursing Measurement*, 28(3), E293–E313. https://doi.org/10.1891/JNM-D-19-00040

National Council of State Boards of Nursing. (n.d.). *Nurse licensure compact.* https://www.ncsbn.org/nlc.htm

Oermann, M. H., & Gaberson, K. B. (2021). *Evaluation and testing in nursing education* (6th ed.). Springer Publishing Company.

Oermann, M. H., Muckler, V. C., & Morgan, B. (2016). Framework for teaching psychomotor and procedural skills in nursing. *The Journal of Continuing Education in Nursing*, 47(6), 278–282. https://doi.org/10.3928/00220124-20160518-10

Oosterbroek, T. A., Younge, O. J., & Myrick, F. (2019). "Everybody knows your name." Belonging in rural preceptorship. *Online Journal of Rural Nursing & Health Care*, 19(1), 64–88. https://doi.org/10.14574/ojrnhc.v19i1.548

Steele-Moses, S., Creel, E., & Carruth, A. (2018). Recruitment attributes important to new nurse graduates employed on adult medical-surgical units. *MEDSURG Nursing*, 27(5), 210–314.

Summers, J. A. (2017). Developing competencies in the novice nurse educator: An integrative review. *Teaching and Learning in Nursing*, 12(2017), 263–276. https://doi.org/10.1016/j.teln.2017.05.001

Ulrich, B. (2019). *Mastering precepting: A nurse's handbook for success* (2nd ed.). Sigma Theta Tau International.

Wang, A. H., Less, C. T., & Espin, S. (2019). Undergraduate nursing students' experiences of anxiety-producing situations in clinical practicums: A descriptive survey study. *Nurse Education Today*, 76(2019), 103–108. https://doi.org/10.1016/j.nedt.2019.01.016

A robust set of instructor resources designed to supplement this text is located at http://connect.springerpub.com/content/book/978-0-8261-6705-7. Qualifying instructors may request access by emailing textbook@springerpub.com.

Process and Models of Clinical Teaching

Clinical teaching is a complex interaction between students and educators. Characteristics of the teacher and learner; the clinical environment and nature of practice within that environment; patients, families, and others for whom students are caring; other healthcare providers; and the inherent nature of clinical practice with its uncertainties all influence the clinical teaching process. This chapter outlines the process of clinical teaching and provides a framework for planning clinical activities appropriate for the competencies to be achieved, guiding students in the practice setting, and evaluating clinical performance. A framework assists clinical teachers in creating an environment and opportunities for students to learn. The outcomes of those experiences, however, may vary considerably among students because many factors in the practice environment influence the learning process. Models of clinical teaching such as traditional, in which one teacher guides the learning of a small group of students; preceptor; and dedicated education units (DEUs), among others, are explained in this chapter.

TEACHING AND LEARNING

Teaching is a complex process intended to facilitate learning. While the goal of teaching is to lead students in discovering knowledge for themselves, the teacher encourages this discovery through deliberate teaching actions that lead in that direction. Clinical teaching involves a sharing and mutual experience on the part of both teacher and student and is carried out in an environment of support and trust. Teaching is not telling, it is not dispensing information, and it is not merely demonstrating skills. Instead, teaching is *involving* the student as an active participant in this learning. The teacher is a resource person with knowledge and skills to share to facilitate learning.

Learning is a process through which people change as a result of their experiences. Some of these changes are observable and measurable; for example, the student can explain the evidence base of an intervention or can accurately perform a procedure. In clinical practice, however, new insights, ideas, and perspectives may be as critical to the student's learning and development as overt and measurable behaviors. Learning, therefore, may be a change in observable behavior or performance, or it may reflect a new perception and insight.

The teaching–learning process is a complex interaction of these processes. When students are actively involved in their learning and perceive a positive teacher–student relationship, they can be honest about their learning needs and how clinical educators can help them in developing their competencies. Active learning may also foster students' higher level thinking as they reflect on patient problems and possible approaches, and consider multiple options (Hong & Yu, 2017; Li et al., 2019; Oermann & Gaberson, 2021).

Although teaching and learning are interrelated processes, each may occur without the other. Significant learning may result from the student's clinical activities without any teacher involvement. Similarly, the teacher's carefully planned assignments and learning activities for students may not lead to new learning or development of competencies. The goal of clinical teaching is to create the *environment and activities for learning*, recognizing that each student will gain different insights and outcomes from them.

PROCESS OF CLINICAL TEACHING: FIVE COMPONENTS

The process of clinical teaching includes five steps:

1. Identifying the clinical competencies,
2. Assessing learning needs,
3. Planning clinical learning activities,
4. Guiding learners, and
5. Evaluating clinical learning and performance.

This process is not linear; instead, each component influences others. For example, clinical evaluation provides data on further learning needs of students that in turn suggest new learning activities. Similarly, as the teacher works with students, observations of performance may alter the assessment and suggest different learning activities.

Identifying the Clinical Competencies

The first step in clinical teaching is to identify the clinical competencies to be achieved in the course or practicum. These competencies suggest areas for assessment, provide guidelines for teaching, and are the basis for evaluating learning. There are many definitions of competencies. The American Association of Colleges of Nursing (AACN) defines competencies as the observable abilities of students— their knowledge, skills, and attitudes (AACN, 2021). In some nursing programs, rather than clinical competencies, faculty identify the outcomes of learning or objectives to be achieved by students in the clinical course or at the end of a specific clinical practicum or set of learning activities.

Exhibit 5.1 provides examples of clinical competencies in 10 broad areas of clinical learning. In some courses, students need to demonstrate learning and performance in all of these areas of learning as well as others specific to the clinical specialty or setting. Other courses may focus on only a few of these areas. Clinical competencies may be stated broadly, similar to most of the examples in Exhibit 5.1, or they can be more specific, such as, "Assess patients' and families' health literacy." The AACN *Essentials* identify competencies and sub-competencies at two levels (entry and advanced).

EXHIBIT 5.1 Examples of Clinical Competencies

1. Concepts, theories, and other knowledge for clinical practice:

   Analyzes the pathophysiology related to common patient conditions.

   Applies concepts of person-centered care to critically ill patients.

2. Use of research and other evidence in clinical practice:

   Uses evidence on pain management interventions in planning care for patients.

   Evaluates evidence for use in long-term care of patients with chronic health problems.

3. Assessment, diagnosis, plan, interventions, and evaluation of outcomes:

   Collects data that are developmentally and age appropriate for healthy and ill children.

   Considers multiple nursing interventions for care of patients with complex health problems.

4. Psychomotor and technological skills, other types of interventions, and informatics competencies:

   Demonstrates skill in conducting a health history and physical examination in role of advanced practice nurse (APN).

   Uses health information technology to retrieve critical information for decision making.

5. Values related to care of patients, families, and communities and other dimensions of healthcare:

   Recognizes personal values that might conflict with professional nursing values.

   Demonstrates respect for diversity and differences in values among patients and healthcare providers.

6. Communication skills, ability to develop interpersonal relationships, and skill in collaboration with others.

   Collaborates with healthcare team in planning interventions for patients.

   Communicates effectively with patients, families, and others, and within the healthcare team.

7. Development of knowledge, skills, and values essential for continuously improving the quality and safety of healthcare:

   Identifies issues with quality of care in a clinical setting using relevant measures.

   Participates in analyzing system errors and designing unit-based improvements.

8. Management of care, leadership abilities, and role behaviors:

   Manages care effectively for a group of patients.

   Demonstrates the role and behaviors of the nurse as leader.

9. Accountability and responsibility of the learner:

   Accepts responsibility for own actions and decisions.

   Is accountable for professional behavior and performing within ethical and legal standards.

10. Self-development and continued learning:

    Identifies own learning needs in clinical practice.

    Seeks learning opportunities to develop clinical competencies.

The clinical competencies should be observable and achievable by students, considering their prior knowledge, skills, and experiences. Learning opportunities should be available in the clinical setting, simulation, or through other experiences. The competencies should be communicated clearly to students, in written form, and understood by them. Similarly, the teacher has an important responsibility in *discussing* these competencies and related clinical activities with agency personnel, not *telling* them. Agency personnel need input into decisions about clinical learning activities. With this input, the teacher may need to alter the clinical activities and plan simulations and other types of learning opportunities for students. Students also should have input into the clinical competencies: There may be some already achieved by students and others to be added to meet their individual learning needs and goals. There should be some flexibility as long as students demonstrate the competencies and achieve the essential knowledge and skills for progressing through the nursing program.

It is important for all clinical teachers—full and part time, adjunct, and preceptors—to understand the competencies students should develop in a course or clinical practicum. The course leader is responsible for ensuring that all educators and preceptors in a course, no matter what their role, use the competencies to guide their selection of patients and other learning activities for students and to assess performance.

Assessing Learning Needs

Teaching begins at the level of the learner. The teacher's goal, therefore, is to assess the student's present level of knowledge and skill and other characteristics that may influence achieving the clinical competencies. The first area of assessment involves collecting data on whether the student has the prerequisite knowledge and skills for the clinical situation at hand and for completing the learning activities. For instance, if the learning activities focus on interventions for health promotion, students first need some understanding of health and wellness. Changing a sterile dressing requires an understanding of principles of asepsis. The teacher's role in assessment of the learner is important so that students engage in learning activities that build on their present knowledge and skills. When students lack the prerequisites, then the instruction can remedy these and more efficiently move students forward in their learning.

Not every student will enter the clinical practicum with the same prerequisite knowledge and skills, depending on past learning and clinical experiences. The teacher, therefore, should not expect the same entry competencies for all students. Assessment reveals the point at which the instruction should begin and does not imply poor performance for students, only that some learners may need different types of learning activities. Assessment may also indicate that some students have already attained certain clinical competencies and can progress to new areas of learning.

The second area of assessment relates to individual characteristics of students that may influence their learning and clinical performance. Students and nurses today represent a diverse group of learners with varied cultural and ethnic backgrounds, ages, learning styles, and other characteristics. Students bring with them a wealth of life, work, and other experiences. These differences may affect students' interactions with educators, patients, and healthcare providers; ways of approaching patient care; clinical judgment; and comfort and skill with technology, among other areas (Lasater et al., 2019; Wang et al., 2019; Williamson & Muckle, 2018).

In addition, many students combine their nursing education with other role responsibilities, such as family and work. Information about these characteristics gives the teacher a better understanding of the students and their responses to different learning situations. Faculty members and clinical educators need to assess individual differences among students and use this knowledge in planning their learning activities.

Planning Clinical Learning Activities

Following assessment of learner needs and characteristics, the teacher plans and then delivers the instruction. In planning the learning activities, the main considerations are the competencies to be developed in the clinical practicum and individual learner needs. Other factors that influence decisions on clinical activities include evidence of the effectiveness of the clinical teaching method and learning activities being considered, characteristics of the clinical learning environment, and availability of the educator, preceptor, or other clinician to guide learners.

CLINICAL COMPETENCIES

Clinical learning activities are selected to facilitate students' developing the clinical competencies or to meet the outcomes of the clinical practicum, depending on how these are stated in the course. The learning activities may include patient care assignments, but care of patients is not the only learning activity in which students engage in the practice setting. The specific competencies to be achieved in that course should guide selection of learning activities. If the competencies focus on communication skills, then the learning activities may involve interviews with patients and others, papers analyzing those interactions, role-play, and simulated patient–nurse interactions rather than providing direct care.

LEARNER NEEDS

While the competencies provide the framework for planning the learning activities, the other main consideration is the needs of the student. Some students may have already met some of the competencies and can then progress to other types of learning activities. The activities should build on the student's present knowledge and skills and take into consideration other learner characteristics. Each student does not have to complete the same learning activities; the teacher is responsible for individualizing the clinical activities so that they best meet each student's needs while promoting achievement of the competencies. Learning activities also build on one another. Planning includes organizing the activities to provide for the progressive development of knowledge, skills, and attitudes for each learner.

EVIDENCE ON EFFECTIVENESS OF TEACHING METHODS

Decisions about the teaching methods to use and types of activities in which students will participate in the clinical setting should be based on evidence about what works best for promoting student learning. Nurse educators should review the literature to identify evidence to support the teaching methods they are planning and to get ideas about other strategies and activities for students that might be as or more effective. The evidence will also guide how a teaching method is implemented—for example, how to debrief after a simulation and the level of questions to ask to promote higher-level thinking. Evidence-based clinical nursing education involves four phases: (a) asking questions about best practices in teaching students in the clinical setting, (b) searching for research and other evidence to answer those questions, (c) evaluating the quality of the evidence and whether it is ready to be used in clinical teaching, and (d) deciding whether the findings are applicable to one's own clinical course, students, and setting (Oermann, 2022a, 2022b).

CHARACTERISTICS OF THE CLINICAL SETTING

The size of the clinical setting, the patient population, the educational level and preparation of nurses, their availability and interest in working with students, other types of healthcare providers in the setting, and other characteristics of the clinical environment should be considered in planning the learning activities. These characteristics are considered in choosing a clinical site for use in a course, as discussed in Chapter 3, and they also guide the faculty in planning learning activities.

AVAILABILITY OF EDUCATOR TO GUIDE STUDENTS' LEARNING

The availability of the clinical nurse educator, preceptor, or another clinician to guide students' learning in the clinical setting is an important consideration in planning the learning activities. Nursing students perceive the teacher's availability as one of the qualities of an effective clinical teacher (Sweet & Broadbent, 2017). The number and level of students in a clinical group, for instance, may influence the type of learning activities planned for a course. Beginning students and nurses new to a clinical practice area may require more time and guidance from the teacher than experienced students and nurses.

Guiding Learners in Clinical Practice

The next step in the process of clinical teaching is guiding learners to acquire the essential knowledge, skills, and attitudes for practice. Guiding is a facilitative and supportive process that leads the student toward achievement of the competencies. It is a process of supporting and coaching students in their learning. Guiding is not supervision; supervision is a process of overseeing. Effective clinical teaching requires that clinical educators guide students in their learning, not oversee their work.

This is the instructional phase in the clinical teaching process—the actual teaching of students in the clinical setting either on site or at a distance. For distance education courses, the instructional phase may be carried out by preceptors, APRNs in the clinical setting, and other providers depending on the course outcomes. With some learning activities, the teacher has a direct instructional role—for instance, demonstrating an intervention to students and questioning them to expand their understanding of a clinical situation. Other teaching activities, though, may be indirect, such as giving feedback on papers and preparing preceptors for their role, among others.

Clinical education provides the avenue for acquiring the knowledge and behaviors for practice in a particular role, whether it is a beginning professional nurse or new role such as APRN. This process requires learning about the role as the initial step and observing and working with nurses in that role as the second step. In clinical instruction, the teacher guides the student in learning about the role and role behaviors of the nurse, and models important values and attributes of the professional in that role. Socialization comes from an integration of clinical and other experiences, not only from the guidance of the teacher. The experiences of students with preceptors and the healthcare team contribute to this socialization process.

SKILL IN OBSERVING PERFORMANCE

In the process of guiding learners, the teacher needs to be skilled in: (a) observing clinical performance, arriving at sound judgments about that performance, and planning additional learning activities if needed, and (b) questioning students to promote their thinking and clinical judgment. Observing students as they learn to care for patients, families, and community members and to interact with others allows the teacher to identify continued areas of learning. This information, in turn, suggests new learning activities for clinical practice.

Observations of students may be influenced by the teacher's values and biases, which may affect *what they see* as they observe a student's performance and their *impressions* of the quality of that performance. All educators should know their own values and biases that might influence their observations of student performance in clinical practice and judgments about student performance of the competencies. Guidelines for observing students are summarized in Exhibit 5.2.

EXHIBIT 5.2 Guidelines for Observing Students in Clinical Practice

Examine your values and biases that may influence observations of students in clinical practice and judgments about clinical performance.

Do not rely on first impressions for these might change significantly with further observations of the student.

Make a series of observations before drawing conclusions about clinical performance.

Share with students on a continual basis observations made of clinical performance and judgments about whether students are meeting the clinical competencies.

Focus observations on the competencies to be achieved.

When the observations reveal other aspects of performance that need further development, share these with students and use the information as a way of providing feedback on performance.

Discuss observations with students, obtain their perceptions of performance, and be willing to modify judgments when a different perspective is offered.

Source: Adapted from Oermann, M. H., & Gaberson, K. B. (2021). *Evaluation and testing in nursing education* (6th ed.). Springer Publishing Company.

SKILL IN QUESTIONING STUDENTS

The second skill needed by the educator to effectively guide clinical learning activities is an ability to ask thought-provoking questions without students feeling that they are being interrogated. The ability to think critically and make sound clinical judgments are integral to providing quality care. These skills can be encouraged by asking students to clarify, relate, think beyond the obvious, and connect (Dinkins & Cangelosi, 2019; Makhene, 2019; Phillips et al., 2017). Open-ended questions about students' thinking and the rationale they used for arriving at clinical judgments foster development of higher level cognitive skills.

Nurse educators, however, tend to ask low-level questions that focus on recall of information rather than ones that foster critical thinking (Phillips et al., 2017). When questioning students in clinical practice, the teacher should assess understanding of related knowledge and concepts and how they apply to patient care. Other questions can ask students about different approaches and decisions possible in a clinical situation, consequences of each decision, what they would do, and their rationale; possible problems, interventions, and their evidence base; and assumptions underlying their thinking. Questions should encourage learners to think beyond the obvious.

The way in which questions are asked is also significant. The purpose of questioning is to encourage students to consider other perspectives and possibilities, not to drill them and create added stress. In the beginning of a clinical course, and particularly in the beginning of the nursing program, the educator should discuss the purpose of questioning and its relationship to developing thinking and clinical judgment skills. The teacher can demonstrate the type of questions that will be asked in the course and emphasize that the goal is to help students learn and begin to think like a nurse.

Because questioning is for instructional purposes, students need to be comfortable that their responses will not influence their clinical grades. Instead, the questions asked and answers given are an essential part of the teaching process, to promote learning and development of higher level thinking skills, not for grading purposes. Only with this framework will students be comfortable in responding to questions and evaluating alternative perspectives, using the teacher as a resource.

Evaluating Clinical Learning and Performance

The remaining component of the clinical teaching process is evaluation. Clinical evaluation serves two purposes: formative and summative. Through formative evaluation, the teacher monitors student progress toward achieving the competencies for clinical practice. Formative evaluation provides information about further learning needs of students and where additional clinical instruction is needed. Clinical evaluation that is formative is not intended for grading purposes; instead, it is designed to diagnose learning needs as a basis for further instruction.

Summative evaluation, in contrast, takes place at the end of the learning process to ascertain whether the student developed the essential competencies or achieved the outcomes (Oermann & Gaberson, 2021). Summative evaluation provides the basis for determining grades in clinical practice or certifying competency. It occurs at the completion of a course, an educational program, orientation, and other types of programs. This type of clinical evaluation determines what *has been* learned rather than what *can be* learned.

There are many clinical evaluation strategies that can be used in nursing courses. These are discussed and examples are provided in Chapter 12.

QUALITIES OF EFFECTIVE CLINICAL TEACHERS

Clinical teaching requires an educator who is knowledgeable about the clinical practice area, is clinically competent, knows how to teach, relates effectively to students, and is enthusiastic about clinical teaching. The teacher also serves as a role model for students or selects clinicians who will model important professional behaviors. There has been much research in nursing education on characteristics and qualities of an effective clinical teacher. Every clinical teacher should be aware of behaviors that promote learning in the practice setting and ones that impede student learning.

Knowledge

Teachers in nursing, as in any field, need to have expertise in the subject they are teaching. In clinical teaching, this means that educators are knowledgeable about patient conditions and populations, interventions, new treatments and technologies in patient care, and related research. Teachers must be up-to-date in the area of clinical practice in which they are working with students. This is particularly true in the traditional model of clinical teaching, in which the teacher is responsible for planning and guiding student learning in practice.

Clinical Competence

Teachers cannot guide student learning in clinical practice without being competent themselves. Clinical competence is an important characteristic of effective clinical teaching in nursing (Lovric et al., 2015). Teachers need to be experts in the area of clinical practice in which they are teaching, maintain their clinical skills, be able to explain and demonstrate nursing care in a real situation, and guide students in developing essential clinical competencies. This quality of teaching may be problematic for faculty members who teach predominantly in the classroom or change practice settings frequently and do not keep current in an area of clinical practice. It is up to the teacher to maintain clinical expertise and skills.

Skill in Clinical Teaching

Skill in clinical teaching includes the ability of the educator to assess learning needs, plan instruction that meets those needs and guides students in developing the clinical competencies, and evaluate learning fairly. These teaching skills are described more specifically in Exhibit 5.3.

The clinical teacher needs to know *how to teach*. While this seems obvious, in some settings, clinical nurse educators, preceptors, and others working with students are not prepared educationally for their roles. They have limited knowledge about how to guide students' learning in the clinical setting and assess their performance.

EXHIBIT 5.3 Clinical Teaching Skills

Assesses learning needs of students, recognizing and accepting individual differences.

Plans assignments that help in transfer of learning to clinical practice, meet learning needs, and promote development of competencies.

Communicates clearly to students the clinical competencies to be achieved and expectations of students in practice.

Considers student goals and needs in planning the clinical activities.

Structures clinical learning activities so they build on one another.

Explains clearly related knowledge, concepts, and theories applicable to patient care.

Demonstrates effectively clinical skills, procedures, and use of technology.

Provides opportunities for practice of clinical skills, procedures, and technology and recognizes differences among students in the amount of practice needed.

Is well prepared for clinical teaching.

Develops clinical teaching strategies that encourage students to problem solve and make sound clinical judgments.

Asks higher level questions that assist students in thinking through complex clinical situations.

Encourages students through teaching and assessment to think independently and beyond accepted practices and to try out new interventions.

Varies clinical teaching strategies and learning activities to stimulate student interest and meet individual needs of students.

Is available to students in clinical practice when they need assistance.

Serves as a role model for students.

Provides specific, timely, and useful feedback on student progress.

Shares observations of clinical performance with students on a continual basis.

Encourages students to assess their own performance.

Corrects mistakes without belittling students.

Exhibits fairness in evaluation.

Being an expert clinician is not enough. In a study by Lovric et al. (2015), students rated teaching ability among the most important competencies of a clinical nurse educator.

Skills in evaluating clinical performance both formatively, for feedback, and summatively, at the end of a period of time in the clinical course, are critical for effective teaching. Research has shown that effective teachers are fair in their evaluations of students, correct student errors without belittling students and diminishing their self-confidence, and give prompt feedback that promotes further learning and development.

Interpersonal Relationships With Students

The ability of the clinical teacher to interact with students, both on a one-to-one basis and in a group, is another important teacher behavior. Qualities of an effective teacher in this area are showing confidence in students, respecting students, being honest and direct, supporting students and demonstrating caring behaviors, being approachable, and encouraging students to ask questions and seek guidance when needed. Considering the demands on students as they learn to care for patients, students need to view the teacher as someone who supports them in their learning.

Personal Characteristics of the Clinical Teacher

Personal attributes of the teacher also influence teaching effectiveness. These attributes include enthusiasm, a sense of humor, willingness to admit limitations and mistakes honestly, patience, and flexibility when working with students in the clinical setting. Students often describe effective teachers as ones who are friendly and provide an opportunity for them to share feelings and concerns about patients. An effective clinical teacher is approachable (Sweet & Broadbent, 2017). The teacher should develop an atmosphere of trust and mutual respect for students to engage in open discussions about care and clinical situations. For these discussions to occur, the student needs to feel safe to share views and opinions.

In clinical teaching, educators need to self-assess and recognize areas of teaching to be improved. They should be willing to reflect on their teaching and evaluation practices and consider better ways of designing clinical activities and guiding students in their learning. Good teachers, like good scholars, strive to perfect their teaching skills over time and avoid stagnation in their teaching approaches.

STRESSES OF STUDENTS IN CLINICAL PRACTICE

Clinical practice is stressful for both prelicensure nursing students and graduate students preparing for advanced practice. In the clinical setting, students face uncertainties and unique situations that they may not have encountered in their prior learning. For some students, clinical practice is stressful because they are unsure about approaches and interventions to use. Interacting with the teacher, other healthcare providers, the patient, and family members may also contribute to the stress that students experience in clinical practice.

Other stresses, from the students' perspective, relate to the changing nature of patient conditions, a lack of knowledge and skill to provide care to patients, excessive workload, unfamiliarity in the clinical setting, working with difficult patients, developing technological skills, and being observed and evaluated by the teacher (Bhurtun et al., 2019; McCarthy et al., 2018; Wang et al., 2019). In a study of 93 undergraduate nursing students in the final year of their nursing program, students reported three situations that were most anxiety producing in the clinical practicum: fear of making a mistake, being observed by the clinical instructor, and their initial clinical experience on a unit (Wang et al., 2019). Learning in clinical practice occurs in public under the watchful eye of the teacher, the patient, and others in the setting. By keeping the nature of clinical learning in mind and using supportive behaviors when interacting with students, the teacher can reduce some of the stress that students naturally feel in clinical practice.

STRESSFUL NATURE OF CLINICAL TEACHING

Clinical teaching can be stressful for the teacher. First, it is time consuming. In many schools, a three-credit theory or online course requires 3 hours per week of instruction, 50 min for each credit hour not including preparation time. However, a three-credit clinical course may require 6 to 9 hours of clinical teaching a week, 2 to 3 clinical practice hours per credit hour, and even more in some nursing education programs. This time commitment for clinical teaching may create stress for faculty who also do academic advisement of students and are responsible for writing grant proposals, conducting research, writing for publication, serving on committees, providing community service, and maintaining a clinical practice. These multiple roles are demanding for clinical educators.

In addition to demands associated with the multiple roles of a nursing faculty member, other aspects of clinical teaching may be stressful. These include:

- Coping with the many expectations associated with clinical teaching.
- Feeling exhausted at the end of a clinical teaching experience with students.
- Too heavy a workload.
- Pressure to maintain clinical competence or a clinical practice without time to do so.
- Feeling unable to satisfy the demands of students, clinical agency personnel, patients, and others.
- Teaching inadequately prepared students.

For some new clinical teachers, their stress relates to a lack of preparation for their role. While clinicians have expert knowledge and skills in their specialty area, they may have limited knowledge of how to teach. As clinicians are recruited to academic positions, schools of nursing need comprehensive plans and education to prepare them for their role as a faculty member and teacher (Fitzwater et al., 2021; Jarosinski et al., 2020; Muirhead et al., 2021; Rogers et al., 2020). The aim of the Eastern Shore Faculty Academy and Mentorship Initiative, a collaboration among three nursing programs, was to facilitate the transition of expert clinicians to part-time clinical educators to meet the needs for faculty in the region. The initiative addressed the nursing faculty shortage by developing a pool of highly qualified and diverse part-time clinical nurse educators who are shared across programs (Hinderer et al., 2016).

Novice faculty members and teachers new to a nursing education program should find a mentor in the school who can support them as they learn the educator role in that setting. Mentors can be good sources of guidance on how to balance clinical teaching with other roles. Adjunct and part-time clinical educators also need a mentor to help them develop as effective clinical teachers. The mentor can be a resource for the clinical teacher and provide a link to the nursing program.

MODELS OF CLINICAL TEACHING

There are different models of clinical teaching: traditional, in which the teacher is directly responsible for guiding students in the clinical setting; preceptor or mentoring; and partnerships, including DEUs. In the preceptor and partnership models, preceptors and others in the clinical setting provide the clinical instruction, with the faculty member responsible for overall planning, coordinating the experience, grading clinical practice, and assuming other course-related responsibilities.

Traditional Model

In the traditional model of clinical teaching, the educator provides the instruction and evaluation for a small group of nursing students and is on site during the clinical experience. Students learn to provide care as they engage in practice themselves.

The traditional model of clinical teaching has been used in nursing education for decades (Giddens & Caputi, 2020). A benefit of this model is the opportunity to assist students in applying the knowledge and concepts learned in class, through online instruction, in readings, and through other learning activities in class to patient care. If the clinical educator is also involved with the course and curriculum overall, the clinical activities can be carefully selected to provide exemplars of the concepts that students are learning in the course. Although this is the most commonly used model, surprisingly there are few studies that document the outcomes of this model (Leighton et al., 2021).

Disadvantages are the large number of students for whom the educator may be responsible; not being accessible to students when needed because of demands of other students in the group; teaching procedures, clinical skills, and use of technologies for which the educator faculty member may lack expertise; the time commitment of providing on-site clinical instruction for faculty members with multiple other roles; and high costs for the nursing program. Clinical nurse educators who are part time or adjunct may not be sufficiently familiar with the philosophy and goals of the program, overall curriculum, clinical competencies developed prior to and following the course in which they are teaching, and other program characteristics, which may affect their planning of clinical activities for students and their expectations of students in the course. It is critical for the full-time faculty to prepare and orient part-time and adjunct faculty members involved in clinical teaching, so they are not only aware of their role and responsibilities but also understand how their course relates to the overall nursing curriculum.

In the traditional model, students may have unproductive time waiting for the educator or another clinician to answer their questions and guide their learning, or in the community, patients and families may not be available at the time students have their assigned clinical practice. Patients' conditions may deteriorate, resulting in students lacking the requisite knowledge and skills to care for them.

Another disadvantage of the traditional model of clinical teaching is that the educator and students may not be part of the healthcare system in which students have clinical practice. They are outsiders to the clinical setting and may not understand the system of care in that setting and its culture. In these situations, educators should work closely with the managers and clinical nursing staff to ensure an effective clinical experience for students. It is up to the educator to develop working relationships with the staff, which is essential to create an environment for learning and take advantage of activities that could be available for students in the setting. In the traditional model of clinical teaching, educators who are not also practicing in the clinical setting often invest extensive time in developing and maintaining these relationships.

The relationships that nursing faculty members develop in the clinical setting are not only with nursing staff but also involve other healthcare providers. With the emphasis on interprofessional practice and team-based care, nursing students need clinical learning activities in which they examine their own role in relationship to other providers, collaborate with other healthcare professionals, and learn to work as a productive member of the healthcare team. This learning also can occur with simulations that involve nursing, medical, pharmacy, and students in other professions. Simulations provide a way for students to learn to collaborate and gain an understanding of different perspectives to patient care. Interprofessional education with simulation is an effective strategy to teach students about collaborative models of care delivery and prepare future health professionals to work effectively within teams (Buhse & Della Ratta, 2017; Horsley et al., 2016; Lapierre et al., 2020; Reed et al., 2016; Zook et al., 2018).

Preceptor or Mentoring Model

In the preceptor model, an expert nurse in the clinical setting works with the student usually on a one-to-one basis in the clinical setting. Preceptors are staff nurses and other nurses employed by the clinical agency who, in addition to their ongoing patient care responsibilities, provide clinical instruction for students and new graduate nurses. In addition to one-to-one teaching, the preceptor guides and supports learners and serves as a role model. In this model, the faculty member from the nursing program serves as the coordinator, liaison between the nursing education program and clinical setting, and resource person for the preceptor. The faculty member, however, is typically not on site during the clinical practicum. The preceptor model involves sharing clinical teaching responsibilities between nursing program faculty and expert clinicians from the practice setting.

One strength of the preceptor model is the consistent one-to-one relationship of the student and preceptor, providing an opportunity for the student to work closely with a role model. This close relationship promotes professional socialization and enables students to gain an understanding of how to function in the role for which they are being prepared. By working closely with a clinical expert in the field, students improve their critical thinking and decision-making skills, develop clinical competencies, build their confidence, and improve readiness for practice as an RN or APRN (Edward et al., 2017; Fowler et al., 2018; Kantar, 2021; Lafrance, 2018).

Potential disadvantages of the preceptor model are lack of integration of didactic learning and clinical practice; lack of flexibility in reassigning students to other preceptors if needed; and time and other demands made on the preceptors. Preceptors must be well prepared for their roles and be competent in clinical teaching as well as patient care. For effective teaching, the preceptor must be skilled as a teacher with the same qualities as other clinical educators described earlier in this chapter. An entire chapter (Chapter 11) describes the use of preceptors in clinical teaching in both prelicensure and APRN programs.

Partnership Model

There are varied types of partnerships in nursing education. Some of these are the result of nursing programs searching for ways to increase student enrollment and cope with budgetary constraints, a nursing faculty shortage, and not enough clinical sites; others are intended to address the gap in preparation for practice readiness (Gorton, 2022; Luckenbach et al., 2021; Mennenga et al., 2021).

SHARING OF FACULTY AND CLINICIANS

Partnerships vary widely. In some programs, the partnership model is a collaborative relationship between a clinical site and nursing program that involves sharing a clinician and academic faculty member. The clinician teaches students in the clinical setting, with the faculty member serving as course coordinator, and the faculty member in turn contributes to the clinical agency—for example, by conducting research and serving as a consultant, or practicing as an APRN in the agency.

Expertise and services are shared between the partners. In this type of partnership, the clinician may work with a prelicensure or graduate nursing student on an individualized basis or may teach a small group of students, as in the traditional model.

Luckenbach et al. (2021) used a mixed-methods approach to examine the outcomes of their affiliate faculty model for clinical teaching, developed as a partnership between the academic health center and school of nursing. An affiliate faculty member is a staff nurse who teaches clinical students one day per week but continues to maintain full-time status in the healthcare system. This partnership model allowed the school of nursing to decrease its student-to-faculty ratio and orientation for clinical nurse educators because they are already employees of the health system. Seventy-two students and 25 affiliate faculty participated in the study (Luckenbach et al., 2021). They agreed that affiliate faculty prepared students to provide safe care, helped them connect classroom learning to clinical practice, were effective educators, supported students at the bedside, and enjoyed teaching. This model, in use for 7 years, is a viable and sustainable partnership model for clinical education.

CLINICAL SCHOLAR MODEL

Another example of a partnership for clinical teaching is the clinical scholar model, which originated in 1984 as a joint initiative between the University of Colorado College of Nursing and University of Colorado Hospital. In this model, clinical nurse experts coordinate student placements and learning experiences, provide consistent instruction for nursing students, and contribute to the evaluation of students' clinical competencies. These clinical experts are masters prepared in nursing and have a minimum of 5 years of experience in a nursing specialty practice and 2 years of employment in the healthcare agency (Gorton, 2022). This model gives students an opportunity to be taught by expert clinicians practicing in the setting.

DEDICATED EDUCATION UNIT

Another type of partnership is the DEU, which is a unit within a clinical site that is dedicated to teaching nursing students. A DEU is a triad of students, clinicians, and faculty members who collaborate to create a learning environment for students. While there are varied DEU models in the United States and other countries, a common element is the active engagement of nursing and other staff in the education of students. In these models, nurse clinicians serve as clinical teachers with academic faculty members in the role as liaison, guiding the clinician to ensure a quality clinical experience and that course outcomes are met (Bittner et al., 2021; Pedregosa et al., 2020; Rusch et al., 2018; Schoening et al., 2021).

In a systematic review, Pedregosa et al. (2020) reported that DEUs and other partnership models improved the clinical learning environment and teaching process for students, and also had benefits for clinicians. Both students and staff report satisfaction with this model of clinical teaching. Another benefit of a DEU is that the clinical partner can often reduce orientation and on-boarding time for new graduate nurses who had DEU clinical experiences in the setting. Other outcomes also are reported with DEUs. Bittner et al. (2021) measured the critical thinking ability of 179 students on non-DEU units and compared this to 64 students on DEUs. There were significant increases in total critical thinking scores for the DEU (intervention) group.

DEUs have been used in a wide range of settings. For example, Schoening et al. (2021) evaluated the outcomes of a psychiatric mental health DEU. Recognizing the need for nurses in rural health and limited availability of clinical sites, Goslee et al. (2020) developed a partnership between an associate degree nursing program and a rural primary care clinic. In this partnership, RNs in the clinic served as clinical nurse educators. Positive outcomes were reported by both RNs and students.

Selecting a Clinical Teaching Model

There is no one model that meets the needs of every nursing education program, clinical course, or group of students. The teacher should select a model considering these factors:

- Educational philosophy of the nursing program
- Philosophy of the faculty about clinical teaching
- Clinical competencies to be developed
- Intended outcomes of the clinical course
- Level of nursing student
- Type of clinical setting
- Availability of preceptors, expert nurses, and other people in the practice setting who can provide clinical instruction
- Willingness of clinical site personnel and partners to participate in teaching students and other educational activities

SUMMARY

The process of clinical teaching begins with identification of the clinical competencies to be achieved and proceeds through assessing the learner, planning clinical learning activities, guiding students, and evaluating clinical learning and performance. The clinical competencies, outcomes to be met in the course, and expectations of students should be communicated clearly to students, in written form, and understood by them. Similarly, the teacher has an important responsibility in discussing these competencies and related clinical activities with clinical site personnel.

Teaching begins at the level of the learner. The teacher's goal, therefore, is to assess the student's present level of knowledge and skill and other characteristics that may influence developing the clinical competencies. Following assessment of learner needs, the teacher plans learning activities and guides learners to acquire essential knowledge, skills, and attitudes to achieve the competencies. In this process of guiding learners, the teacher needs to be skilled in: (a) observing clinical performance, arriving at sound judgments about that performance, and planning additional learning activities if needed, and (b) questioning learners to encourage higher level thinking but without interrogating them. The last component of the clinical teaching process is evaluation.

Teaching in the clinical setting requires an educator who is knowledgeable, is clinically competent, knows how to teach, relates effectively to students, and is enthusiastic about clinical teaching. The research in nursing education over the years has substantiated that these qualities are important in clinical teaching.

Clinical practice is stressful for students. Students have identified dimensions of clinical learning that often produce anxiety, such as fear of making a mistake that would harm the patient; interacting with the patient, the teacher, and other health-care providers; the changing nature of patient conditions; a lack of knowledge and skill for giving care to patients; and working with difficult patients, among others. In some research studies, students have reported that the teacher is a source of added stress for them. These findings highlight the need for the teacher to develop supportive and trusting relationships with students in the clinical setting and to be aware of the stressful nature of this learning experience. A climate that supports the process of learning in clinical practice is dependent on a caring relationship between teacher and student rather than an adversarial one.

The teacher chooses a model for clinical teaching: traditional, preceptor, or partnership, including the DEU model. In the traditional model, the clinical educator teaches a group of students and is on site for the practicum. In the preceptor model of clinical teaching, an expert nurse in the clinical setting works with the student typically on a one-to-one basis. The partnership model varies with the academic institution but is generally a collaborative relationship between the nursing program and a clinical site. One type of partnership is the DEU, in which agency nursing staff teach nursing students with the unit assuming responsibility for creating a supportive learning environment. In these models, clinicians serve as clinical teachers with academic faculty members in the role of liaison, guiding the clinician to ensure a quality clinical experience and that course outcomes are met.

CNE® EXAMINATION TEST BLUEPRINT CORE COMPETENCIES

1. **Facilitate Learning**
   A. Implement a variety of teaching strategies appropriate to
      1. content
      2. setting (clinical)
      3. learner needs
      4. learning style
      5. desired learner outcomes
      6. method of delivery
   B. Use teaching strategies based on
      1. educational theory
      2. evidence-based practices related to education
   C. Modify teaching strategies and learning experiences based on consideration of
      1. cultural background
      2. past clinical experiences
      3. past educational and life experiences
   G. Model reflective thinking practices, including critical thinking
   H. Create opportunities for learners to develop their own critical thinking skills
   I. Create a positive learning environment that fosters a free exchange of ideas
   J. Show enthusiasm for teaching, learning, and the nursing profession that inspires and motivates students
   K. Demonstrate personal attributes that facilitate learning (e.g., caring, confidence, patience, integrity, respect, and flexibility)
   L. Respond effectively to unexpected events that affect instruction
   M. Develop collegial working relationships with clinical agency personnel to promote positive learning environments
   N. Use knowledge of evidence-based practice to instruct learners

O. Demonstrate ability to teach clinical skills
P. Act as a role model in practice settings
Q. Foster a safe learning environment

2. **Facilitate Learner Development and Socialization**
   A. Identify individual learning styles and unique learning needs of learners
   B. Provide resources for diverse learners to meet their individual learning needs
   C. Advise learners in ways that help them meet their professional goals
   D. Create learning environments that facilitate learners' self-reflection, personal goal setting, and socialization to the role of the nurse
   E. Foster the development of learners in these areas
      1. cognitive domain
      2. psychomotor domain
      3. affective domain
   F. Assist learners to engage in thoughtful and constructive self and peer evaluation
   H. Encourage professional development of learners

5. **Pursue Systematic Self-Evaluation and Improvement in the Academic Nurse Educator Role**
   A. Engage in activities that promote one's socialization to the role
   F. Manage the teaching, scholarship, and service demands as influenced by the requirements of the institutional setting
   I. Mentor and support faculty colleagues in the role of an academic nurse educator
   J. Engage in self-reflection to improve teaching practices

6. **Engage in Scholarship, Service, and Leadership**
   B. Engage in scholarship of teaching
      2. Use evidence-based resources to improve and support teaching
      4. Share teaching expertise with colleagues and others
   C. Function effectively within the organizational environment and academic community
      3. Integrate the values of respect, collegiality, professionalism, and caring to build an organizational climate that fosters the development of learners and colleagues

CNE®cl EXAMINATION TEST BLUEPRINT CORE COMPETENCIES

1. **Function within the Education and Health Care Environments**
   A. Function in the Clinical Educator Role
      1. Bridge the gap between theory and practice by helping learners to apply classroom learning to the clinical setting
      5. Act as a role model of professional nursing within the clinical learning environment
      6. Demonstrate inclusive excellence (e.g., student-centered learning, diversity)
   B. Operationalize the Curriculum
      1. Assess congruence of the clinical agency to curriculum, course goals, and learner needs when evaluating clinical sites
      2. Plan meaningful and relevant clinical learning assignments and activities
      3. Identify learners' goals and outcomes

4. Prepare learners for clinical experiences (e.g., facility, clinical expectations, equipment, and technology-based resources)
5. Structure learner experiences within the learning environment to promote optimal learning
8. Implement assigned models fo clinical teaching (e.g., traditional, preceptor, simulation, DEU)
C. Abide by Legal Requirements, Ethical Guidelines, Agency Policies, and Guiding Framework
2. Assess learner abilities and needs prior to clinical learning experiences
3. Facilitate learning activities that support the mission, goals, and values of the academic institution and the clinical agency
4. Inform others of program and clinical agency policies, procedures, and practices
5. Adhere to program and clinical agency policies, procedures and practices when implementing clinical experiences

2. **Facilitate Learning in the Health Care Environment**
A. Implement a variety of clinical teaching strategies appropriate to learner needs, desired learner outcomes, content, and context
F. Create a positive and caring learning environment
G. Develop collegial working relationships with learners, faculty colleagues, and clinical agency personnel
H. Demonstrate enthusiasm for teaching, learning, and nursing to help inspire and motivate learners

3. **Demonstrate Effective Interpersonal Communication and Collaborative Interprofessional Relationships**
B. Foster a shared learning community and cooperate with other members of the healthcare team
N. Communicate performance expectations to learners and agency staff

5. **Facilitate Learner Development and Socialization**
G. Create learning environments that are focused on socialization to the role of the nurse

REFERENCES

American Association of Colleges of Nursing. (2021). *The essentials: Core competencies for professional nursing education.* https://www.aacnnursing.org/Portals/42/AcademicNursing/pdf/Essentials-2021.pdf
Bhurtun, H. D., Azimirad, M., Saaranen, T., & Turunen, H. (2019). Stress and coping among nursing students during clinical training: An integrative review. *Journal of Nursing Education, 58*(5), 266–272. https://doi.org/10.3928/01484834-20190422-04
Bittner, N. P., Campbell, E., & Gunning, T. (2021). Impact of a dedicated education unit experience on critical thinking development in nursing students. *Nurse Educator.* https://doi.org/10.1097/NNE.0000000000000966
Buhse, M., & Della Ratta, C. (2017). Enhancing interprofessional education with team-based learning. *Nurse Educator, 42*(5), 240–244. https://doi.org/10.1097/nne.0000000000000370
Dinkins, C., & Cangelosi, P. (2019). Putting Socrates back in Socratic method: Theory-based debriefing in the nursing classroom. *Nursing Philosophy, 20*(2), e12240. https://doi.org/10.1111/nup.12240

Edward, K. L., Ousey, K., Playle, J., & Giandinoto, J. A. (2017). Are new nurses work ready–The impact of preceptorship. An integrative systematic review. *Journal of Professional Nursing, 33*(5), 326–333. https://doi.org/10.1016/j.profnurs.2017.03.003

Fitzwater, J., McNeill, J., Monsivais, D., & Nunez, F. (2021). Using simulation to facilitate transition to the nurse educator role: An integrative review. *Nurse Educator.* https://doi.org/10.1097/NNE.0000000000000961

Fowler, S. M., Knowlton, M. C., & Putnam, A. W. (2018). Reforming the undergraduate nursing clinical curriculum through clinical immersion: A literature review. *Nurse Education in Practice, 31*, 68–76. https://doi.org/10.1016/j.nepr.2018.04.013

Giddens, J. F., & Caputi, L. (2020). Conceptual teaching strategies for clinical education. In J. F. Giddens, L. B. Caputi, & B. Rodgers (Eds.), *Mastering concept-based teaching* (pp. 101–117). Elsevier.

Gorton, K. (2022). Partnerships with clinical settings: Roles and responsibilities of nurse educators. In M. H. Oermann, J. C. De Gagne, & B. C. Phillips (Eds.), *Teaching in nursing and role of the educator: The complete guide to best practice in teaching, evaluation, and curriculum development* (3rd ed., pp. 231–254). Springer Publishing Company.

Goslee, E., Chesak, S., Forsyth, D. M., Foote, J., & Bergen, S. (2020). Implementation of a dedicated education unit model for ADN students in a rural primary care setting. *Nurse Educator, 45*(2), 97–101. https://doi.org/10.1097/NNE.0000000000000711

Hinderer, K. A., Jarosinski, J. M., Seldomridge, L. A., & Reid, T. P. (2016). From expert clinician to nurse educator: Outcomes of a faculty academy initiative. *Nurse Educator, 41*(4), 194–198. https://doi.org/10.1097/nne.0000000000000243

Hong, S., & Yu, P. (2017). Comparison of the effectiveness of two styles of case-based learning implemented in lectures for developing nursing students' critical thinking ability: A randomized controlled trial. *International Journal of Nursing Studies, 68*, 16–24. https://doi.org/10.1016/j.ijnurstu.2016.12.008

Horsley, T. L., Reed, T., Muccino, K., Quinones, D., Siddall, V. J., & McCarthy, J. (2016). Developing a foundation for interprofessional education within nursing and medical curricula. *Nurse Educator, 41*(5), 234–238. https://doi.org/10.1097/nne.0000000000000255

Jarosinski, J. M., Seldomridge, L. A., Reid, T. P., & Hinderer, K. A. (2020). "Learning how to teach" in nursing: Perspectives of clinicians after a formal academy. *Nurse Educator, 45*(1), 51–55. https://doi.org/10.1097/NNE.0000000000000662

Kantar, L. D. (2021). Teaching domains of clinical instruction from the experiences of preceptors. *Nurse Education in Practice, 52*, 103010. https://doi.org/10.1016/j.nepr.2021.103010

Lafrance T. (2018). Exploring the intrinsic benefits of nursing preceptorship: A personal perspective. *Nurse Education in Practice, 33*, 1–3. https://doi.org/10.1016/j.nepr.2018.08.018

Lapierre, A., Bouferguene, S., Gauvin-Lepage, J., Lavoie, P., & Arbour, C. (2020). Effectiveness of interprofessional manikin-based simulation training on teamwork among real teams during trauma resuscitation in adult emergency departments: A systematic review. *Simulation in Healthcare : Journal of the Society for Simulation in Healthcare, 15*(6), 409–421. https://doi.org/10.1097/SIH.0000000000000443

Lasater, K., Holloway, K., Lapkin, S., Kelly, M., McGrath, B., Nielsen, A., Stoyles, S., Dieckmann, N. F., & Campbell, M. (2019). Do prelicensure nursing students' backgrounds impact what they notice and interpret about patients? *Nurse Education Today, 78*, 37–43. https://doi.org/https://doi.org/10.1016/j.nedt.2019.03.013

Leighton, K., Kardong-Edgren, S., McNelis, A. M., Foisy-Doll, C., & Sullo, E. (2021). Traditional clinical outcomes in prelicensure nursing education: An empty systematic review. *Journal of Nursing Education, 60*(3), 136–142. https://doi.org/10.3928/01484834-20210222-03

Li, S., Ye, X., & Chen, W. (2019). Practice and effectiveness of "nursing case-based learning" course on nursing student's critical thinking ability: A comparative study. *Nurse Education in Practice, 36*, 91–96. https://doi.org/10.1016/j.nepr.2019.03.007

Lovric, R., Prlic, N., Zec, D., Puseljic, S., & Zvanut, B. (2015). Students' assessment and self-assessment of nursing clinical faculty competencies: Important feedback in clinical education? *Nurse Educator*, *40*, E1–E5. https://doi.org/10.1097/nne.0000000000000137

Luckenbach, A., Nelson-Brantley, H., & Ireland-Hoffmann, G. (2021). Affiliate faculty in nursing clinical education: Student and faculty perceptions. *Nurse Educator*, *46*(4), 245–249. https://doi.org/10.1097/NNE.0000000000000925

Makhene, A. (2019). The use of the Socratic inquiry to facilitate critical thinking in nursing education. *Health SA Gesondheid*, *24*, a1224. https://doi.org/10.4102/hsag.v24i0.1224

McCarthy, B., Trace, A., O'Donovan, M., Brady-Nevin, C., Murphy, M., O'Shea, M., & O'Regan, P. (2018). Nursing and midwifery students' stress and coping during their undergraduate education programmes: An integrative review. *Nurse Education Today*, *61*, 197–209. https://doi.org/10.1016/j.nedt.2017.11.029

Mennenga, H. A., Brown, R. J., Horsley, T. L., Abuatiq, A. A., & Plemmons, C. (2021). Collaborating with rural practice partners to provide a primary care experience for prelicensure nursing students. *Nurse Educator*, *46*(2), E14–E17. https://doi.org/10.1097/NNE.0000000000000876

Muirhead, L., Brasher, S., Vena, C., Hall, P., & Cadet, A. (2021). Assimilation of expert clinician into the academy: A competency-based faculty development plan. *Nurse Educator*, *46*(2), 121–125. https://doi.org/10.1097/NNE.0000000000000859

Oermann, M. H. (2022a). Evidence-based teaching in nursing. In M. H. Oermann, J. C. De Gagne, & B. C. Phillips (Eds.), *Teaching in nursing and role of the educator: The complete guide to best practice in teaching, evaluation, and curriculum development* (3rd ed., pp. 377–393). Springer Publishing Company.

Oermann, M. H. (2022b). Innovative, evidence-based approaches to facilitate and evaluate learning. In M. H. Adams & T. Valiga (Eds.), *Achieving distinction in nursing education* (pp. 73–85). National League for Nursing/Wolters Kluwer.

Oermann, M. H., & Gaberson, K. B. (2021). *Evaluation and testing in nursing education* (6th ed.). Springer Publishing Company.

Pedregosa, S., Fabrellas, N., Risco, E., Pereira, M., Dmoch-Gajzlerska, E., Şenuzun, F., Martin, S., & Zabalegui, A. (2020). Effective academic-practice partnership models in nursing students' clinical placement: A systematic literature review. *Nurse Education Today*, *95*, 104582. https://doi.org/10.1016/j.nedt.2020.104582

Phillips, N. M., Duke, M. M., & Weerasuriya, R. (2017). Questioning skills of clinical facilitators supporting undergraduate nursing students. *Journal of Clinical Nursing*, *26*(23–24), 4344–4352. https://doi.org/10.1111/jocn.13761

Reed, T., Horsley, T. L., Muccino, K., Quinones, D., Siddall, V. J., McCarthy, J., & Adams, W. (2016). Simulation using TeamSTEPPS to promote interprofessional education and collaborative practice. *Nurse Educator*, *42*(3), E1–E5. https://doi.org/10.1097/nne.0000000000000350

Rogers, J., Ludwig-Beymer, P., & Baker, M. (2020). Nurse faculty orientation: An integrative review. *Nurse Educator*, *45*(6), 343–346. https://doi.org/10.1097/NNE.0000000000000802

Rusch, L. M., McCafferty, K., Schoening, A. M., Hercinger, M., & Manz, J. (2018). Impact of the dedicated education unit teaching model on the perceived competencies and professional attributes of nursing students. *Nurse Education in Practice*, *33*, 90–93. https://doi.org/10.1016/j.nepr.2018.09.002

Schoening, A. M., Williams, J., & Saldi, D. (2021). Developing a psychiatric mental health dedicated education unit: Student, staff nurse, and patient experience. *Nurse Educator*, *46*(2), 106–110. https://doi.org/10.1097/NNE.0000000000000875

Sweet, L., & Broadbent, J. (2017). Nursing students' perceptions of the qualities of a clinical facilitator that enhance learning. *Nurse Education in Practice*, *22*, 30–36. https://doi.org/10.1016/j.nepr.2016.11.007

Wang, A. H., Lee, C. T., & Espin, S. (2019). Undergraduate nursing students' experiences of anxiety-producing situations in clinical practicums: A descriptive survey study. *Nurse Education Today*, *76*, 103–108. https://doi.org/10.1016/j.nedt.2019.01.016

Williamson, K. M., & Muckle, J. (2018). Students' perception of technology use in nursing education. *Computers, Informatics, Nursing, 36*(2), 70–76. https://doi.org/10.1097/cin.0000000000000396

Zook, S. S., Hulton, L. J., Dudding, C. C., Stewart, A. L., & Graham, A. C. (2018). Scaffolding interprofessional education: Unfolding case studies, virtual world simulations, and patient-centered care. *Nurse Educator, 43*(2), 87–91. https://doi.org/10.1097/nne.0000000000000430

A robust set of instructor resources designed to supplement this text is located at http://connect.springerpub.com/content/book/978-0-8261-6705-7. Qualifying instructors may request access by emailing textbook@springerpub.com.

Ethical and Legal Issues in Clinical Teaching

Clinical teaching and learning take place in a social context. Teachers, students, staff members, and patients have roles, rights, and responsibilities that are sometimes in conflict. These conflicts create legal and ethical dilemmas for clinical teachers. This chapter discusses some ethical and legal issues related to clinical teaching and offers suggestions for preventing, minimizing, and managing these difficult situations.

USE OF SOCIAL MEDIA

Online social networking is a useful and popular means of communication and collaboration. Social media forms include Facebook, Twitter, LinkedIn, Instagram, Myspace, YouTube, Pinterest, Yelp, and Foursquare, among others. Many nursing students at every educational level are active users of social media, especially members of the millennial generation who are "digital natives." Healthcare professionals' conduct both on and off the job is held to ethical and legal standards and guidelines; personal and professional identities overlap and are difficult to separate. Nursing students may be unaware of their responsibilities with regard to social media use in the context of nurse–patient relationships and as members of the profession of nursing. Therefore, nursing faculty members and students may encounter ethical and legal consequences of social media misuse (Daigle, 2020; De Gagne et al., 2018).

Misuse of social media becomes a source of regulatory concern when role boundary violations occur (De Gagne et al., 2018). The American Nurses Association (ANA) *Code of Ethics for Nurses with Interpretative Statements* (2015) emphasizes the obligation of nurses to act within the professional role and to maintain role boundaries in relationships with patients. Boundary violations can occur when students "friend" or "follow" patients or former patients on social media, resulting in harm to patients.

The *Code of Ethics* (ANA, 2015) also specifically mentions social media in emphasizing the nurse's obligation to maintain patient privacy. Confidentiality can be breached when information about patients is posted on social media sites, even without revealing a patient's name. Patients have a right to privacy, and sometimes information can be pieced together from various postings (possibly by different people) resulting in the identification of a specific patient. Such disclosures often are unintentional, but they can have serious consequences for patients.

In addition to potential harm to patients, social media misuse can have serious consequences for nursing students, nursing education programs, and healthcare facilities. While nursing students cannot be disciplined by state boards of nursing, they may face disciplinary action, including course failure or dismissal, by the nursing education program. Additionally, nursing education programs' working relationships with clinical agencies could be damaged by students' boundary violations and breaches of confidentiality, and future nursing students could lose valuable clinical learning opportunities in those settings. Healthcare facilities can face fines for student violations of the U.S. Health Insurance Portability and Accountability Act (HIPAA) of 1996 (discussed later in this chapter), and students could be subject to private legal actions by patients or consequences for violating laws.

Nursing education programs should develop and enforce explicit policies regarding the use of electronic communication and social media, including specific consequences for policy violations. Professional guidelines such as the ANA's *Code of Ethics* (2015), *ANA's Principles for Social Networking and the Nurse* (2011), and the National Council of State Boards of Nursing's (NCSBN) *A Nurse's Guide to the Use of Social Media* (2018) can be referenced in these policies. Students may be required to sign documents affirming that they have reviewed and agree to adhere to the nursing education programs social media use policies (Daigle, 2020; De Gagne et al, 2018).

Nursing faculty members should discuss guidelines for nurses' appropriate use of social media with students. These guidelines include:

▪ *Conduct Standards:* Nursing students are held to the same professional, legal, and ethical behavior as licensed nurses. While engaged in clinical learning activities, they are subject to agency policies and requirements. Conduct outside of class and clinical practica may be evaluated according to the same professional standards.
▪ *Protecting Patient Privacy:* Do not post or transmit individually identifiable patient information, including names, images, or any information that can reasonably be used to identify patients. Do not transmit patient information to anyone who does not have a legitimate care-based or legal need to know.
▪ *Maintaining Nurse–Patient Boundaries:* Establish, communicate, and enforce professional boundaries with patients in social media. Nurses should not participate in online social relationships with patients or former patients.
▪ *Viewing by Others:* Evaluate all online communication and behavior with the understanding that it could be viewed by patients, educators, colleagues, and employers or potential employers. Even if later deleted, the data remain on a server and could be retrieved by others or discovered by a court of law.
▪ *Separate Online Personal and Professional Information:* Use the privacy settings on social media sites to keep personal and professional online activities separate. However, these precautions do not guarantee that information will not be disseminated by others in less protected formats.
▪ *Response to Questionable Content:* Take appropriate action regarding the posting of social media content that reflects incompetent, unethical, illegal, or impaired practice. Bring questionable content to the attention of colleagues who posted it so that they may take appropriate action. If the posted content poses a risk to patient safety or privacy, report it to a supervisor or teacher and, if action is not taken, to the appropriate external authorities.

- *Development of Policy:* Participate in the development of institutional policy concerning online conduct that raises legal and ethical concerns. Such policies should address remedial action for patients and nonpunitive correction and training for nurses whose questionable online conduct is unintentional.
- *Respect for Colleagues and Employers:* Avoid discussing school- or work-related issues online, including complaints about classmates, teachers, clinical agencies, or the educational institution. Do not make disparaging, threatening, harassing, derogatory, or other offensive comments about others. These activities may constitute cyber-bullying. Such behavior also may be detrimental to effective healthcare team functioning, with patient safety ramifications, and may result in sanctions against the nurse. (ANA, 2011; De Gagne et al., 2018; NCSBN, 2018)

Faculty members should review the ethical and legal standards and guidelines for social media use with students regularly (e.g., yearly or every semester) and may reinforce these concepts using case studies or simulations (Daigle, 2020). Table 6.1 provides a summary of the implications of these principles for nursing students.

TABLE 6.1 GUIDELINES FOR APPROPRIATE USE OF SOCIAL MEDIA WITH STUDENTS

Guideline	Implications for Nursing Students
Maintain standards of conduct	Students are held to the same professional, legal, and ethical behavior as licensed nurses In clinical learning activities, students need to follow agency policies and requirements Students' conduct outside of the course and clinical practicum may be evaluated based on the same professional standards
Protect the privacy of patients	Students cannot post or transmit individually identifiable patient information (names, images, or other information that can be used to identify patients) Students cannot share patient information unless the individual requesting it has a legitimate care-based or legal need to know
Maintain nurse–patient boundaries	Students should maintain professional boundaries with patients in social media
Evaluate all online communication	Students, faculty, and others need to evaluate their online communication because it *could* be viewed by others (patients, nurse educators, colleagues, employers, or potential employers)
Separate online personal and professional information	Set the privacy settings on social media sites (to keep personal and professional online activities separate)

(continued)

TABLE 6.1	GUIDELINES FOR APPROPRIATE USE OF SOCIAL MEDIA WITH STUDENTS (*CONTINUED*)
Guideline	**Implications for Nursing Students**
Respond to questionable content	Students, educators, and others should take action if they find social media content that reflects incompetent, unethical, illegal, or impaired practice Bring questionable content to the attention of the colleagues who posted it and if the content poses a risk to patient safety or privacy, report it to a supervisor or faculty member
Develop policies about online content	Educators, administrators in healthcare systems, and others need an institutional policy about online conduct that raises legal and ethical concerns
Respect colleagues and employers	Students and faculty should not discuss school- or work-related issues online, including complaints about peers, faculty, clinical agencies, or the educational institution

ETHICAL ISSUES

Ethics are standards of conduct based on beliefs about what is good and bad, obligations related to good and bad acts, and principles underlying decisions to conform to these standards. Ethical standards make it possible for nurses, patients, teachers, and students to understand and respect each other. Contemporary bioethical standards are related to respect for human dignity, autonomy, and freedom; beneficence; justice; veracity; privacy; and fidelity (Oermann & Gaberson, 2021). These standards are important considerations for all parties involved in clinical teaching and learning.

Learners in a Service Setting

If the word *clinical* means "involving direct observation of the patient," clinical activities must take place where patients are. Traditionally, learners encounter patients in healthcare service settings, such as acute care, extended care, and rehabilitation facilities. With the increasing focus on controlling healthcare costs and primary prevention, however, patients increasingly receive healthcare in the home, community, and school environments. Whatever the setting, patients are there to receive healthcare, staff members have the responsibility to provide care, and students are present to learn. Are these purposes always compatible?

Although it has been more than three decades since Corcoran (1977) raised ethical questions about the use of service settings for learning activities, those concerns still are valid. In the clinical setting, nursing students or new staff members are learners who are somewhat less skilled than experienced practitioners. Although their activities are observed and guided by clinical teachers, learners are not expected to provide cost-effective, efficient patient care services. On the other hand, patients expect quality service when they seek healthcare; providing learning opportunities for students is not usually their priority. The ethical standard of *beneficence* refers to the duty to help, to produce beneficial outcomes, or at least to do no harm. Is this standard violated when the learners' chief purpose for being in the clinical environment is to learn, not to give care?

Patients who encounter learners in clinical settings may feel exploited or fear invasion of their privacy; they may receive care that takes more time and creates more discomfort than if provided by expert practitioners. The presence of learners in a clinical setting also requires more time and energy from staff members, who are usually expected to give and receive reports from students, answer their questions, and demonstrate or help with patient care. These activities may divert staff members' attention from their primary responsibility for patient care, interfere with their efficient performance, and affect their satisfaction with their work.

Because achieving the desired outcomes of clinical teaching requires learning activities in real service settings, teachers must consider the rights and needs of learners, patients, and staff members when planning clinical learning activities. The clinical teacher is responsible for making the learning objectives clear to all involved persons and for ensuring that learning activities do not prevent the achievement of service goals. Patients should receive adequate information about the presence of learners in the settings where they are receiving care before giving their informed consent to participate in clinical learning activities. Teachers should ensure learners' preparation and readiness for clinical learning as well as their own presence and competence as instructors, as discussed in Chapter 4.

Student–Faculty Relationships

RESPECT FOR PERSONS

As discussed in Chapter 1, an effective and beneficial relationship between clinical teacher and student is built on a base of mutual trust and respect. Although both parties are responsible for maintaining this relationship, the clinical teacher must initiate it by demonstrating trust and respect for students. A trusting, respectful relationship with students demonstrates the teacher's commitment to ethical values of respect for human dignity and autonomy. Because civil behavior is learned, teachers must model discretion, attentiveness, respectful communication, and professional behavior in all encounters with students, colleagues, patients, and staff members in the clinical setting.

Incivility is a form of disrespect for persons. Uncivil behavior and extreme rudeness unfortunately are pervasive in contemporary society and increasingly are manifest on college campuses (Stalter et al., 2019). Both nursing faculty members and nursing students perceive incivility to be a growing concern in nursing education. Academic incivility is behavior in the form of words, actions, or gestures that is intended to be rude or disrespectful, that interferes with the teaching–learning process, and that leads to mental and physical distress among those in that environment. It can span a broad continuum of behaviors including lack of preparation for learning activities, unwillingness to engage in the learning process, tardiness, unauthorized use of cell phones or other devices, distracting side conversations, insulting the instructor, intimidation, physical aggression against other students or teachers, and making direct threats of violence. In clinical practice, uncivil behavior can negatively affect patient safety by disrupting interdisciplinary team functioning and hampering clear, timely communication of patient information.

If nursing students do not learn civil interaction with patients, team members, and those in authority, they are likely to become uncivil employees in the healthcare system (Luparell & Frisbee, 2019).

Student factors that may contribute to incivility include high levels of academic stress and anxiety as well as competing demands of occupational workload and family responsibilities, financial stress, time management challenges, and mental health and personal issues (Luparell & Frisbee, 2019). These stressors exhaust students' adaptive coping mechanisms, resulting in fear, desperation, and intense frustration manifested in the form of anger, impulsivity, impaired judgment, and incivility.

Faculty conduct may exacerbate academic incivility, including teaching behaviors that perpetuate or amplify student anxiety, such as arrogance, superiority, and abuse of authority; gossip about students; expression of anger; threats regarding grades; publicly embarrassing or ridiculing students in clinical settings; lack of clarity in the course syllabus about expectations for student performance, evaluation, and conduct; perceived favoritism toward some students; and inability to manage or overlooking uncivil student behavior (Holtz et al., 2018). Student anxiety is magnified by teachers whose teaching practices gravitate toward opposite ends of the spectrum. Some teachers fail to clearly communicate their expectations, while others use rigid and oppressive pedagogies that lack caring and respect.

The most effective approach to managing incivility in clinical teaching focuses on prevention while simultaneously specifying and implementing progressive disciplinary measures if the proactive methods fail. The faculty must establish clear policies about the administration of each course (e.g., attendance, unsafe clinical practice) and expectations for student performance, evaluation, and behavior, including the repercussions of uncivil behavior. These expectations should be included in course syllabi and discussed with students at the beginning of the academic term. A set of behavioral standards to which students and faculty must adhere minimizes misunderstandings and misalignment of expectations. These standards may be developed collaboratively by teachers and students, regularly reviewed with students, and referenced in course syllabi. As previously mentioned, teachers must consistently adhere to such behavioral standards and model the civil behavior they wish to see in students (Stalter et al., 2019).

In addition to setting and clearly communicating a set of conduct standards, the faculty and administration must develop a well-written policy and procedures that promote the consistent handling of academic incivility. This protocol should also be shared with students so that they are aware that a standardized approach to conduct violations will be used by faculty members and administrators. The protocol should clearly specify progressive discipline for infractions, which may include an oral or written warning or reprimand, removal from the clinical environment for a specified period of time, a disciplinary hearing, or dismissal from the nursing education program, depending on the severity of the infraction. As is the case for all such policy development, the faculty is advised to seek guidance from the institution's legal counsel to make sure that student rights are protected and that the policy and procedures are consistent with those of the governing institution. Additionally, a carefully crafted and publicized protocol has no power unless it is consistently applied by all faculty members with support from program administrators.

FAIRNESS AND JUSTICE

The ethical standard of justice refers to fair treatment—judging each person's behavior by the same standards. Clinical teachers must evaluate each student's performance by the same standard. Students may perceive a clinical teacher's behavior as unfair when the teacher appears to favor some students by praising, supporting, and offering better learning opportunities to them more than others. Developing social relationships with some students could be perceived as favoritism by other students. Teachers often find it challenging to set appropriate role boundaries for teacher–student relationships. While their primary role is that of teacher, they also want to model caring behavior to students, be supportive to students who are struggling, and be approachable and student-friendly. Clinical teachers should maintain professional boundaries with students with regard to social media use; professional integrity can be jeopardized by becoming involved in students' personal lives on social media. Maintaining healthy boundaries that facilitate student success through a professional open relationship is essential (Daigle, 2020).

As previously discussed, nurse educators should be prudent about their use of social networking sites such as Facebook and Twitter. Faculty members have used Twitter to communicate with students, build relationships with them, and enhance their learning. However, these uses of social networking sites should be separate from the teacher's personal use of these technologies. Befriending students on their Facebook page and following them on Twitter raises faculty–student boundary issues and implies an egalitarian relationship that does not acknowledge the power advantage that faculty members hold (Oermann & Gaberson, 2021). Inviting students to sign up as friends or followers to a Facebook or Twitter account that the teacher uses for social interaction with peers invites their discovery of information that the teacher might prefer to be private.

Students' Privacy Rights

When students have a succession of clinical instructors, it is common for the instructors to communicate information about student performance. Learning about the students' levels of performance in their previous clinical assignment helps the next instructor to anticipate their needs and to plan appropriate learning activities for them. Although students usually benefit when teachers share such information about their learning needs, personal information that students reveal in confidence should not be shared with other teachers. The U.S. Family Educational Rights and Privacy Act of 1974, as amended, restricts disclosure of students' academic information to individuals who have a legitimate need to know; written permission from students is necessary to discuss their performance with anyone else. Evaluative statements about student performance should not be shared with other faculty members, but information about a student's need for a particular learning activity or more practice with a specific skill is necessary for a teacher to provide the appropriate guidance.

Additionally, when sharing information about students, teachers should focus on factual statements about performance without adding personal judgments. Characterizing or labeling students is rarely helpful to the next instructor, and such behavior violates ethical standards of privacy as well as respect for persons.

Because clinical teachers in nursing education programs are professional nurses, they sometimes experience conflict regarding their knowledge of students' health problems. As nurses, they might tend to respond in a therapeutic way if a student revealed personal information about a health concern, but as teachers, their primary obligation is to a teacher–student relationship. Absent any existing institutional policy or compelling evidence that the personal information should be disclosed to protect the safety of the student or other person, educators should follow the principle of what action would best promote student learning.

Clinical teachers who are aware of a student's health problem should also avoid making special exceptions for this student that would not be available to other students. Students who need special accommodations because of a health problem should request them from the institution's disability services officer. If accommodations are granted, the clinical teacher should discuss with the student how they will be made available. See the discussion on students with disabilities later in this chapter.

Competent Teaching

Applying the ethical standard of beneficence to teaching, students have a right to expect that their clinical teachers are competent, responsible, and knowledgeable. As discussed in Chapter 5, clinical competence, including expert knowledge and clinical skill, is an essential characteristic of effective clinical teachers. In addition, clinical teachers must be competent in facilitating students' learning activities, including planning appropriate assignments and giving specific, timely feedback on individual student performance. Examples of unethical behavior related to clinical teacher competence include not being available for guidance in the clinical setting and not planning sufficiently for a clinical learning activity that maximizes student learning.

Academic Dishonesty

As discussed in Chapter 2, although cheating and other forms of dishonest behavior are believed to be common in the classroom environment, academic dishonesty can occur in clinical settings as well. Academic dishonesty is defined as intentional participation in deceptive practices regarding the academic work of self or others. Dishonest acts include lying, cheating, plagiarizing, altering or forging records, falsely representing oneself, and knowingly assisting another person to commit a dishonest act (McClung & Gaberson, 2021). While we discuss academic dishonesty as an ethical violation, it can also be classified as a legal issue when it serves as the basis of a disciplinary action.

Examples of academic dishonesty in the clinical setting include:

- *Cheating:* A student copies portions of a classmate's case study analysis and presents the assignment as her own work. Similarly, a student who asks for a staff member's assistance to calculate a medication dose but tells the instructor that he did the work alone is also cheating.
- *Lying:* A student tells the instructor that she attempted a home visit to a patient but the patient was not at home. In fact, the student overslept and missed the scheduled time of the visit.
- *Plagiarism:* While preparing materials for a patient-teaching project, a student paraphrases portions of a published teaching pamphlet without citing the source.

■ *Altering a document:* A staff nurse orientee appends information to the documentation of nursing care for a patient on the previous day without noting it as a late addition.

■ *False representation:* As a family nurse practitioner student begins a physical examination, the patient addresses the student as "doctor." The student continues with the examination and does not tell the patient that he is a nurse.

■ *Assisting another in a dishonest act:* Student A asks Student B to cover for her while she leaves the clinical agency to run a personal errand. The teacher asks Student B if he has seen Student A; Student B says that he thinks she has accompanied a patient to the physical therapy department.

Although some of the previous examples may appear to be harmless or minor infractions, dishonest acts should be taken seriously because they can have harmful effects on patients, learners, faculty–student relationships, and the educational program. Clinical dishonesty can jeopardize patient safety if learners fail to report errors or do not receive adequate guidance because their competence is assumed. Mutual trust and respect form the basis for effective teacher–learner relationships, and academic dishonesty can damage a teacher's trust in students. Dishonest acts that are ignored by teachers contribute to an environment that supports academic dishonesty, conveying the impression to students that this behavior is acceptable or at least excusable. Additionally, honest students resent teachers who fail to deal effectively with cheating.

Students who are dishonest in school may be more likely to conceal or deny errors in the workplace or violate professional conduct standards. For this reason, most nurse faculty members are conscientious about holding students accountable to standards of integrity and imposing severe consequences as permitted by policy. However, student appeals of these decisions are often overturned or modified by grade appeal panels comprising faculty members from nonclinical disciplines who may not understand the serious implications for patient safety.

Clinical academic dishonesty usually results from one or more of the following factors:

■ *Competition, desire for good grades, and heavy workload:* Competition for good grades in clinical nursing courses may result from student misunderstanding of the evaluation framework. If students believe that a limited number of good grades are available, they may compete fiercely with their classmates, sometimes leading to deceptive acts in an attempt to earn the highest grades. Additionally, many nursing students have additional pressures related to employment and family responsibilities; they may feel overloaded and unable to meet all of the demands of a rigorous nursing education program without resorting to cheating. In an increasingly high-stakes postsecondary education environment, academic success affects students' retention in, progression through, or graduation from a program; ability to obtain or retain scholarships and loans; and ability to gain or maintain family approval and support.

■ *Emphasis on perfection:* As discussed in Chapter 2, clinical teachers often communicate the expectation that good nurses do not make mistakes. Although nurse educators attempt to prepare practitioners who will perform carefully and skillfully, a standard of perfection is unrealistic. Students naturally make mistakes in the process of learning new knowledge and skills, and punishment for mistakes, in the form of low grades or a negative performance evaluation, will not prevent these errors. In fact, it is the fear of punishment that often motivates students to conceal errors, and errors that are not reported are often harmful to patient safety (McClung & Gaberson, 2021).

■ *Poor role modeling:* The influence of role models on behavior is strong. Nursing students and novice staff nurses who observe dishonest behavior of teachers and experienced staff members may emulate these examples, especially when the dishonest acts have gone unnoticed, unreported, or unpunished (McClung & Gaberson, 2021).

Clinical teachers can use a variety of approaches to discourage academic dishonesty. They should be exemplary role models of honest behavior for learners to emulate. They should acknowledge that mistakes occur in the learning process and create a learning climate that allows students to make mistakes in a safe environment with guidance and feedback for problem solving.

However, students need reassurance that, if humanly possible, teachers will not allow them to make errors that would harm patients. Finally, each nursing education program should develop a policy that defines academic dishonesty and specifies appropriate penalties for violations. This policy should be communicated to all students, reviewed with them at regular intervals, and applied consistently and fairly to every violation.

When enforcing the academic integrity policy, it is important to apply ethical standards to protect the dignity and privacy of students. A public accusation of dishonesty that is found later to be ungrounded can damage a student's reputation. The teacher should speak with the student privately and calmly, describe the student's behavior and the teacher's interpretation of it, and provide the student with an opportunity to respond to the charge. It is essential to keep an open mind until all available evidence is evaluated, because the student may be able to supply a reasonable explanation for the behavior that the teacher interpreted as cheating.

LEGAL ISSUES

It is beyond the scope of this book to discuss and interpret all federal, state, and local laws that have implications for clinical teaching and evaluation, and the authors are not qualified to give legal advice to clinical teachers regarding their practice. We recommend that clinical teachers refer questions about the legal implications of policies and procedures to the legal counsel for the institution in which they are employed; concerns about a teacher's legal rights in a specific situation are best referred to the individual's attorney. However, this section discusses common legal issues that often arise in the practice of clinical teaching.

Students With Disabilities

Two federal laws have implications for the education of learners with disabilities. The Rehabilitation Act of 1973, Section 504, prohibits public postsecondary institutions that receive federal funding from denying access or participation to individuals with disabilities. The Americans with Disabilities Act (ADA) of 1990 and the ADA Amendment Act of 2008 guarantee persons with disabilities equal access to educational opportunities if they are otherwise qualified for admission. A qualified individual with a disability is one who has a physical or mental impairment that substantially limits one or more of that individual's major life activities, or that the individual has a record of or is regarded as having such impairment.

In the ADA amendments, the definition of disability did not change, but the interpretation of disability is more expansive, providing protection to a wider range of individuals with disabilities. In determining whether an individual is disabled, the following three conditions apply:

1. The effects of ameliorating agents cannot be considered. For example, a person with epilepsy whose seizures are controlled by medications or one who uses a hearing aid to correct hearing loss is still considered to have a qualifying condition if one or more life activities are affected.
2. Conditions that are in remission or episodic are considered to be disabilities if, when they are active, they have a similar effect on one or more life activities.
3. The term "life activities" is now more broadly defined to include "seeing, hearing, eating, smelling, sleeping, breathing, walking, speaking, bowel and bladder control, learning, reading, writing, spelling, concentrating, thinking, communicating, perceiving and other neurologic functions, working, performing self-care and other manual tasks" (Southern Regional Education Board [SREB], 2016).

In nursing education programs, qualified individuals with disabilities are those who meet the essential eligibility requirements for participation, with or without modifications (Glasgow et al., 2021; SREB, 2016). A common goal of nursing education programs is to produce graduates who can function safely and competently in the roles for which they were prepared. For this reason, it is appropriate for those who make admission decisions to determine whether applicants could be reasonably expected to develop the necessary competence. The first step in this decision process is to define the core performance standards necessary for participation in the program. Because nursing is a practice discipline, core performance standards include cognitive, sensory, affective, and psychomotor competencies. The SREB recommended that core performance standards be published in catalogs, on websites, in application materials, and in program descriptions for the state board of nursing and accrediting bodies. They should also be made available to students, faculty members, staff members, and agencies in which students have clinical learning activities. All applicants to nursing education programs should be informed of the core performance standards to allow them to make initial judgments about their qualifications. Under the ADA as amended, nursing education programs cannot base admission or progression decisions on the core performance standards. Instead, the standards should be used to assist applicants and students to determine their need for accommodations (SREB, 2016).

Persons with disabilities who are admitted to nursing education programs are responsible for informing the institution of the disability and requesting reasonable accommodations. An institution is not required to provide specific accommodations requested by a student with a disability, and it does not need to make an accommodation that would cause it undue hardship. For example, an accommodation that would substantially alter the nursing education program would create an undue hardship (Glasgow et al., 2021). Each institution must determine on an individual basis whether the necessary modifications can be made reasonably. The nursing faculty, administration, and staff should cooperate with other institutional units to identify auxiliary aids and services, such as building accessibility and assistive devices, that students with identified disabilities may need. Reasonable accommodations for participating in clinical learning activities might include (SREB, 2016):

- Allowing additional time for a student with a qualified learning disability to complete an assignment.
- Allowing additional time to complete the program.
- Scheduling clinical learning activities in facilities that are readily accessible to and usable by individuals with disabilities.
- Providing the use of an amplified stethoscope for a student with a hearing impairment.
- Providing qualified readers or interpreters.

Another example of a reasonable accommodation in a clinical setting is the use of a service animal by a student with a disability (Silbert-Flagg et al., 2020). A service animal, usually a dog, is individually trained to perform specific tasks for a person with a disability, and it is considered a general accommodation under the ADA. Understandably, many people are concerned about the presence of a service animal in a healthcare facility, but with adequate planning by faculty members, students, and clinical practice site personnel, these concerns can be allayed. Although individuals with a service animal have the right to access all areas of a facility that are open to the public, not all areas within a healthcare facility are classified as such, including operating rooms, sterile supply processing and storage areas, intensive care units, and medication preparation areas. For this reason, clinical learning activities for a student using a service animal may need to be modified to avoid these areas. Adequate precautions to protect patients, agency personnel, and the animal should be taken, including proper grooming of the animal, identifying areas in a patient room where the animal remains while the student interacts with the patient, keeping the animal on a leash, providing breaks for the student to toilet the animal, and providing personal protective equipment to anyone with an animal dander allergy who must interact with the animal (Silbert-Flagg et al., 2020).

Reasonable accommodations do not include lowering academic standards or eliminating essential technical performance requirements. However, nurse educators need to distinguish essential from traditional functions by discussing such philosophical issues as whether individuals who will never practice bedside nursing in the conventional manner should be admitted to nursing education programs.

Disabilities may be visible (e.g., limited mobility, visual or hearing deficit, physical or functional loss of a limb) or invisible (e.g., learning disability, behavioral or mental health problem, chronic illness). Learning disabilities currently are the most commonly identified disability among nursing students (Yarbrough & Welch, 2021). As previously discussed, clinical teachers should not attempt to determine whether accommodation is indicated, nor should they decide on the specific type of accommodation necessary. The disabilities services officer of the educational institution determines whether the student is a qualified individual with a disability and, if so, whether the disability requires accommodations. This officer then issues a formal, written description of the required clinical accommodations, usually to the student, who decides whom to share it with. Accommodation statements should not be shared with others without the student's written permission. The purpose of accommodation is to provide the student with a disability the means to compensate for it so that full participation in the clinical learning activity is possible. Reasonable accommodation practices promote inclusive nursing education environments and ensure equal opportunities for students with documented disabilities. For students with learning disabilities, promoting inclusiveness involves reducing stigma by keeping accommodations private to the extent possible (Yarbrough & Welch, 2021).

Many nursing faculty members voice concerns about the capacity of students with physical disabilities to perform physical tasks associated with nursing practice. A clinical teacher of a student with a physical disability should carefully analyze a planned learning activity to identify the essential elements necessary to produce desired outcomes, keeping in mind that much of the professional nurse's work is intellectual. Is it more important for a nursing student to demonstrate the ability to reposition a patient or to demonstrate the ability to assess the patient's skin integrity and pulmonary and circulatory function, recognize the need for repositioning, delegate the task to a licensed or unlicensed staff member and supervise that person as necessary, and evaluate the patient outcomes?

Students with disabilities are the best sources of information about their disabilities and the limitations that they present, adaptations they have learned to compensate for them, and what accommodations have worked in the past. Disabilities services staff members may have experience identifying institutional academic accommodations resources for students in classroom settings but may not have much experience suggesting appropriate accommodations for students with disabilities in clinical settings. Clinical teachers often have the most realistic understanding of the context for clinical learning and the essential elements of safe nursing practice. Collaboration among students, disabilities services staff members, and clinical teachers is necessary to explore options that would meet each student's individual needs for accommodations in clinical learning environments. This often is a lengthy process, and students need to be advised to identify their needs for accommodations well before the beginning of a clinical practicum so that appropriate resources can be identified and implemented in a timely fashion.

After appropriate accommodations are provided, students with disabilities must be evaluated according to the same criteria as other students. In cases where students with disabilities are at risk of clinical failure, it is important that faculty members and administrators have clearly and consistently documented any offer and provision of accommodations and the students' subsequent use or non-use of them. Evaluations should be based on a genuine substantive assessment of the students' performance with any appropriate accommodations. Students must have been notified, orally and in writing, about their clinical practice deficiencies and the related consequences well before grading decision were made. The clinical teacher must have provided constructive feedback about students' performance, suggested specific improvements, and provided a time frame within which those improvements must be made.

Due Process

Another legal issue related to clinical teaching is that of student rights to due process. The 14th Amendment of the U.S. Constitution specifies that the state cannot deprive a person of life, liberty, or property without due process of law. With regard to the rights of students to due process, however, this constitutional protection extends only to those enrolled in public institutions. Students at private institutions may base a claim against the school on contract law. For example, if a private school publishes a code of student rights and procedures for student grievances in its student handbook, those documents may be regarded as part of a contract between the school and the student. In paying and accepting tuition, the student and the school jointly agree to abide by this code of rights and set of procedures. A student may sue on the basis of breach of contract if the school does not follow the stated due process procedures.

Courts hold different standards for due process based on whether it applies to academic or disciplinary decisions. Academic decisions pertain to issues related to performance and academic standing, such as assigning a failing grade in a course, delaying progress, and dismissal from a program because of failure to maintain acceptable academic standing. Academic due process concerns both the *process* used to inform students of their academic standing and the *basis* for a decision regarding academic standing. Thus, *procedural due process* relates to the fairness of the process used to make academic decisions, and *substantive due process* relates to the basis for those decisions. A student appeal of an academic decision may allege a violation of either type of due process rights, but courts usually do not intervene in faculty members' evaluation of student didactic or clinical performance because such academic decisions involve the professional judgment of the faculty (Glasgow et al., 2021). The following legal principles apply to substantive due process:

■ Students must be informed in advance about the academic standards that will be used to judge their performance.
■ Student performance should be evaluated using the stated standards or criteria and grades assigned according to the stated policy. A teacher's academic decision should be based on a genuine substantive evaluation of the student's performance. All students should be evaluated according to the same standards; academic decisions should not be arbitrary or capricious.

If a student believes that a grade or other academic decision is unfair, the stated appeal or grievance process should be followed. Usually, the first level of appeal is to the teacher or group of teachers who assigned the grade. If the conflict is not resolved at that level, the student usually has the right of appeal to the administrator to whom the teacher reports. The next level of appeal is usually to a student standing committee or appeal panel of nursing faculty members. Finally, the student should have the right to appeal the decision to the highest level administrator in the nursing education program and then to the appropriate academic administrators at the parent institution.

Procedural due process concerns the fairness of the process by which academic decisions are made. Students should be notified about their academic deficiencies and the related consequences well before grading decisions are made. Ideally, notification occurs orally and in writing. To further protect students' procedural due process rights, the teacher should provide constructive feedback about their performance, suggest specific improvements, and provide a timeframe within which those improvements must be made. Evaluation of clinical performance is as much an academic decision as is assessment of classroom work, and the same procedural due process protections should be followed.

If students exhaust every level of appeal and are still not satisfied with the outcome, they have the right to seek relief in the court system. It is important to note that the courts will allow such a lawsuit to go forward only if there is evidence that the student has first exhausted all internal school remedies, and the law limits the issues that the court can consider, requiring judges to defer to the expertise of the academic institution in certain key areas such as academic evaluations. With regard to due process for academic decisions, the key to resolving conflict and minimizing faculty liability is in maintaining communication with students whose performance is not meeting standards.

Disciplinary decisions such as dismissal on the basis of misconduct or dishonesty require a higher level of due process than is required for academic actions. Unlike academic decisions that require professional judgments and are therefore beyond the scope of judicial review, disciplinary actions can be reviewed by the courts' traditional fact-finding procedures (Glasgow et al., 2021).

Disciplinary decisions are made when a student violates the law or regulation by engaging in prohibited activity. All colleges and universities have rules, standards, conduct codes, and policies that students are expected to meet, usually published in the institutional catalog and student handbook. Nursing education programs often have specific expectations regarding adherence to professional codes of conduct that are consistent with but go above and beyond the rules and standards of the parent institution. These publications must also explicate the procedures that will be followed if these rules are violated (Glasgow et al., 2021).

Disciplinary due process includes the following components:

- The student is provided with adequate written notice, including specific details concerning the misconduct. For example, a notice may inform a student who failed to attend a required clinical activity that neither the faculty member nor nursing unit secretary was informed of the anticipated absence, in violation of school policy on professional conduct; and that, because this incident represented the third violation of professional conduct standards, the student would be dismissed from the program according to the sanctions provided in the policy.
- The student is provided the opportunity for a fair, impartial hearing on the charges. Students have the right to speak on their own behalf, to present witnesses and evidence, and to question the other participants in the case (usually teachers and administrators). Using the preceding example, the student might present evidence of an attempt to call the faculty member to report the absence; this evidence could include the date and time of the call, the name of the person with whom the student spoke, and a copy of a telephone bill verifying the date, time, and number called. Although the student and the faculty member are entitled to the advice of legal counsel, neither attorney may question or cross-examine witnesses.
- The student has the right to appeal an unfavorable decision by the hearing panel to an appeals panel or a designated administrator. Usually, this administrator or, ultimately, the university or college president has the authority to make the final decision (Glasgow et al., 2021).

If the final decision is to uphold the dismissal, students have the right to seek remedy from the court system if they believe that due process was not followed. However, in disciplinary cases, the burden of proof that due process was denied rests with the student.

Negligence, Liability, and Unsafe Clinical Practice

When determining whether a given action meets the criteria for professional negligence, the overall standard of care is what an ordinary, reasonable, and prudent person would have done in the same context. The standard of care for a nursing student is not what another nursing student would have done; students are held to the same standards of care as RNs. The NCSBN Model Nurse Practice Act (2014), Article V, Section 10 includes the statement that the nurse practice act does not prohibit the practice of nursing by a student in an approved nursing education program as long as the student "is under the auspices of the program [and] . . . acts under the supervision of an RN serving for the program as a faculty member or teaching assistant" (p. 7). Another section of the Model Act (Article VII, Section 2) states that each nurse is required to know and adhere to the requirements of the nurse practice act, that nurses are accountable for their decisions based on their education and experience, and that nurses must practice with reasonable skill and safety. The concept of personal liability also applies to cases of professional negligence. Each person is responsible for their own behavior, including negligent acts. Students are liable for their own actions as long as they are performing according to the usual standard of care for their education and experience, and they seek guidance when they are uncertain what to do. Therefore, it is not true that students practice under the faculty member's license.

Teachers are not liable for negligent acts performed by their students as long as the teacher has (a) selected appropriate learning activities based on objectives; (b) determined that students have prerequisite knowledge, skills, and attitudes necessary to complete their assignments; and (c) provided competent guidance. However, teachers are liable for their negligent actions if they make assignments that require more knowledge and skill than the learner has developed or if they fail to guide student activities appropriately. The NCSBN Model Rules (2017) include statements about the grounds for disciplining an RN. These include failure to competently guide student clinical learning activities as a clinical teacher. Even if the clinical teacher was not negligent in making assignments or guiding student learning, the clinical teacher is likely to be named as a defendant in any lawsuit arising from a nursing student's alleged negligence or malpractice. For this reason, clinical teachers should carry sufficient individual professional liability insurance to cover the costs of defending themselves, even if their employers provide insurance coverage for faculty members.

If a student demonstrates clinical performance that is potentially unsafe, the student and the teacher who made the assignment may be liable for any subsequent injury to the patient. However, because time for learning must precede time for evaluation, is it fair for the teacher to assign a failing grade in clinical practice before the end of the course, when to do so would prevent the students' access to learning opportunities for which they have paid tuition? In this case, denying access to clinical learning activities because of unsafe practice or inadequate clinical reasoning should not be considered an academic grading decision. Instead, it is an appropriate response to protecting the rights of patients to safe, competent care—a disciplinary decision.

The teacher's failure to take such protective action potentially places the teacher and the educational program at risk for liability. Instead of denying the student access to all learning opportunities, removal from the clinical setting should be followed by a substitute assignment that would help the student to remove the deficiency in knowledge, skill, or attitude. For example, the student might be given a library assignment to acquire the information necessary to guide safe patient care, or an extra skills laboratory session could be arranged to allow more practice of psychomotor skills. A set of standards of safe clinical practice and a program policy that enforces the standards are helpful guides to faculty decision making and action while protecting student and faculty rights. Exhibit 6.1 is an example of safe clinical practice standards, and Exhibit 6.2 is an example of a policy that enforces these standards.

EXHIBIT 6.1 Standards of Safe Clinical Practice

XXXXXX UNIVERSITY

SCHOOL OF NURSING

BSN PROGRAM

STANDARDS OF SAFE CLINICAL PRACTICE

In clinical practice, students are expected to demonstrate responsibility and accountability as professional nurses with the goal of health promotion and prevention of harm to self and others. The School of Nursing faculty believes that this goal will be attained if each student's clinical practice adheres to the Standards of Safe Clinical Practice. Safe clinical performance always includes, but is not limited to, the following behaviors:

1. Practice within boundaries of the nursing student role and the scope of practice of the RN.
2. Comply with instructional policies and procedures for implementing nursing care.
3. Prepare for clinical learning assignments according to course requirements and as determined for the specific clinical setting.
4. Demonstrate the application of previously learned skills and principles in providing nursing care.
5. Promptly report significant client information in a clear, accurate, and complete oral or written manner to the appropriate person or persons.

ACKNOWLEDGMENT

I have read the XXXXXX University School of Nursing Standards of Safe Clinical Practice and I agree to adhere to them. I understand that these standards are expectations for my clinical practice and will be incorporated into the evaluation of my clinical performance in all clinical courses. Failure to meet these standards may result in my removal from the clinical area, which may result in clinical failure due to inability to achieve the required learning outcomes.

_____   _____

Signature   Date

EXHIBIT 6.2 Policy on Safe Clinical Practice

XXXXXX UNIVERSITY

SCHOOL OF NURSING

BSN PROGRAM

SAFE CLINICAL PRACTICE POLICY

POLICY

During enrollment in the XXXXXX University School of Nursing BSN Program, all students, in all clinical activities, are expected to adhere to the Standards of Safe Clinical Practice. Failure to abide by these standards will result in disciplinary action, which may include dismissal from the nursing program.

(continued)

EXHIBIT 6.2 Policy on Safe Clinical Practice (*continued*)

PROCEDURES

1. Students will receive a copy of the Standards of Safe Clinical Practice, and they will be reviewed during the Annual Nursing Assembly at the beginning of each academic year. At that time, students will be required to sign an agreement to adhere to the standards. Each student will retain one copy of the agreement, and one copy will be retained in the student's file.
2. Violation of these standards will result in the following disciplinary action:
   a. First violation
      1. Student will be given an immediate oral warning by the faculty member. The incident will be documented by the faculty member on the Violation of Standards of Safe Clinical Practice form. One copy of this form will be given to the student, and one copy will be kept in the student's record.
      2. At the discretion of the faculty member, the student may be required to leave the clinical setting for the remainder of that day. The student may be given an alternative assignment.
      3. If this violation is of a serious nature, it may be referred to the associate dean and the dean of nursing for further disciplinary action as in b and c below.
   b. Second violation
      1. The faculty member will document the incident on the Violation of Safe Clinical Practice form. Following discussion of the incident with the student, the faculty member will forward a copy of the form to the associate dean for review and recommendation regarding further action.
      2. The recommendation of the associate dean will be forwarded to the dean of nursing for review and decision regarding reprimand or dismissal. This disciplinary action process will be documented and placed in the student's record.
   c. If the student has not been dismissed and remains in the program following the above disciplinary action, any additional violation will be documented and referred as above to the associate dean and the dean of nursing for disciplinary action, which may include dismissal from the program.
   d. The rights of students will be safeguarded as set forth in the XXXXXX University Code of Student Rights, Responsibilities, and Conduct published in the current XXXXXX University Student Handbook.

Documentation and Record Keeping

Teachers should keep records of their evaluations of student clinical performance. These records may include anecdotal notes, summaries of faculty–student conferences, progress reports, and summative clinical evaluations. These records are helpful in documenting that students received feedback about their performance, areas of teacher concern, and information about student progress toward correcting deficiencies.

An anecdotal note is a narrative description of the observed behavior of the student in relation to a specific learning objective. The note may also include the teacher's interpretation of the behavior, recorded separately from the description. Limiting the description and optional interpretation to a specified clinical objective avoids recording extraneous information, which is an ineffective use of the teacher's time. Anecdotal notes should record both positive and negative behaviors so as not to give the impression that the teacher is biased against the student. Students should review these notes and have an opportunity to comment on them; used in this way, anecdotal notes are an effective means of communicating formative evaluation information to students (Oermann & Gaberson, 2021). Some sources recommend that both teacher and student sign the notes.

Writing anecdotal notes for every student, every day, is unnecessarily time consuming. An effective, efficient approach might be to specify a minimum number of notes to be written for each student in relation to specified objectives. A student whose performance is either meritorious or cause for concern might prompt the instructor to write more notes.

Records of student–teacher conferences are likewise summaries of discussions that focused on areas of concern, plans to address deficiencies, and progress toward correcting weaknesses. These conferences should take place in private and should address the teacher's responsibility to protect patient safety, concern about the student's clinical deficiencies, and a sincere desire to assist the student to improve. During the conference, the student has opportunities to clarify and respond to the teacher's feedback. At times, an objective third party such as a department chairperson or program director may be asked to participate in the conference to witness and clarify the comments of both teacher and student. The conference note should record the date, time, and place of the conference; the names and roles of participants; and a summary of the discussion, recommendations, and plans. The note may be signed only by the teacher or by all participants, according to institutional policy or guidelines.

Because they contain essentially formative evaluation information, anecdotal notes and conference notes should not be kept in the student's permanent record. Teachers should keep these documents in their private files, taking appropriate precautions to ensure their security, until there is no reasonable expectation that they will be needed. In most cases, when the learner successfully completes the program or withdraws in good academic standing, these records can be discarded (again, taking appropriate security precautions). It is unlikely that successful learners will appeal favorable academic decisions. However, it is recommended that anecdotal records and conference notes be kept for longer periods when there is a chance that the learner may appeal the grade or other decision. The statute of limitations for such an appeal is a useful guide to deciding how long to keep those materials. It is recommended that teachers consult with legal counsel if there is a question about institutional policy on retention of records.

Patient Privacy Laws

HIPAA, created in 1996, affirms patients' fundamental right to privacy for their personal health information. HIPAA privacy rules apply to "covered entities" such as hospitals, clinics, and rehabilitation centers. Nursing education programs that place students at these sites for clinical learning activities usually are not considered covered entities but "business associates" that are bound by the same privacy standards. Nursing students thus are subject to HIPAA rules while engaged in clinical learning activities at these facilities. Additionally, they should understand that HIPAA rules apply to their private conduct outside of their clinical practice.

The 2009 Health Information Technology for Economic and Clinical Health (HITECH) Act is another federal law that protects patient information. It includes a requirement for patient notification of any breach of confidentiality and a tiered structure of civil penalties for violations (What is the HITECH Act?, n.d.).

Additionally, there may be state laws protecting patient information, enabling patients to file civil lawsuits for breach of confidentiality. According to common law doctrine, patients also have a right to sue for "invasion of privacy" on the basis of harm resulting from disclosure of personal information.

Patient privacy laws, while protecting patient rights, have created new challenges for clinical nurse educators. Because of privacy concerns regarding disclosure of individually identifiable health information, many healthcare facilities have adopted policies and procedures that may pose barriers to clinical teaching and learning.

Most healthcare organizations require nursing education programs to provide documentation that their students have been oriented to the requirements of HIPAA. If numerous clinical sites are used by a program, this requirement can be onerous if each agency requires students to attend or complete its own HIPAA orientation. Nursing education administrators may be able to negotiate with all clinical agencies to agree on the basic content of the required orientation, recognizing that the requirement could be met in various ways. Students are typically asked to sign a verification that they have been oriented to HIPAA requirements and that they agree to abide by those requirements. This orientation and verification should be repeated at regular intervals (e.g., yearly or each semester).

As previously discussed, social media use also can result in HIPAA violations, sometimes inadvertently. Students should adhere to professional guidelines for social media use, including not posting or transmitting information that might be used to identify patients to anyone who does not have a legitimate right to know. Students may be required to sign documents affirming that they have been informed of HIPAA requirements and that they agree to adhere to them.

Because healthcare agencies also usually require nursing education programs to provide verification that nursing students have met specified health requirements, this verification process may create HIPAA concerns. If the nursing education program collects, receives, or transmits students' individually identifiable health information, it could be deemed responsible for maintaining reasonable and appropriate administrative, technical, and physical safeguards to ensure the integrity and confidentiality of the information and to protect against any reasonably anticipated threats to the security of the information and unauthorized uses or disclosures of it. Some clinical agencies request specific health data as evidence that students have met clinical health requirements, such as a rubella titer result. However, if the nursing education program complies with this request and the agency misuses the information in any way, both the education program and the clinical agency risk claims of unauthorized release or use of protected information about individual students.

Many nursing education programs avoid these potential complications by requiring a licensed healthcare provider to verify that a student has met all specified clinical health requirements. This verification, including dates for immunizations and a signed statement that the student's general health is adequate to allow full participation in the nursing program, is kept in the nursing education program files, but the raw data remain the property of the student and the student's healthcare provider. Another approach to resolving these concerns is to have all nursing students examined and tested by the student health service of the parent institution, with the raw data stored in that office and notification to the nursing education program that the clinical health requirements have or have not been met. It is wise to seek the advice of the school, college, or university counsel about how requirements for verification of students' health status by clinical agencies should be handled so that an appropriate policy can be developed and implemented.

During the recent global COVID-19 pandemic, healthcare facilities transformed their internal operations as well as the roles of staff members to manage the rapid and extreme changes in numbers and acuity of patients. Many acute care institutions determined that they could no longer accommodate the placement of health professional students for clinical practica. To address the sudden need for alternative clinical learning placements, nursing leaders developed a model for practice-academic partnerships (NCSBN, 2020), recommending that nursing students be employed in healthcare facilities as support workers and be given academic credit for doing so (Benton et al., 2020). If a nursing education program implements this model, students would be required to adhere to the health requirements of the agency in which they are employed as support workers, including requirements for COVID-19 testing and vaccination. That health information, like the previously described health requirement data, may be directly collected from students by the agency because of the students' special status as temporary employees. If not, the nursing education program would be responsible for ensuring that the students' protected health information is properly handled to avoid claims of unauthorized release or use of protected information. Nursing education programs or their governing institutions also may institute policies requiring COVID-19 testing or vaccination or both. Students who do not meet these requirements may not be permitted to complete in-person learning activities, which may result in failure to demonstrate the intended learning outcomes of the clinical practicum.

SUMMARY

Because clinical teaching and learning take place in a social context, the rights of teachers, students, staff members, and patients are sometimes in conflict. These conflicts create legal and ethical dilemmas for clinical teachers. This chapter discussed selected ethical and legal issues related to clinical teaching.

Online social networking is a useful and popular means of communication and collaboration, but nursing faculty members and students may encounter ethical and legal consequences of social media misuse. The ANA *Code of Ethics for Nurses with Interpretative Statements* emphasizes the obligation of nurses to act within the professional role and to maintain role boundaries in relationships with patients. Boundary violations can occur when students "friend" or "follow" patients or former patients on social media. Nurses also have an obligation to maintain patient privacy; confidentiality can be breached when information about patients is posted on social media sites, sometimes inadvertently. Social media misuse can have serious consequences for patients, nursing students, nursing education programs, and healthcare facilities. Nursing education programs should develop and enforce explicit policies regarding the use of electronic communication and social media, including specific consequences for policy violations; professional guidelines for use of social media can be used to inform policy development. Guidelines for appropriate use of social media should be reviewed regularly with students; examples of these guidelines were provided in the chapter.

Ethical standards such as respect for human dignity, autonomy, and freedom; beneficence; justice; veracity; privacy; and fidelity are important considerations for all parties involved in clinical teaching and learning. Students must learn to apply these standards to nursing practice, and teachers must apply them in their relationships with students as well as their teaching and evaluation responsibilities. Incivility in nursing education was discussed, with suggestions for how to prevent it and manage it.

Specific ethical issues related to clinical teaching and learning include the presence of learners in a service setting, the need for faculty–student relationships to be based on justice and respect for persons, students' privacy rights, teaching competence, and academic dishonesty.

Legal issues that have implications for clinical teaching and learning include educating students with disabilities, student rights to due process for academic and disciplinary decisions, standards of safe clinical practice, student and teacher negligence and liability, documentation and record keeping regarding students' clinical performance, and potential violations of HIPAA requirements with regard to student health information.

Suggestions were offered for preventing, minimizing, and managing these difficult ethical and legal situations. Laws and institutional policies often provide guidelines for action in specific cases. However, these suggestions should not be construed as legal advice, and teachers are advised to seek legal counsel in regard to specific questions or problems.

CNE® EXAMINATION TEST BLUEPRINT CORE COMPETENCIES

1. **Facilitate Learning**
   E. Practice skilled oral and written (including electronic) communication that reflects an awareness of self and relationships with learners (e.g., evaluation, mentorship, and supervision)
   K. Demonstrate personal attributes that facilitate learning (e.g., caring, confidence, patience, integrity, respect, and flexibility)
   P. Act as a role model in practice settings
2. **Facilitate Learner Development and Socialization**
   A. Identify individual learning styles and unique learning needs of learners with these characteristics:
      4. At-risk (e.g., educationally disadvantaged, learning and/or physically challenged, social, and economic issues)
   B. Provide resources for diverse learners to meet their individual learning needs
   D. Create learning environments that facilitate learners' self-reflection, personal goal setting, and socialization to the role of the nurse
   E. Foster the development of learners in these areas:
      3. affective domain
3. **Use Assessment and Evaluation Strategies**
   B. Enforce nursing program standards related to
      1. admission
      2. progression
      3. graduation

K. Advise learners regarding assessment and evaluation criteria
L. Provide timely, constructive, and thoughtful feedback to learners
5. **Pursue Systematic Self-Evaluation and Improvement in the Academic Nurse Educator Role**
H. Practice according to legal and ethical standards relevant to higher education and nursing education
6. **Engage in Scholarship, Service, and Leadership**
C. Function effectively within the organizational environment and the academic community
3. Integrate the values of respect, collegiality, professionalism, and caring to build an organizational climate that fosters the development of learners and colleagues

CNE®cl EXAMINATION TEST BLUEPRINT CORE COMPETENCIES

1. **Function within the Education and Health Care Environments**
A. Function in the Clinical Educator Role
5. Act as a role model of professional nursing within the clinical learning environment
6. Demonstrate inclusive excellence (e.g., student-centered learning, diversity)
C. Abide by Legal Requirements, Ethical Guidelines, Agency Policies, and Guiding Framework
1. Apply ethical and legal principles to create a safe clinical learning environment
4. Inform others of program and clinical agency policies, procedures, and practices
5. Adhere to program and clinical agency policies, procedures, and practices when implementing clinical experiences
6. Promote learner compliance with regulations and standards of practice
7. Demonstrate ethical behaviors

2. **Facilitate Learning in the Health Care Environment**
E. Promote a culture of safety and quality in the healthcare environment
F. Create a positive and caring learning environment
G. Develop collegial working relationships with learners, faculty colleagues, and clinical agency personnel

3. **Demonstrate Effective Interpersonal Communication and Collaborative Interprofessional Relationships**
D. Support an environment of frequent, respectful, civil, and open communication with all members of the healthcare team
E. Act as a role model showing respect for all members of the healthcare team, professional colleagues, clients, family members, as well as learners
G. Listen to learner concerns, needs, or questions in a non-threatening way
I. Manage emotions effectively when communicating in challenging situations
J. Effectively manage conflict
K. Maintain an approachable, non judgmental, and readily accessible demeanor
M. Demonstrate effective communication in clinical learning environments with diverse colleagues, clients, cultures, healthcare professionals, and learners
N. Communicate performance expectations to learners and agency staff

5. **Facilitate Learner Development and Socialization**
   A. Mentor learners in the development of professional nursing behaviors, standards, and codes of ethics
   B. Promote a learning climate of respect for all
   C. Promote professional integrity and accountability
   D. Maintain professional boundaries
   G. Create learning environments that are focused on socialization to the role of the nurse
   H. Assist learners to develop the ability to engage in constructive peer feedback

6. **Implement Effective Clinical Assessment and Evaluation Strategies**
   D. Maintain integrity in the assessment and evaluation of learners
   E. Provide timely, objective, constructive, and fair feedback to learners
   J. Document learner clinical performance, feedback, and progression

REFERENCES

American Nurses Association. (2011). *ANA's principles for social networking and the nurse: Guidance for registered nurses.* https://www.nursingworld.org/~4af4f2/globalassets/docs/ana/ethics/social-networking.pdf

American Nurses Association. (2015). *Code of ethics for nurses with interpretive statements.* http://nursingworld.org/DocumentVault/Ethics-1/Code-of-Ethics-for-Nurses.html

Benton, D. C., Alexander, M., Fotsch, R., & Livanos, N. (2020, August 12). Lessons learned and insights gained: A regulatory analysis of the impacts, challenges, and responses to COVID-19. *OJIN: The Online Journal of Issues in Nursing, 25*(3). https://doi.org/10.3912/OJIN.Vol25No03PPT51

Corcoran, S. (1977). Should a service setting be used as a learning laboratory? An ethical question. *Nursing Outlook, 25*, 771–774.

Daigle, A. (2020). Social media and professional boundaries in undergraduate nursing students. *Journal of Professional Nursing, 36*(2), 20–23.

De Gagne, J. C., Yamane, S. S., Conklin, J. L., Chang, J., & Kang, H. S. (2018). Social media use and cybercivility guidelines in U.S. nursing schools: A review of websites. *Journal of Professional Nursing, 34*(1), 35–41. https://doi.org/10.1016/j.profnurs.2017.07.006

Family Educational Rights and Privacy Act, 20 U.S.C. § 1232g; 34 CFR Part 99 (1974).

Glasgow, M. E., Dreher, H. M., Dahnke, M. D., & Gyllenhammer, J. (2021). *Legal and ethical issues in nursing education: An essential guide.* Springer Publishing Company.

Health Insurance Portability and Accountability Act (HIPAA) of 1996. Public Law 104–191.

Holtz, H., K., Rawl, S. M., & Draucker, C. (2018). Types of faculty incivility as viewed by students in bachelor of science in nursing programs. *Nursing Education Perspectives, 39*(2), 85–90.

Luparell, S., & Frisbee, K. (2019). Do uncivil nursing students become uncivil nurses? A national survey of faculty. *Nursing Education Perspectives, 40*(6), 322–327. https://doi.org/10.1097/01.NEP.0000000000000491

McClung, E. L., & Gaberson, K. B. (2021). Academic dishonesty among nursing students: A contemporary view. *Nurse Educator, 46*(2), 111–115. https://doi.org/10.1097/NNE.0000000000000863

National Council of State Boards of Nursing. (2014). *NCSBN model act.* https://www.ncsbn.org/14_Model_Act_0914.pdf

National Council of State Boards of Nursing. (2017). *NCSBN model rules.* https://www.ncsbn.org/17_Model_Rules_0917.pdf

National Council of State Boards of Nursing. (2018). *A nurse's guide to the use of social media.* [Brochure]. https://www.ncsbn.org/NCSBN_SocialMedia.pdf

National Council of State Boards of Nursing. (2020). *Policy brief: U.S. nursing leadership supports practice/academic partnerships to assist the nursing workforce during the COVID-19 crisis.* https://www.ncsbn.org/Policy_Brief_US_Nursing_Leadership_COVID19.pdf

Oermann, M. H., & Gaberson, K. B. (2021). *Evaluation and testing in nursing education* (6th ed.). Springer Publishing Company.

Silbert-Flagg, J., Shilling, S. D., Lucas, L., Nolan, M. T., Lin, L., Bellefeuille, P., Foley, M., Mallareddy, D., Baker. D., & D'Aoust, R. (2020). Preparing for a student with a service animal. *Journal of Professional Nursing, 36*(6), 458–461. https://doi.org/10.1016/j.profnurs.2020.03.001

Southern Regional Education Board. (2016). *The Americans with Disabilities Act: Implications for nursing education.* http://www.sreb.org/publication/americans-disabilities-act

Stalter, A. M., Phillips, J., M., Ruggiero, J. S., Wiggs, C. M., Brodhead, J., & Swanson, K. (2019). Systems perspective for incivility in academia: An integrative review. *Nursing Education Perspectives, 40*(3), 144–150. https://doi.org/10.1097/01.NEP.0000000000000466

What is the HITECH Act? (n.d.). *HIPAA Journal.* https://www.hipaajournal.com/what-is-the-hitech-act/

Yarbrough, A. E., & Welch, S. R. (2021). Uncovering the process of reasonable academic accommodations for prelicensure nursing students with learning disabilities. *Nursing Education Perspectives, 42*(1), 5–10. https://doi.org/10.1097/01.NEP.0000000000000666

Strategies for Effective Clinical Teaching

Clinical Teaching Methods and Crafting Clinical Learning Assignments

One of the most important responsibilities of the clinical educator is selecting teaching methods and crafting clinical assignments that are related to the competencies to be developed, appropriate to students' levels of knowledge and skill, and challenging enough to motivate learning. Although having students provide comprehensive nursing care to one or more patients is a typical clinical assignment, it is only one of many possible assignments and not always the most appropriate choice. This chapter presents clinical teaching methods—clinical assignments and options for these assignments (skill vs. total care focus, student–patient ratio options, management activities, guided observation, and service learning); discussion; clinical conferences; and written assignments. The chapter provides a framework for planning clinical assignments for learners.

FACTORS AFFECTING SELECTION OF CLINICAL TEACHING METHODS AND ASSIGNMENTS

The selection of teaching methods and learning activities within the context of the clinical teaching process was discussed in Chapter 5. Clinical activities help learners to apply knowledge to practice, develop skills, cultivate professional values, and form the role of the professional nurse. Some of these activities may be assignments in which students provide complete care to one or more patients. However, other assignments may involve specific learning activities such as medication administration for a large group of patients or interviews of providers because these are the best strategies to help students achieve the specific competencies or outcomes and apply the concepts being examined in class to practice, or because they will meet students' individual learning needs. As explained in Chapter 5, clinical teaching methods and learning activities, which may include patient assignments, are selected according to the competencies to be developed or outcomes to be met in the clinical practicum, individual learner needs, evidence of the effectiveness of the teaching methods and learning activities being considered, characteristics of the clinical learning environment, and availability of the educator, preceptor, or other clinician to guide learners.

In addition to these factors, two other considerations are the needs of patients and other individuals for whom the students are providing care or interacting with and timing of the activities and availability of learning opportunities. Educators should consider if the nursing care and learning activities present enough of a challenge for learners, or if they might be too complex for the student to manage. Some patients, family members, and other caregivers may not want care from a nursing student or to complete other activities with students. Nursing staff members and others in the clinical agency can often help the teacher determine whether student learning needs and specific patient needs can both be met through a particular clinical assignment.

Because the purpose of clinical learning is to foster application of theory to practice, clinical learning activities should be related to what is being taught in the classroom. Ideally, activities are planned so that learners can make immediate transfer and application of knowledge to nursing practice. However, this is usually difficult to do. The availability of clinical sites and learning opportunities in those settings affects assignments and other learning activities. For example, if one of the outcomes of the practicum is for students to "Identify significant data about patients' conditions from the electronic health record (EHR)," students may be restricted from accessing the EHR or may have limited opportunities to gain access to patient records at change of shift when other providers are documenting care. Thus, planning for simulated experiences in an academic EHR application or scheduling learners to arrive at the clinical site at midmorning may be more appropriate.

Some clinical settings, such as outpatient clinics, may be available to both patients and students only on a daytime, Monday through Friday, schedule. In other settings, scheduling learning activities during evening or night-time hours or in the community may offer students better opportunities to meet certain outcomes. If students are learning about health teaching, they can develop these skills in a wide range of clinical settings, in simulation, and through other learning activities. By knowing the concepts that students are learning in the classroom, the clinical teacher can identify learning activities to help students apply those concepts in patient care. For example, if the focus is wound healing, students could have learning activities involving patients with postoperative wounds, pressure ulcers, traumatic wounds, or arterial or venous chronic leg ulcers. It is not necessary for every student to have a similar learning opportunity if all learning activities enable students to apply the same concept in practice. In a postclinical conference, students can discuss the various ways in which they applied a particular concept, identifying similarities and differences among the various patient responses to a common alteration in health status.

CLINICAL ASSIGNMENTS

When planning clinical assignments, teachers typically think about patients for whom students will provide care. The primary role of the student in the clinical setting, however, is that of learner, not nurse. Although students need contact with patients to apply classroom learning to clinical practice, caring for patients is not synonymous with learning. Safe, competent nursing practice requires students to integrate theory with practice and develop clinical reasoning and judgment skills

(Nielsen et al., 2020). Practice in clinical settings provides experiences for students with concepts they are learning about in class. As students gain knowledge about concepts such as fluid and electrolyte balance and pain management in class, they can engage in a wide range of learning activities in the clinical setting in which they apply this knowledge to patient care. A complete patient assignment may not be the most appropriate learning activity.

Options for Clinical Assignments

Several options are available for making clinical assignments for nursing students. Although it is the teacher's responsibility to specify the clinical competencies and learning outcomes to be met, students should have choices of learning activities that will help them develop the competencies. Having a choice of assignment or at least a choice between options selected by the teacher motivates students to be responsible for their own learning and fully engage in the learning activity. Allowing learners to participate in selecting their own assignments may also reduce student anxiety.

The teacher should offer guidance to students in selecting appropriate learning activities. Sometimes teachers need to be more directive: A student may choose an assignment that clearly requires more knowledge or skill than the student has developed. In this case, the teacher should intervene to protect patient safety and help the student make realistic plans to acquire the necessary competencies. Other students may choose assignments that do not challenge their abilities. The teacher's role is to support and encourage such students to take advantage of opportunities to achieve higher levels of knowledge and skill.

SKILL FOCUS VERSUS TOTAL CARE FOCUS

The traditional clinical assignment for nursing students is to give total care to one or more patients. However, many outcomes to do not require students to practice total patient care. For example, if the goal is for students to assess patient and family preparation for discharge, the student does not have to provide total care to the postoperative patient. The student could develop this skill by interviewing a patient or family member, observing a case manager's assessment of the patient's and family's readiness for discharge, reviewing a physical therapist's assessment of the patient's ability to perform activities at home, collecting data from the EHR, or participating in a simulation. Additionally, total patient care is an integrative activity that can be accomplished effectively only when students are competent in performing the component skills.

As previously discussed, all students do not need to be engaged in the same learning activities at the same time. Depending on their individual learning needs, some students might be engaged in activities that focus on developing a particular skill, while others could be practicing more integrative activities such as providing total patient care. One advantage to assigning some students to learning activities that do not involve total patient care is that the clinical educator is more available for closer guidance of students when they are learning to care for patients with complex needs. Staggering assignments in this way helps the teacher better meet the learning needs of all students.

STUDENT–PATIENT RATIO OPTIONS

Although the traditional clinical assignment takes the form of one student to one patient, there are other assignment options. These options include:

- *One student/one patient or multiple patients:* One student is responsible for certain aspects of care or for comprehensive care for one or more patients. The student works alone to plan, implement, and evaluate nursing care. This type of assignment is advantageous when the outcome is to integrate multiple aspects of care.
- *Multiple students/one patient:* Two or more students are assigned to plan, implement, and evaluate care for one patient. Each learner has a defined role, and all collaborate to provide care. This assignment strategy is particularly useful when patients have complex needs that are beyond the capability of one student, although it can be used in any setting with a large number of students and a low patient census. Other advantages include reducing student anxiety and teaching teamwork and collaborative learning.
- *Multiple students–patient aggregate:* A group of students is assigned to complete activities related to a community or population at risk for certain health problems. For example, a small group of students might be assigned to conduct a community assessment. Clinical activities would include interviewing community residents, identifying environmental health hazards, and documenting the availability of social and healthcare services. The student group would then analyze the data and prepare a report on their findings.

MANAGEMENT ACTIVITIES

Some clinical assignments are chosen to enable learners to meet outcomes related to nursing leadership, management, quality improvement, and healthcare organizational goals. For example, a student at the end of the prelicensure program may enact the role of team leader for other nursing students who are assigned to provide care for individual patients. The student team leader may receive handoff reports about the group of patients from agency staff, plan assignments for the other students, give reports to those students, supervise and coordinate work, and communicate patient information to staff members.

GUIDED OBSERVATION

Observation is an important skill in nursing practice, and teachers should provide opportunities for learners to develop this skill systematically. Observing patients to collect data is a prerequisite to problem solving and clinical judgment. To make accurate and useful observations, the student should have knowledge of the patient's condition or the related concept. As a clinical learning assignment, observation should not be combined with an assignment to provide care. If students do not have concurrent care responsibilities, they are free to choose the times and sometimes the locations of their observations. The focus should be on observing purposefully to develop this skill.

Observation also provides opportunities for students to learn through modeling. By observing another person interacting with and caring for patients and others in the clinical setting or community, the learner forms an image of the role of that individual and how interventions are to be performed. For this reason, it may be helpful to schedule learners to observe in a clinical setting before they are assigned to practice activities. However, scheduling an observation before the learner has acquired the prerequisite knowledge is unproductive: the student may not be able to make meaning out of what is observed.

Written observation guidelines can be used effectively to prepare learners for the activity and to guide their attention to important data during the observation. Exhibit 7.1 is an example of a guide to prepare students for an observation activity in an operating room. The guide includes the expectation that, before the observation, students read and anticipate what they will see. Students may be asked to evaluate the observation activity by identifying what they did and did not learn from the activity. Exhibit 7.2 is a sample evaluation tool for an observation activity.

EXHIBIT 7.1 Example of an Observation Guide

OPERATING ROOM OBSERVATION GUIDE

Purposes of the Observation Activity

1. To gain an overview of perioperative nursing care in the intraoperative phase.
2. To observe application of principles of surgical asepsis in the operating room.
3. To distinguish among roles of various members of the surgical team.

General Information

You are expected to prepare for this observation and to complete an observation guide after observing the surgical procedure. Please read your medical–surgical nursing textbook, pp. 195 to 200, for a general understanding of nursing roles in the intraoperative phase. Bring this observation guide on the day of your observation. The guide will be collected and reviewed by the instructor at the end of the observation activity.

Preparation of the Patient

1. Who is responsible for obtaining the consent for the surgical procedure? Why?
2. Who identifies the patient when they are brought into the operating room? Why?
3. What other patient data should be reviewed by a nurse when the patient is brought to the operating room (sign-in protocol)? Why?
4. Who transfers the patient from transport bed to the operating room bed? What safety precautions are taken during this procedure?
5. What is the nurse's role during anesthesia induction?
6. What team members participate in the time-out protocol? Identify elements of the protocol that protect the safety of this patient.
7. When is the patient positioned for the surgical procedure? Who does this? What safety precautions are taken? What special equipment may be used?
8. What is the purpose of the preoperative skin preparation of the operative site? When is it done? What safety precautions are taken?
9. What is the purpose of draping the patient and equipment? What factors determine the type of drape material used? What safety precautions are taken? Who does the draping? Why?

(continued)

EXHIBIT 7.1 Example of an Observation Guide (*continued*)

Preparation of Personnel

1. Apparel: Who is wearing what? What factors determine the selection of apparel? How and when do personnel don and remove apparel items? What personal protective equipment is used and why?
2. Hand antisepsis: Which personnel use hand antisepsis techniques to prepare for the procedure? When? Which method is used?
3. Gowning and gloving: What roles do the scrub person and the circulator play?

Roles of Surgical Team Members: Record observations of personnel (role and tasks of each).

Maintenance of Aseptic Technique

1. Movement of personnel
2. Sterile areas and items
3. Nonsterile areas and items
4. Handling of sterile items

Equipment: Identify equipment in the room and its use.

Conclusion of Procedure

1. What elements of the sign-out protocol are implemented at this time?
2. How is the patient handoff communication conducted? What personnel are involved? Were the essential elements included?
3. What patient problems are likely to be identified for this patient in the postoperative period?

EXHIBIT 7.2 Example of Student Evaluation of a Guided Observation Activity

STUDENT EVALUATION OF OBSERVATION

1. How would you rate the overall value of this learning activity?
   ___ It was excellent; I learned a great deal.
   ___ It was very good; I learned more than I expected to.
   ___ It was good; I learned about as much as I expected to.
   ___ It was fair; I didn't learn as much as I expected to.
   ___ It was poor; I didn't learn anything of value.
2. How would you rate the value of the observation guide in helping you to prepare for and participate in the observation?
   ___ Extremely helpful in focusing my attention on significant aspects to be observed.
   ___ Very helpful in guiding me to observe activities.
   ___ Helpful in guiding my observations.
   ___ Only a little helpful; it seemed like a lot of work for little benefit.
   ___ Not at all helpful; I did not learn anything by completing the observation guide.
3. What was the most meaningful part of this learning activity for you? What was the most important or surprising thing you learned?
4. What was the least meaningful part of this observation activity? If there is something that you would change, suggest a specific change to improve the experience.

SERVICE LEARNING

Another option for clinical learning assignments is service learning. Service learning differs from volunteer work, community service, fieldwork, and internships. Volunteer and community service focus primarily on the service that is provided to the recipients, and fieldwork and internships primarily focus on benefits to student learning. Service learning benefits the community and students, and allows students to see the value of service to vulnerable populations (Baker et al., 2020; Beauvais et al., 2015; Gresh et al., 2021; Velez & Koo, 2020). Service learning is an academic credit-earning learning activity in which students:

- Participate in an organized service activity that meets identified community needs
- Reinforce course content
- Reflect on the service activity to gain a deeper understanding of the nurse's role in society

Benefits of service learning to students include developing skills in communication, critical thinking, and collaboration; a community perspective and commitment to health promotion and health equity in the community; an awareness of diversity and cultural dynamics; and leadership abilities and professional identity (Taylor & Leffers, 2016; Thompson et al., 2013; Velez & Koo, 2020). Benefits to the community include having control of the service provided and recipients of the service.

As nursing education programs include more community-based learning activities, opportunities to incorporate service learning increase. Meaningful community-based service-learning opportunities are based on relationships between the academic unit and the community to be served. For such partnerships to work effectively, there must be a good fit between the academic unit's mission and goals and the needs of the community. A key element of service learning is the community partner's identification of need (Taylor & Leffers, 2016).

As is true for any other clinical learning activity, planning for a service-learning activity begins with the teacher's decision that these activities would help students to achieve one or more course outcomes. The success of service learning depends on the embedding of this pedagogy in an existing academic course with clearly defined outcomes (Taylor & Leffers, 2016). The teacher should determine how much time to allot to this activity, keeping in mind that the time spent in service learning would replace and not add to the total time available for other clinical activities for that course.

Before students participate in a service-learning activity, they should prepare a learning contract that includes:

- The name of the community agency or group
- The clients or recipients of that agency's or group's services
- The services to be provided by the student
- A service objective related to a need that has been identified by the community or the community recipient of the proposed service
- A learning objective that is related to a course outcome or competency that the activity would help the student to achieve

The educator should identify agencies and groups appropriate for service learning in a specific course from among those with which the educational institution has formed an academic–practice partnership. Examples of community settings, programs, and agencies that would be appropriate for service learning include day care centers, extended care or assisted living centers, senior centers, food delivery programs, the American Red Cross, health screening programs, vaccine clinics, health outreach or shelter programs for homeless individuals and families, and camps for children, among many others.

As another option, a group of students enrolled in the same course could be placed in a community setting to participate in a designated population-based project relevant to the course objectives. For example, Decker et al. (2016) described a service-learning activity in which nursing students implemented a bystander intervention on their college campus. Findings from 118 students over a 2-year period showed that students helped improve campus safety while growing as professionals. The students' service was part of their community clinical nursing course.

The role of the clinical teacher as facilitator is critical to the success of service learning. The teacher needs to structure pre-engagement, on-site, and post-engagement student learning activities to ensure the achievement of desired outcomes (Taylor & Leffers, 2016). Because service learning is more than expecting students to use some of their clinical practice hours for service projects, clinical teachers should plan to spend as much time planning these activities as they do traditional clinical learning activities. Students' reflection on their experiences is an essential component of service learning, differentiating it from a volunteer experience.

DISCUSSIONS

Discussions between teacher and student, and preceptor and orientee, occur frequently but do not always promote learning. These discussions often involve the teacher telling the learner what to do or not to do for a patient. Discussions, though, should be an exchange of ideas through which the teacher, by asking open-ended questions and supporting learner responses, encourages students to arrive at their own decisions or to engage in self-assessment about clinical practice. Discussions are not intended to be an exchange of the teacher's ideas to the students. In a discussion, both teacher and student actively participate in sharing ideas and considering alternative perspectives.

Discussions give learners an opportunity to interact with one another, critique each other's ideas, and learn from others. For that reason, discussions are an effective method for promoting critical thinking and clinical judgment (Berkstresser, 2016; Hensel & Billings, 2020). The teacher can ask open-ended and thought-provoking questions, which encourage higher-level thinking if students perceive that they are free to discuss their own ideas and those of others involved in the discussion. The teacher is a resource for students, giving immediate feedback and further instruction as needed. Discussions also provide a forum for students to explore feelings associated with their clinical practice and simulation experiences, clarify values and ethical dilemmas, and learn to interact in a group format. Those outcomes are not as easily met in a large group setting. Over a period of time, students learn to collaborate with peers in working toward solving clinical problems.

Creating a Climate for Discussions

An important role of the teacher is to develop a climate in which students are comfortable discussing concepts and issues without fear that the ideas expressed will affect the teacher's evaluation of their performance and subsequent clinical grade. Discussions should be carried out in an atmosphere in which learners feel comfortable to express their own opinions and ideas and to question others' assumptions. Discussions are for formative, not summative, evaluation. Without this climate for exchanging ideas, though, discussions cannot be carried out effectively, because students fear that their comments may influence their clinical evaluation and grade—or, for nurses, their performance ratings.

Guidelines for Discussions

Discussions can be face-to-face in the clinical setting or conducted online (Hannans, 2019). They can be carried out individually with learners or in a small group. The size of the group for a discussion can range from 2 to 10 people. A larger group makes it difficult for each person to participate. An effective teacher keeps the discussion focused; avoids talking too much, with students in a passive role; and avoids side-tracking. While the teacher may initiate the discussion, the interaction needs to revolve around the students, not the teacher. Rephrasing students' questions for them to answer suggests that the teacher has confidence in students' ability to arrive at answers and provides opportunities for students to think aloud and share their reasoning. Open-ended questions without one specific answer encourage higher level thinking. Exhibit 7.3 summarizes the roles of the teacher and students in clinical discussions.

EXHIBIT 7.3 Roles of Teacher and Student in Discussions

1. Teacher
   Plans discussion
   Presents problem, issue, case for analysis, or asks students to do this
   Develops questions for discussion
   Facilitates discussion with students as active participants
   Develops and maintains atmosphere for open discussion of ideas and issues
   Monitors time
   Avoids side-tracking
   Provides feedback
2. Student
   Prepares for discussion
   Participates actively in discussion
   Works collaboratively with group members to arrive at solutions and decisions
   Examines different points of view,
   Is willing to modify own view and perspective to reach group consensus
   Reflects on clinical experiences and simulation
3. Teacher and Student
   Summarize outcomes of discussion and learning
   Identify implications of discussion for other clinical situations

These guidelines also apply to online discussions about clinical practice. Instead of a face-to-face postclinical conference, the conference can be held online at a later time (Berkstresser, 2016; Hannans, 2019). With an online discussion or forum following the clinical experience, students have time for reflection about the care they provided and their interactions with patients and others in the clinical setting. Online discussions about clinical practice promote learning by allowing students to view and respond to the thinking of their peers, similar to face-to-face postconferences. It is critical that no information is shared about patients and others in the clinical setting, and students need to be told this prior to beginning the practicum. An online discussion can refer to "a patient" or "a staff member with whom I interacted."

The teacher can post higher level questions to begin the discussion and specify when students need to post their answers. Similar to a face-to-face discussion, the teacher's role is to facilitate the discussion with prompts and responses to stimulate further thinking but not to dominate with their own comments. Consistent with other discussion forums, there needs to be a set time frame for the discussion, for example, one week. With online discussions the teacher can prepare questions to help students relate their learning from class to clinical practice, reflect on their care and interactions, identify other perspectives and approaches, and seek further evidence that is relevant to their patient care. Online discussions may also promote affective learning because students may be more comfortable sharing their feelings and values online than in person. For students who are quiet and are hesitant to participate in face-to-face discussions, online ones may build their confidence.

Purposes of Discussions

Discussions promote several types of learning depending on the goals and structure:

- Development of problem-solving, higher level thinking, and clinical judgment skills
- Debriefing of clinical experiences and following simulations
- Development of cooperative learning and group process skills
- Assessment of own learning
- Development of oral communication skills

Every discussion will not necessarily promote each of these learning outcomes. The teacher should be clear about the intent of the discussion so it may be geared to the particular outcomes to be achieved. For instance, discussions for critical thinking require carefully selected questions that examine alternative possibilities and "what if" types of questions. This same type of questioning, however, may not be necessary if the goal is to develop cooperative learning or group process skills.

DEVELOPMENT OF COGNITIVE SKILLS

An important purpose of discussions is to promote development of problem-solving, higher level thinking, and clinical judgment skills. Discussions are effective because they provide an opportunity for the teacher to gear the questioning toward these skills. Not all discussions, though, lead to these higher levels of thinking. The key is the type of questions asked by the teacher or discussed among students—questions need to encourage students to examine alternative perspectives and points of view in a given situation and to provide a rationale for their thinking.

Exhibit 7.4 presents strategies for directing discussions toward development of higher-level cognitive skills.

Discussions are valuable to help students think through clinical situations and develop their clinical judgment skills. Questions in a discussion can be used as prompts to lead students through this process. Prompts are planned questions about clinical judgment to make the students' thinking and decision making visible (Billings, 2019; Hensel & Billings, 2020). The questions in Table 7.1 are examples of prompts for the development of clinical judgment.

EXHIBIT 7.4 Discussions for Cognitive Skill Development

Ask students to:
Identify problems in a real or hypothetical clinical situation.
Identify possible alternative problems.
Assess the problem and clinical situation further.
Differentiate relevant and irrelevant information for the problem or issue being discussed.
Discuss their own point of view and others' points of view.
Examine their own assumptions and those of other students.
Identify different solutions and interventions that might be used and why.
Compare possible alternatives and defend the choice of one particular action over another.
Take a position about an issue and provide a rationale both for and against that position.
Reflect on own biases, values, and beliefs that influence thinking.
Evaluate the effectiveness of interventions and approaches to solving problems.

TABLE 7.1 PROMPTS TO TEACH CLINICAL JUDGMENT

Steps of Clinical Judgment	Possible Prompts
Recognizing Cues	What cues did you recognize?
	What are the most significant findings?
	What information was less important or distracting?
Analyzing Cues	What findings did you expect based on the client's diagnosis/concern?
	Are there any findings that seem contradictory?
	What other information can you gather to help you determine the significance of the cues?
	What set of cues are most concerning?
Generating Hypothesis	What is most likely occurring?
	What makes you say that?
	What will happen if this is not treated?
	What else could be going on?
	Which hypothesis is the most important and the nurse should manage first?
	What are the risks for ignoring other hypotheses?

(continued)

Steps of Clinical Judgment	Possible Prompts
Generating Solutions	What are the desired outcomes related to your hypothesis? (Give at least 2) What interventions are indicated? What interventions should be avoided?
Taking Action	What intervention(s) are needed immediately? What interventions can you delegate and to whom? What are the mechanisms of actions of any medications, and what are their major nursing considerations? What specific items will you teach the client? What information would you include in a SBAR report for handoff and any referrals?
Evaluating Outcomes	What follow up data are needed? What findings would show an intervention is working? What findings show an intervention is not effective? Are there any critical values to monitor?

TABLE 7.1 PROMPTS TO TEACH CLINICAL JUDGMENT (*CONTINUED*)

SBAR, Situation, Background, Assessment, Recommendation.

From Hensel, D., & Billings, D. M. (2020). Strategies to teach the National Council of State Boards of Nursing clinical judgment model. *Nurse Educator*, *45*(3), 130. https://doi.org/10.1097/nne.0000000000000773. Reprinted by permission Wolters Kluwer Health.

DEBRIEFING OF CLINICAL EXPERIENCES

Debriefing is the practice of engaging learners in a reflective discussion after a learning experience (Vihos et al., 2017). While debriefing has been examined most frequently in the context of simulation, postclinical conferences are a form of debriefing. These discussions provide an opportunity for students to describe and reflect on their care. In these discussions, students receive feedback from the teacher and also from peers about their decisions and other possible approaches they could use. Debriefing also provides an opportunity to share feelings about clinical practice and interactions with other healthcare providers. These discussions are particularly valuable in helping students analyze ethical dilemmas, consider different points of view, and explore their own values and beliefs.

DEVELOPMENT OF COOPERATIVE LEARNING SKILLS

Group discussions are effective for promoting cooperative learning skills. In cooperative learning, students work in small groups to meet particular learning outcomes related to the course. Students are actively involved in their learning and foster the learning of others in the group. Discussions using cooperative learning strategies begin with the teacher planning the discussion and presenting a task to be completed by the group, problem to be solved, or case to be analyzed. Students work cooperatively in groups (or pairs) and present the results of their discussions to the rest of the students.

ASSESSMENT OF OWN LEARNING

Discussions provide a means for students to assess their own learning, identify gaps in their understanding, and learn from others in a nonthreatening environment. Students can ask questions of the group and use the teacher and peers as resources for their learning. If the teacher is effective in developing an atmosphere for open discussion, students, in turn, will share their feelings, concerns, and questions as a beginning to their continued development.

DEVELOPMENT OF ORAL COMMUNICATION SKILLS

The ability to present ideas orally, as well as in written form, is an important outcome to be achieved by students in clinical courses. Discussions provide opportunities for students to present ideas to a group, explain concepts clearly, handle questions raised by others, and refine presentation style. Participation in a discussion requires formulating ideas and presenting them logically to the group.

Students may make formal presentations to the clinical group as a way of developing their oral communication skills. They may lead a discussion and present on a specific topic related to the outcomes of the clinical course. Discussion provides an opportunity for peers and the teacher to give feedback to students on how well students communicated their ideas to others and to improve their communication techniques.

CLINICAL CONFERENCES

Clinical conferences are discussions in which students share information about their clinical experiences, engage in thinking about and reflecting on clinical practice, lead others in discussions, and give formal presentations to the group. Clinical conferences can be face-to-face in the clinical or academic setting, or they can be conducted online. There are many types of clinical conferences.

Preclinical conferences are small group or one-to-one discussions with the clinical nurse educator or preceptor that precede clinical learning activities. In preclinical conferences, students ask questions about their patients or other aspects of clinical practice. An important role of the teacher in preclinical conferences is to ensure that students have the essential knowledge and competencies to complete their clinical activities. In many instances, the teacher needs to instruct students further and fill in the gaps in students' learning.

Postclinical conferences are held at the conclusion of clinical learning activities. Postclinical conferences provide a forum for analyzing patient care and exploring other options, thereby facilitating critical thinking. Postclinical conferences may be used for peer review and critiquing each other's work. They are not intended as substitutes for classroom instruction with the teacher lecturing and presenting new content to students. A similar problem often occurs with guest speakers who treat the conference as a class, lecturing to students about their area of expertise rather than encouraging group discussion and student reflection.

Clinical conferences can also focus on ethical and professional issues associated with clinical practice. Conferences of this type encourage critical thinking about issues that students have encountered or may in the future. In these conferences, students can analyze events that occurred in the clinical setting, ones in which they were personally involved or learned about through their clinical experience. A student can present the situation to the group for analysis and discussion. The discussion should focus on varied approaches that might be used and how to decide on the best strategy.

Debates provide a forum for analyzing problems and issues in depth, considering opposing viewpoints, and defending a position. Students can examine a topic from different angles and gain depth in their understanding of an issue (George et al., 2020). Debates developed around clinical issues give students an opportunity to prepare an argument for or against a particular position and to take a stand on an issue.

WRITTEN ASSIGNMENTS

Written assignments for clinical learning have four main purposes: (a) assist students in understanding concepts, theories, and other content that relate to care of patients; (b) develop higher level thinking skills; (c) examine their own feelings, beliefs, and values generated from their clinical learning experiences; and (d) develop writing skills. In choosing written assignments for clinical courses, the teacher should first consider the outcomes to be met through the assignments and the competencies that students need to develop in the course and nursing program. Writing assignments should build on one another to progressively develop students' skills. Another consideration is the number of assignments to be completed. How many assignments are needed to demonstrate mastery? It may be that one assignment well done is sufficient for meeting the outcomes, and students may then progress to other learning activities. Teachers should avoid using the same written assignments repeatedly throughout a clinical practicum and should instead choose assignments for specific learning outcomes.

Promote Understanding

In written assignments, students can describe concepts and other information relevant to the care of their patients and can explain how that knowledge guides their clinical decisions and judgments. Assignments for this purpose need a clear focus to prevent students from merely summarizing and reporting what they read. Shorter assignments that direct students to apply particular concepts to clinical practice may be of greater value in developing higher level thinking skills than longer assignments for which students summarize readings without any analysis of them.

Examples of written assignments to promote understanding of concepts and other information related to clinical practice are:

- Compare, in no more than three pages, two interventions appropriate for your patient in terms of their rationale and evidence. How will you evaluate their effectiveness?
- Read a research article related to care of one of your patients, critique the article, report on the analysis, and explain why the research findings are or are not applicable to the patient's care.
- Compare data collected from your patient with the description of that condition in your textbook or other readings. What are similarities and differences? Why?
- Develop a concept map (a graphic arrangement of key concepts related to your patient's care) and provide a written description of the relationships among the concepts in your map.

- Investigate the process used in your clinical setting for handoff. Write a summary report. How does the handoff process relate to concepts you learned in your course about communicating patient information between providers?

Develop Higher Level Thinking Skills

Written assignments provide an opportunity for students to analyze patient and other problems they have encountered in clinical practice, evaluate their interventions, and propose new approaches. In writing assignments, students can analyze data and clinical situations, identify additional assessment data needed for decision-making, identify patient needs and problems, propose approaches, compare interventions based on evidence, and evaluate the effectiveness of care. Writing assignments are particularly valuable for learning about evidence-based practice (EBP). Students can search for and examine the evidence underlying different interventions and make decisions about the best approaches to use with their patients. Students can identify assumptions they made about patients' responses that influenced their clinical decisions, critique arguments, take a stand about an issue and develop a rationale to support it, and draw generalizations about patient care from different clinical experiences.

Written assignments for developing higher level thinking skills can be short, ranging from one to two paragraphs to a few pages. In developing these assignments, the teacher should avoid activities in which students merely report on the ideas and thinking of others. Instead, the assignment should ask students to consider an alternative point of view or a different way of approaching an issue. Short assignments also provide an opportunity for teachers to give prompt feedback to students.

The writing assignment should focus on meeting a particular learning outcome and should have specific directions to guide students' writing. For example, students may be asked to prepare a one-page paper comparing the physiological processes of asthma and bronchitis. Rather than writing on everything they read about asthma and bronchitis, students can focus their papers on the physiology of these two conditions.

Examples of written assignments for developing higher level cognitive skills follow:

- Describe in one paragraph significant information you collected from your patient and why it is important to your decisions about approaches to use with that patient.
- Select one need or problem you identified for your patient and provide a rationale for it. What is one alternative need or problem you might also consider and why? Complete this assignment in two typed pages.
- Identify a near miss (close call) or an unsafe practice that you experienced or observed in your clinical setting. Analyze what went wrong and practices that should have been used. Prepare a response integrating the concept of just culture.
- Identify an issue affecting the community. Provide a rationale for actions to be taken and role of the nurse.
- Identify a procedure you performed in your clinical setting. Find the policy. Was your performance consistent with that policy? Why or why not? Are there

deviations or workarounds you observed on the unit with that procedure? Write a report about what you learned.

■ Identify a patient you cared for in this or a prior course. Briefly describe the patient. What were the most important contributors to that person's health? How do they relate to the social determinants of health?

Examine Feelings, Beliefs, and Values

Written assignments help learners examine feelings generated from caring for patients and reflect on their beliefs and values that might influence that care. Journals, for instance, provide a way for students to record their feelings about a patient or clinical activity and later reflect on these feelings. Assignments may be developed for students to identify their own beliefs and values and analyze how they affect their interactions with patients, families, and staff. Value-based statements may be given to students for written critique, or students may be asked to analyze an ethical issue, propose alternative courses of actions, and take a stand on the issue.

Examples of writing assignments that help students explore their feelings, beliefs, and values are:

■ Identify an issue that affects healthcare. Read about the issue and write an op-ed (opinion piece) that describes how you would address the issue.
■ In your journal, write about your feelings about caring for your patient and other patients in this setting. In what way do those feelings influence your care?
■ A peer tells you they forgot to re-order a patient's PRN (pro re nata, as needed) medications but is not telling the nurse practitioner who is serving as the preceptor. The patient never asked about these medications. What would you say to this individual? Why did you choose this approach?
■ Think about the community in which your patients live. How does that community influence their health?

Develop Writing Skills

An important outcome of writing assignments is the development of skill in communicating ideas in written form. Assignments help students learn how to organize thoughts and present them clearly. This clarity in writing develops through planned writing activities integrated in the nursing program. As a skill, writing ability requires practice, and students need to complete writing assignments across clinical courses. All too often, writing assignments are not sequenced progressively across courses or levels in the program; students, then, do not have the benefit of building writing skills sequentially.

A benefit of this planned approach to teaching writing is faculty feedback, provided through drafts and rewrites of papers. Drafts are essential to foster development of writing skill. Drafts should be critiqued by faculty members for accuracy of content, development of ideas, organization, clarity of expression, and writing skills such as sentence structure, punctuation, and spelling (Oermann & Hays, 2019).

Small group critique of each other's writing is appropriate particularly for formative purposes. Small group critique provides a basis for subsequent revisions and gives feedback to students about both content and writing style. Although students may not identify every error in sentence structure and punctuation, they can provide valuable feedback on content, organization, how the ideas are developed, and clarity of writing. Peer review should be used for giving feedback only, not for determining a grade for the assignment.

Types of Writing Assignments for Clinical Learning

Many types of writing assignments are appropriate for enhancing clinical learning. Some assignments help students learn the content they are writing about but do not necessarily improve writing skill, and other assignments also promote competency in writing. For example, structured assignments such as care plans provide minimal opportunity for freedom of expression, originality, and creativity. Other assignments, though, such as term papers on clinical topics, promote understanding of new content and its use in clinical practice as well as writing ability. Types of written assignments for clinical learning include concept map, short written assignments, nursing care plan, analysis of cases, EBP papers, teaching plan, reflective journal, group writing, and electronic portfolio.

CONCEPT MAP

A concept map is a graphic or pictorial arrangement of key concepts related to a patient's care, which shows the interrelationships of those concepts. By developing a concept map, students can visualize how assessment data, problems, interventions, medications, and other aspects of a patient's care relate to one another.

Concept maps have many uses in clinical learning. First, students may complete a concept map from their readings to assist them in applying new information to their patients. The readings that students complete for clinical practice, and in nursing courses overall, contain vast amounts of facts and specific information. Concept maps help students process this information in a meaningful way, linking new, and existing ideas.

Second, concept maps are useful in helping students prepare for clinical practice. They can be developed prior to or at the beginning of a clinical experience as a way of organizing assessment information, relating it to the patient's needs and problems, and planning nursing care. In preclinical conferences, students can present the maps for feedback from the teacher and from peers. Students can modify the maps as they provide care for patients.

Third, concept maps may be developed collaboratively by students in clinical conferences. For this purpose, students may present a patient for whom they have provided care, and the clinical group then develops a concept map about that patient's care, or the clinical group may develop a concept map about conditions they are learning about in the course. As another strategy, students can present the concept maps they developed for their patients, and the group can analyze and discuss them. Critiquing each other's concept maps enhances students' thinking, learning from one another, and group process; it also allows for feedback from the teacher and peers.

SHORT WRITTEN ASSIGNMENTS

Short written assignments in clinical courses are valuable for promoting higher level thinking and helping students apply what they are learning in class to clinical practice. Short assignments avoid students' reporting on and summarizing what others have written without thinking critically about the content themselves. With a short assignment, students can analyze patient problems, compare interventions with their evidence, explore decisions that might be made in a clinical situation, analyze an issue and approaches, and analyze a case scenario. Sample assignments are found in Exhibit 7.5.

NURSING CARE PLAN

Nursing care plans enable students to analyze patients' health problems and design plans of care. With care plans, students can record assessment data, identify patient needs and problems, select evidence-based interventions, and identify outcomes to be measured. Care plans should be usable—they should guide students' planning of their patients' care and be realistic.

EXHIBIT 7.5 Examples of Short Written Assignments for Clinical Courses

The unit clerk is slow about notifying nursing staff when patients use their call bells. It appears that only the assigned staff will answer the call bells; other nurses and staff who happen to be close by the patient's room will not respond. Develop a quality improvement project to address this issue.

Select an intervention or treatment you used in patient care. Search for evidence related to that intervention or treatment. What were your sources of evidence? Summarize the strength of the evidence and discuss what it means for patient care.

Read the article on loneliness. In no more than one page, explain how you would use that concept in an assessment.

Describe patient-centered care and key attributes.

In the handoff, the nurse reports that your patient "had no pain and walked twice around the room." When you assess the patient, he complains of severe pain and says he has not been out of bed for 24 hours. What are two different ways of approaching this situation? What would you do next and why?

The nurse practitioner who is serving as your preceptor makes a decision to admit a patient with heart failure. The patient is agitated, is short of breath, and has swelling of his ankles and legs. What additional data would you collect? Explain why this information is important and would support readmission.

Identify a decision you made in clinical practice involving either patients or staff. Describe the situation and why you responded that way. Propose another approach that could have been used.

Describe the process on your unit for handoff at the end of the shift. What changes would you propose in that process and why?

Completing a written care plan may help the student identify nursing and other interventions for specific problems, but whether that same care plan promotes problem-solving learning and higher level thinking is questionable. Often students develop care plans from their textbook or the literature without thinking about the content. Even if the care plan is an appropriate written assignment for the outcomes, the question remains as to how many care plans students need to complete in a clinical course to meet the outcomes. Once these have been achieved, then other written assignments may be more effective for clinical learning.

EVIDENCE-BASED PRACTICE PAPERS

Assignments in clinical courses can guide students' learning about EBP and its use in patient care. Clinical assignments that are integrated in courses throughout the nursing program prepare students with the skills they need to search for and use evidence in their future practice. Through these assignments, students can learn the steps of the EBP process, beginning with recognizing the need for evidence to guide decisions and writing a clinical question, through evaluating the outcomes of practice decisions and disseminating evidence (Melnyk & Fineout-Overholt, 2019). These steps can be used as a framework for planning learning activities for students and assignments in clinical courses. By using a framework such as this one or another EBP model, teachers can plan assignments for each clinical course in the curriculum, systematically developing students' understanding and skills and avoiding repetition of assignments. Exhibit 7.6 provides sample clinical assignments for learning about EBP and steps in the process.

EXHIBIT 7.6 Sample Clinical Assignments for Learning About Evidence-Based Practice

---

DEVELOP QUESTIONS ABOUT CLINICAL PRACTICE

1. Write a clinical question using patient, intervention, comparison, outcome, and time (PICOT) format.
2. Think about a patient for whom you cared this week. Identify a question you had about that patient's care and write the question in PICOT format. List two sources of information you could consult to answer that question with a rationale for why these are appropriate. Discuss your question with a peer during postclinical conference. Is your question specific enough to guide a search? If not, revise it.
3. Identify a change in practice needed on your unit. Why is it needed? What led you to this decision? Write a short paper (no more than one page).

Search for Evidence

1. Conduct a search using your PICOT question. Identify key words or terms to search for an answer. Go to the Cumulative Index to Nursing and Allied Health Literature (CINAHL) and modify your key words as needed. Complete the search in CINAHL, mapping out your search strategy. Summarize your findings. What would you do differently with this search the next time? Write a two- to three-page paper on this search and what you found.
2. Conduct the same search in PubMed (MEDLINE). What are the differences, if any, in the results of your search? What did you learn about these two databases? Present in clinical conference.

(continued)

EXHIBIT 7.6 Sample Clinical Assignments for Learning About Evidence-Based Practice (*continued*)

3. Conduct another search using your PICOT question. What evidence did you find related to your PICOT question?

Critically Appraise the Evidence

1. Identify a PICOT question or a change in practice that might be indicated. Search for evidence and record your search strategy and results. What studies are relevant for inclusion in your review and why? Critique the evidence (consider validity, relevance, and applicability). Summarize your findings and develop a written proposal for use of this evidence to guide practice or why a practice change is not indicated.
2. Discuss how you can use the Cochrane Database of Systematic Reviews (www.cochranelibrary. com/cdsr/about-cdsr) in your patient care. Select a nursing intervention and locate information about this intervention in Cochrane. Write a three- to four-page report on your findings.
3. Select one of your PICOT questions and searches. Critique the evidence you found in that search. Use an established evidence hierarchy and rate the strength of the evidence. Discuss the implications of the evidence for nursing practice.

Use the Evidence in Clinical Practice

1. How do the nurse's clinical expertise and the patient's preferences and values interface with evidence-based practice? Should the evidence be weighed more heavily in decisions than patient preferences? Lead a discussion on this topic in the discussion forum.
2. List interventions for one of your patients. What is the evidence base for each of these? Provide a rationale for their use based on the strength of the evidence. Include the sources of information you used to determine the evidence base. What evidence is missing, and what do you propose?
3. Review your patient's care. Select one problem not adequately met with current practices. Search for evidence to suggest a change in practice, evaluate the evidence, and write a paper about how you would change practice based on your review. What would you do differently the next time you care for that patient or patients with similar problems?
4. Select an intervention and find evidence using resources from the Joanna Briggs Institute or similar resource. Describe the evidence you located. Did it help you make a decision about the effectiveness of the intervention? Why or why not? How would you use this information in your clinical practice? Prepare a short paper.

Evaluate Outcomes of Practice Decisions

1. For a practice change or evidence-based intervention you proposed in an earlier assignment, plan how you would evaluate its effect on patient outcomes. Present in online discussion.
2. Implement an evidence-based intervention in patient care and evaluate its outcomes. Write a short (no more than two pages) report on your findings.

REFLECTIVE JOURNALS

Journal writing assists students in relating theory to clinical practice, linking their classroom and online instruction to care of patients, and reflecting on their clinical learning activities. When students re-examine their clinical decisions and propose alternative actions, journaling also encourages the development of higher level thinking skills and clinical judgment. Reflective journals are particularly valuable for students to examine their own values that can affect patient care and interactions with others and reflect on their experiences in clinical practice.

There are different ways of structuring journals, and the decision should be based on the intended outcomes of using the journal in the clinical practicum. The first step for the teacher is to identify the learning outcomes to be met through journal writing, such as reflecting on clinical decisions or describing feelings in caring for a patient, and then how journal entries should be made. Journals are not intended for grading but provide an opportunity for giving feedback to learners and developing a dialogue with them.

GROUP WRITING

Not all writing assignments need to be done by students individually. There is much to be gained with group writing exercises as long as the groups are small, and the exercises are carefully focused. Short written assignments may be completed in clinical conferences or done online in small groups. These group assignments provide opportunities for students to express their ideas to others in the group and work collaboratively to communicate the results of their thinking as a group in written form. Strategies for grading group writing assignments are discussed in Chapter 12.

ELECTRONIC PORTFOLIO

An electronic portfolio (e-portfolio) provides an opportunity for students to present projects and other materials they developed in their clinical practicum to document the competencies they achieved (Oermann & Gaberson, 2021). Portfolios can represent a student's best work for evaluation or can illustrate the growth and development of competencies over a period of time. These can be prepared using commercially available software, or students can upload their e-portfolios in the course management system or at a website for this purpose.

The content of the e-portfolio depends on its purpose. Examples of these materials include documents that students developed for patient care, papers written about clinical practice, selected journal entries, reports of activities in the clinical setting, group work and products, reflections of experiences, self-assessment, and other products (referred to as artifacts) that demonstrate students' clinical competencies and what they learned in the course. Planning for this type of assignment as part of the evaluation is described in Chapter 12.

SUMMARY

The chapter provided a framework for planning clinical assignments for learners. Clinical teachers should select assignments that are related to the competencies or desired learning outcomes, appropriate to students' levels of knowledge and skill, and challenging enough to motivate learning. Providing comprehensive nursing care to one or more patients is a typical clinical assignment, but it is not always the most appropriate choice. There are different options for clinical assignments (skill versus total care focus, student–patient ratio options, management activities, guided observation, and service learning), which were presented in the chapter.

The chapter also described and provided examples of other clinical teaching methods—discussions, clinical conferences, and written assignments. Discussions are an exchange of ideas in a small group format. Discussions promote several types of learning: developing higher level thinking skills; debriefing clinical experiences; assessing own learning; and developing oral communication skills. Clinical conferences are discussions in which students analyze patient care and clinical situations, lead others in discussions about clinical practice, present ideas in a group format, and give presentations to the group. Conferences serve the same goals as any discussion.

Written assignments for clinical learning have four main purposes: to learn about concepts, theories, and other content related to clinical practice; develop thinking skills; examine values and beliefs that may affect patient care; and develop writing skills. Not all writing assignments achieve each of these outcomes. The teacher decides first on the outcomes to be met, then plans the writing assignment with these outcomes in mind. Many types of written assignments can be used for clinical learning. Concept map, short written assignment, nursing care plan, EBP papers, reflective journals, group writing, and e-portfolio were presented in this chapter.

CNE® EXAMINATION TEST BLUEPRINT CORE COMPETENCIES

1. **Facilitate Learning**
   A. Implement a variety of teaching strategies appropriate to:
      1. content
      2. setting (i.e., clinical vs. classroom)
      3. learner needs
      4. learning style
      5. desired learner outcomes
   E. Practice skilled oral and written (including electronic) communication that reflects an awareness of self and relationships with learners (e.g., evaluation, mentorship, and supervision)
   F. Communicates effectively orally and in writing with an ability to convey ideas in a variety of contexts
   H. Create opportunities for learners to develop their own critical thinking skills
   I. Create a positive learning environment that fosters a free exchange of ideas
   M. Develop collegial working relationships with clinical agency personnel to promote positive learning environments
   P. Act as a role model in practice settings
2. **Facilitate Learner Development and Socialization**
   B. Provide resources for diverse learners to meet their individual learning needs
   D. Create learning environments that facilitate learners' self-reflection, personal goal setting, and socialization to the role of the nurse
   E. Foster the development of learners in these areas
      1. cognitive domain
      2. psychomotor domain
      3. affective domain
   G. Encourage professional development of learners
3. **Use Assessment and Evaluation Strategies**
   L. Provide timely, constructive, and thoughtful feedback to learners
4. **Participate in Curriculum Design and Evaluation of Program Outcomes**
   H. Collaborate with community and clinical partners to support educational goals

CNE®cl EXAMINATION TEST BLUEPRINT CORE COMPETENCIES

1. **Function within the Education and Health Care Environments**
   A. Function in the Clinical Educator Role
      1. Bridge the gap between theory and practice by helping learners to apply classroom learning to the clinical setting
      4. Value the contributions of others in the achievement of learner outcomes (e.g., health team, families, social networks)
      5. Act as a role model of professional nursing within the clinical learning environment
   B. Operationalize the Curriculum
      2. Plan meaningful and relevant clinical learning assignments and activities
      3. Identify learners' goals and outcomes
      5. Structure learner experiences within the learning environment to promote optimal learning
      7. Provide opportunities for learners to develop problem-solving and clinical reasoning skills related to course objectives (e.g., learning outcomes)
   C. Abide by Legal Requirements, Ethical Guidelines, Agency Policies, and Guiding Framework
      2. Assess learner abilities and needs prior to clinical learning experiences
      5. Adhere to program and clinical agency policies, procedures and practices when implementing clinical experiences
      7. Demonstrate ethical behaviors
2. **Facilitate Learning in the Health Care Environment**
   A. Implement a variety of clinical teaching strategies appropriate to learner needs, desired learner outcomes, content, and context
   B. Ground teaching strategies in educational theory and evidence-based teaching practices
   C. Use technology (e.g., simulation, learning management systems, electronic health records) skillfully to support the teaching-learning process
   D. Create opportunities for learners to develop critical thinking and clinical reasoning skills
   H. Demonstrate enthusiasm for teaching, learning, and nursing to help inspire and motivate learners
4. **Apply Clinical Expertise in the Health Care Environment**
   G. Balance client care needs and student learning needs within a culture of safety

REFERENCES

Baker, H., Pfeiffer, K., Field, M., Nasatir-Hilty, S., Doiev, J., Worland, B. J., Clark-Youngblood, M., Harrell, K., & Mascorro, A. (2021). A substance use disorder service-learning immersion experience for prelicensure nursing students. *Nurse Educator, 46*(5), 273-275. https://doi.org/10.1097/nne.0000000000000952

Beauvais, A., Foito, K., Pearlin, N., & Yose, E. (2015). Service learning with a geriatric population: Changing attitudes and improving knowledge. *Nurse Educator, 40*(6), 318–321. https://doi.org/10.1097/NNE.0000000000000181

Berkstresser, K. (2016). The use of online discussions for post-clinical conference. *Nurse Education in Practice, 16*(1), 27–32. https://doi.org/10.1016/j.nepr.2015.06.007

Billings, D. M. (2019). Teaching nurses to make clinical judgments that ensure patient safety. *Journal of Continuing Education in Nursing, 50*(7), 300–302. https://doi.org/10.3928/00220124-20190612-04

Decker, K., Hensel, D., & Fasone, L. (2016). Outcomes of a bystander intervention community health service-learning project. *Nurse Educator*, *41*(3), 147–150. https://doi.org/10.1097/NNE.0000000000000232

George, T. P., Munn, A. C., & Phillips, T. A. (2021). The use of debates in an online nursing course. *Nurse Educator*, *46*(4), E60–E63. https://doi.org/10.1097/nne.0000000000000922

Gresh, A., LaFave, S., Thamilselvan, V., Batchelder, A., Mermer, J., Jacques, K., Greensfelder, A., Buckley, M., Cohen, Z., Coy, A., & Warren, N. (2021). Service learning in public health nursing education: How COVID-19 accelerated community-academic partnership. *Public Health Nursing*, *38*(2), 248–257. https://doi.org/10.1111/phn.12796

Hannans, J. (2019). Online clinical post conference: Strategies for meaningful discussion using VoiceThread. *Nurse Educator*, *44*(1), 29–33. https://doi.org/10.1097/nne.0000000000000529

Hensel, D., & Billings, D. M. (2020). Strategies to teach the National Council of State Boards of Nursing clinical judgment model. *Nurse Educator*, *45*(3), 128–132. https://doi.org/10.1097/nne.0000000000000773

Melnyk, B. M., & Fineout-Overholt, E. (Eds.). (2019). *Evidence-based practice in nursing and healthcare: A guide to best practice* (4th ed.). Wolters Kluwer.

Nielsen, A., Lanciotti, K., Garner, A., & Brown, L. (2020). Concept-based learning for capstone clinical experiences in hospital and community settings. *Nurse Educator*. Online ahead of print. https://doi.org/10.1097/nne.0000000000000964

Oermann, M. H., & Hays, J. (2019). *Writing for publication in nursing* (4th ed.). Springer Publishing Company.

Taylor, S. L., & Leffers, J. M. (2016). Integrative review of service-learning assessment in nursing education. *Nursing Education Perspectives*, *37*(4), 194–200. https://doi.org/10.1097/01.NEP.0000000000000022

Thompson, L. M., Jarvis, S., Sparacino, P., Kuo, D., & Genz, S. (2013). Perceptions of health equity and subjective social status among baccalaureate nursing students engaged in service-learning activities in Hawai'i. *Hawaii J Med Public Health*, *72*(10), 339–345.

Velez, R., & Koo, L. W. (2020). International service learning enhances nurse practitioner students' practice and cultural humility. *Journal of the American Association of Nurse Practitioners*, *32*(3), 187–189. https://doi.org/10.1097/jxx.0000000000000404

Vihos, J., Pollard, L., Bazin, M., Lozza, D., MacDonald, P., Moniz, N., & Spies, D. (2017). Debriefing in laboratory experiences: A quality improvement project. *Nurse Educator*, *42*(6), 316–319. https://doi.org/10.1097/nne.0000000000000367

A robust set of instructor resources designed to supplement this text is located at http://connect.springerpub.com/content/book/978-0-8261-6705-7. Qualifying instructors may request access by emailing textbook@springerpub.com.

Cases for Clinical Learning

Clinical practice provides opportunities for students to gain the knowledge and skills needed to care for patients; develop values important in professional practice; and develop higher level thinking and clinical judgment skills. Ability to apply concepts to clinical situations, solve problems, arrive at carefully thought out decisions, and provide safe, quality care are essential competencies gained through clinical practice. Case method, case study, and unfolding cases are teaching methods that help students meet these learning outcomes. Case method and case study describe a clinical situation developed around an actual or a hypothetical patient for student analysis. In case method, the case provided for analysis is generally shorter and more specific than in a case study. Case studies are more comprehensive in nature, thereby presenting a complete picture of the patient and clinical situation. With unfolding cases, the scenario changes, presenting new data to students for analysis and integration with prior information about the case. Unfolding cases promote students' thinking and clinical reasoning skills. This chapter describes the development and use of cases as a teaching method with examples.

CASES FOR DEVELOPING COGNITIVE SKILLS

With cases, students can apply concepts and theories to clinical situations, identify patient and other types of problems, propose varied approaches for solving them, weigh them against the evidence, and choose the most appropriate approaches. These methods provide experience for students in analyzing clinical situations and thinking through possible decisions.

Problem Solving

Problem solving is the ability to solve clinical problems, some relating to the patient and others that arise from clinical practice. Problem solving begins with recognizing and defining the problem, gathering data to clarify it further, identifying possible approaches, weighing them against evidence, and choosing the best one considering patient needs and responses (Oermann & Gaberson, 2021). The student does not need to provide hands-on care to develop problem-solving skills. By observing and discussing patients with the clinical nurse educator or preceptor, and by analyzing cases, students can gain experience in thinking through possible problems suggested by the data and arriving at a decision about the most likely problem. This same type of thinking can be done on possible approaches to use. Cases also expose students to clinical situations that they may not encounter in their own clinical practice.

Critical Thinking

Critical thinking enables the nurse to make reasoned and informed judgments in the practice setting and decide what to do in a given situation. There are varied definitions of critical thinking. A key idea across many of these definitions is that critical thinking is a process of analyzing one's own thinking with the goal of improving it. Critical thinking has two components: (a) ability, which includes possessing and using higher level thinking skills such as comprehending, applying, analyzing, evaluating, and synthesizing information, and (b) having the habit or disposition to engage in this type of thinking (Foundation for Critical Thinking, 2019).

Critical thinking can also be viewed as reflective thinking about patient problems when the problem is not obvious, or the nurse knows what is wrong but is unsure what to do. Through critical thinking, the learner considers multiple perspectives to care, weighs possible approaches considering the evidence, and makes a careful and well-thought-out decision about what to do in the situation. With cases, students can practice these skills: They can generate possible alternatives, weigh them using evidence, consider the consequences of each, then arrive at a decision following this analysis. To develop these skills, higher level questions, discussed in Chapter 7, need to be included with these cases. Noone and Seery (2018) suggested that clinically based scenarios with questioning by the educator challenge nursing students and contribute to their critical thinking development. It is important, though, for the nurse educator to first assess if students have the needed knowledge base for critical thinking. Students need to understand the patient situation and have the related knowledge to engage in critical thinking (Von Colln-Appling & Giuliano, 2017).

Clinical Judgment

Early on Tanner (2006) developed a model of clinical judgment in nursing that incorporates concepts of problem solving, decision making, and critical thinking. In this model, clinical judgment involves interpreting a patient's needs and problems and deciding on actions and approaches, taking the patient's responses into consideration. The clinical judgment process includes four aspects: (a) noticing, grasping the situation; (b) interpreting, understanding the situation in order to respond; (c) responding, deciding on actions that are appropriate or that no actions are needed; and (d) reflecting, being attentive to how patients respond to the nurse's actions.

Currently, other frameworks of clinical judgment have been developed. The National Council of State Boards of Nursing (2019) defined clinical judgment as the "observed outcome of critical thinking and decision making" (p. 1). With this process the nurse assesses patients and clinical situations, identifies patient problems and concerns, prioritizes them, considers and implements evidence-based interventions, and evaluates outcomes. The ability to apply clinical judgment is essential to provide safe and effective nursing care to achieve patient outcomes (Sommer et al., 2021).

CASE METHOD AND STUDY

Case method and case study serve similar purposes in clinical teaching: They provide a simulated scenario for student review and critique. In case method, the case provided for analysis is generally shorter and more specific than in case study.

Case Method

In case method, short cases are developed around actual or hypothetical patients followed by higher level questions to encourage students' thinking about the case. Short cases are used to avoid directing students' thinking in advance. Depending on how the case is written, case method is effective for applying concepts and other types of knowledge to clinical practice and for promoting development of cognitive skills. With cases, students can analyze patient data, identify needs and problems, and decide on the best approaches in that situation after weighing the evidence. Cases also assist students in relating course content to clinical practice and integrating different concepts and content areas in a particular clinical situation. Examples of case method are presented in Exhibit 8.1.

EXHIBIT 8.1 Examples of Case Method

Your patient has moderate dementia. She lets the nurse practitioner do a pelvic examination because she has a "woman's problem." The examination shows an anterior wall prolapse. While helping the patient get dressed, the nurse practitioner observes that, as soon as the patient stands up, urine begins leaking onto the floor.
1. List and prioritize this patient's problems. Provide a rationale for how the problems are prioritized.
2. Develop a plan of care.

Your patient is admitted from the ED with severe headache, right-sided weakness, and aphasia. His temperature is normal, pulse 120, respirations 16, and blood pressure 180/120.
1. What are possible reasons for these symptoms? Provide an explanation for your answer.
2. What additional data would you collect on admission to your unit? Why is this information important to planning the patient's care?
3. In postclinical conference, as a group develop this case further. Based on the data you added to the case, what information would you include in a report on this patient to the incoming nurse using SBAR (situation, background, assessment, recommendation)?

Your patient is seen for a prenatal check-up. She is in her 24th week of pregnancy. The nurse practitioner notes swelling of the ankles and around the patient's eyes. The patient says she has not been able to wear rings for a week because of swelling. Her blood pressure is 144/96.
1. What are possible problems that might be going on for this patient? List all problems given the information in the scenario.
2. What additional data should be collected at this time? Why?

You are working in a pediatrician's office. A patient brings in her son for a check-up after a severe asthma attack a month ago that required emergency care. When you ask the mother how her son is doing, she begins to cry softly. She tells you she is worried about his having another asthma attack and this time not recovering from it. When the pediatrician enters the examination room, the mother is still crying. The physician says, "What's wrong? Look at him. He's doing great. There is no reason to worry."
1. What would you say to the mother, if anything, in this situation?
2. What would you say to the pediatrician, if anything?
3. Analyze this case in the context of patient-centered case.

As you record a patient's vital signs in the electronic medical record, the patient asks you to show the computer screen to her husband so he can read about the diagnoses they are ruling out.
1. What would you say to this patient?
2. What principles guide your decision? Provide a rationale for your response.

(continued)

EXHIBIT 8.1 Examples of Case Method (*continued*)

You have a new patient, 81 years old, with heart failure. The referral to your home health agency indicates that the patient has difficulty breathing, tires easily, and has edema in both legs, making it difficult for him to get around. He lives alone.

1. What are problems you anticipate for the patient? Include a rationale for each of these problems.

At your first home visit, you find him sitting in a chair with his feet on the floor. During your assessment, he gets short of breath talking with you and has to stop periodically to catch his breath.

1. Describe at least three different nursing interventions that could be used in this patient's care.
2. Specify outcome criteria for evaluating the effectiveness of the interventions you selected.
3. What would you teach the patient? How could you use the teach-back method in this situation?
4. Select one of your interventions and review the evidence on its use. What are your conclusions about the effectiveness of the intervention?
5. Identify one published research study that relates to this patient's care. Critique the study and describe whether you could use the findings in caring for him and patients with similar problems.

A grandmother brings her 8-year-old granddaughter to the office for her annual visit. In reviewing the immunization record, the nurse notices that the child never received the second dose of the measles, mumps, rubella (MMR) vaccine. The nurse tells the grandmother not to worry: her granddaughter can get the second dose when she is 11 or 12 years old.

1. Do you agree or disagree with the nurse's advice? Provide a rationale for your decision.

Read the following statements: One in three adults and one in five adolescents are overweight. Being overweight is prevalent among certain ethnic groups.

1. What additional information do you need before identifying the implications of this statement for your community?
2. Why is this information important?

The heart failure clinic at your hospital has been effective in reducing the number of readmissions, but to save costs the hospital is closing it. As the nurse practitioner in that clinic, write a report about why the clinic should remain open, with data to support your position. To whom would you send that report and why? Then write a report from the perspective of the hospital administration supporting closure of the clinic.

Case Study

A case study provides an actual or hypothetical patient situation for students to analyze and arrive at varied decisions. Case studies typically are longer and more comprehensive than in case method, providing background data about the patient, family history, and other information for a more complete picture. For this reason, students can analyze case studies in greater depth than with case method and present a more detailed rationale for their analysis. In their critique of the case study, students can describe the concepts that guided their analysis, how they used them in understanding the case, and the literature they reviewed. An example of a case study is presented in Exhibit 8.2.

EXHIBIT 8.2 Example of a Case Study

Your 44-year-old patient is seen in the physician's office with hoarseness and a slight cough. During the assessment, she tells the nurse that she also has shortness of breath, particularly when walking fast and going up the stairs. She has never smoked. Her vital signs are: blood pressure 120/80; heart rate 88 beats per minute; respirations 32 per minute; and temperature 36.6°C (97.8°F).

The patient is married with two teenage daughters. She works part-time as a substitute teacher. She has always been health conscious, watching her weight and eating properly. She tells the nurse how worried she is because she has read about women getting lung cancer even if they never smoked.

1. The physician orders a combined PET/CT scan. What is a PET/CT scan, and why was it ordered?
2. What would you teach the patient about the scan so she understands why it was ordered?
3. Identify a potential diagnosis and add data to the case consistent with that diagnosis. What types of problems would you anticipate for her? Describe nursing management for each of those problems.
4. Add data about the patient and her family to the case. Select a family theory and use it to analyze this family. What did you learn about the family, and how will this influence your care?

Using Cases in Clinical Courses

Short cases and longer case studies can be integrated in clinical courses throughout the curriculum to assist students in applying concepts and knowledge they are learning in their courses to clinical situations of increasing complexity. In beginning courses, teachers can develop cases that present problems that are relatively easy to identify and require standard nursing interventions. At this level, students learn how to apply concepts to clinical situations and think through them. Students can work as a group to analyze cases; explore different perspectives of the case, what students noticed about it, and their interpretations; and discuss possible approaches to use.

In the beginning, the teacher should think aloud, guiding students through the analysis, pointing out significant aspects of the case and their own expectations and interpretations. By thinking aloud, the teacher can model the clinical judgment process step by step through a case. As students progress through the curriculum, the cases can become more complex with varied problems and approaches that could be used in the situation.

Students can analyze cases in a postclinical conference, as an independent activity, or online either individually or in small groups. They can share resources they used to better understand the case. If cases are analyzed individually, further discussion about the case can occur with the clinical group as a whole, or students can post their thoughts and responses online for others to reflect and comment on.

Based on the questions asked about the case, cases can be used to meet many different learning outcomes of a clinical course. For example, if the goal of the case is to guide students in interpreting data, then questions might ask students to identify significant information in the situation and explain what the data mean. Cases are effective as an instructional method, but they also can be graded similar to essay items.

Complexity of Cases for Review

Cases may be of varying levels of complexity. Some cases are designed with the problems readily apparent. With these cases, the problem is described clearly, and sufficient information is included to guide decisions on how to intervene. Brookhart and Nitko (2019) called these cases well structured: They provide an opportunity for students to apply knowledge to a clinical situation and develop an understanding of how it is used in practice. Cases of this type link knowledge presented in class, online, and through readings to practice situations. With well-structured cases, there is usually one correct answer that students can identify based on what they are currently learning in the clinical course or learned in previous courses and experiences.

Well-structured cases are effective for students beginning a clinical course in which they have limited background and experience. These cases give students an opportunity to practice their thinking before caring for an actual patient.

Most patient care situations, however, are not that easily solved. In clinical practice, the problems are sometimes difficult to identify, or the nurse may be confident about the patient's problem but unsure how to intervene. These are problems in Schön's (1990) swampy lowland—ones that do not lend themselves to resolution by a technical and rational approach. These are cases that vary from the way the problems and solutions were presented in class and through readings. For such cases, the principles learned in class may not readily apply, and clinical judgment is required for analysis and resolution.

Brookhart and Nitko (2019) referred to these cases as ill structured, describing problems that reflect real-life clinical situations faced by students. With ill-structured cases, different problems may be possible; there may be an incomplete data set to interpret; or the need and problem may be clear, but multiple approaches may be possible. Exhibit 8.3 presents examples of a well-structured and an ill-structured case.

EXHIBIT 8.3 Well-Structured and Ill-Structured Cases

Well-Structured case

Your patient reports having bad headaches for the last month. The headaches occur about twice weekly usually in the late morning. Initially, the pain began as a throbbing at her right temple. Her headaches now affect either her right or left eye and temple. The pain is so severe that she usually goes to bed. She also describes pain in her neck, and you note tenderness in the posterior neck on palpation.

1. What type or types of headache might this patient be experiencing?
2. Describe additional data that should be collected. Why is this information important to deciding what is wrong with this patient?
3. Select two interventions that might be used. Provide evidence for their use.

Ill-Structured Case

A 55-year-old patient calls for an appointment because he fell yesterday at home. He has a few bruises from his fall and a tingling feeling in his legs. He had been at the eye doctor's office last week because of double vision.

1. What do you think about this patient?
2. What are possible problems this patient might be experiencing?
3. Plan additional data to collect to better understand those problems and explain why that information is important.

Developing Cases

Case method and study have two components: a case description and questions to answer about the case or its analysis. In case method, the situations described are typically short and geared to specific outcomes to be met. Case studies include background information about the patient, family history, and complete assessment data to provide a comprehensive description of the patient or clinical situation.

The case should provide enough information for analysis without directing the students' thinking in a particular direction. The case may be developed first, then the questions, or the teacher may draft the questions first, then develop the case to present the clinical situation. Once students have experience in analyzing cases, another strategy is for students to develop a case scenario based on data provided by the teacher. In this method, students need to think about what patient needs and problems might fit the data, which promotes their thinking.

The questions developed for the case are the key to its effective use. The questions should be geared to the outcomes to be met. For instance, if the intent of the case is for students to analyze laboratory data, apply physiological principles, and use concepts of pathophysiology for the analysis, then the questions need to relate to each of these. Similarly, if the goal is to improve skill in responding to clinical situations, then the questions should ask about possible actions to take for the situation, including no immediate intervention, and evidence to consider in deciding on actions. With most cases, questions should be included that focus on the underlying thought process used to arrive at an answer rather than the answer alone.

GEAR CASE TO PROBLEM SOLVING

Cases can be written for the development of specific cognitive skills. In designing cases to promote problem solving, the teacher should develop a case that asks students to:

- Identify patient and other problems apparent or expected in the case.
- Suggest alternative problems that might be possible if more information were available and identify the information needed.
- Identify relevant and irrelevant information in the case.
- Interpret the information to enable a response.
- Propose different approaches that might be used.
- Weigh approaches against the evidence.
- Select the best approaches for the case situation with a rationale.
- Evaluate the effectiveness of interventions.
- Plan alternative interventions based on analysis of the case.

An example of a case for problem solving is:

A 56-year-old patient with shortness of breath, chest pain, and a dry cough is seen in the clinic. His blood pressure is 144/96.

1. List all possible problems that might be occurring with this patient.
2. What additional data should be collected at this time? Why?

3. Add new information to the scenario and explain how this new information confirms or rules out each of the problems identified earlier.
4. Record your answers and share with a peer for critique.

GEAR CASE TO CRITICAL THINKING

Cases also meet critical thinking outcomes. There are a number of strategies that teachers can use when developing cases that are intended for critical thinking. These are listed in Table 8.1.

An example of a case for critical thinking is:

You are a nurse practitioner (NP) working in a Federally Qualified Health Center. A teenager comes to the Center complaining of nausea and vomiting and feeling bloated. She thinks she might be pregnant and does not want her mother to know.

1. What additional information do you need to make a decision about what to do next?
2. Add that information to the scenario. Considering the original scenario and the new data you added, what are your options at this time?
3. What option would you choose to implement? Why?
4. Choose another option that you listed for question 2. What are the advantages and disadvantages of that approach over your first choice?

TABLE 8.1   STRATEGIES FOR DEVELOPING CASES FOR CRITICAL THINKING

Develop	Ask students to
Present an issue for analysis, a question to be answered that has multiple possibilities, or a complex problem to be solved.	Analyze the case and provide a rationale for the thinking process they used for the analysis. Examine the assumptions underlying their thinking. Describe the evidence on which their reasoning was based. Describe the concepts and theories they used for their analysis and *how* they applied to the case.
Have different and conflicting points of view.	Analyze the case from their own points of view and then analyze the case from a different point of view.
Present complex data for analysis.	Analyze the data and draw possible inferences given the data. Specify additional information needed and why it is important.
Present clinical situations that are unique and offer different perspectives.	Analyze the clinical situation, identify multiple perspectives possible, and examine assumptions made about the situation that influenced thinking.
Describe ethical issues and dilemmas.	Propose alternative approaches and consequences. Weigh alternatives and arrive at a decision. Critique an issue from a different point of view.

GEAR CASE TO CLINICAL JUDGMENT

Cases can also be written with the intent to promote clinical judgment skills. The prompts to teach clinical judgment provided in Table 7.1 can be used when writing questions for these cases. To gear cases to clinical judgment, they should ask students to:

- Recognize Cues in the Scenario: Identify cues, findings that are most significant, additional data to collect, and what information to collect first.
- Analyze Cues: Interpret the meaning of the cues, explain findings expected based on the patient's diagnosis or concern, and identify other information to gather to help determine the significance of the cues.
- Identify Possible Problems/Generate Hypotheses: Explain the patient's condition, identify all possible problems, and decide on the priority problem.
- Identify Interventions and Solutions: Identify possible interventions with evidence to support them, a rationale for taking no action, and how interventions promote intended outcomes.
- Implement Interventions and Actions: Identify the most appropriate interventions, actions to be taken immediately and why, and information to report immediately to others and why.
- Evaluate Outcomes: Explain findings to monitor to determine if the patient is improving; assess if the patient is improving and why or why not; and determine if interventions are effective and, if not, what other interventions and approaches should be considered.

An example of a case for clinical judgment is:

You make a home visit to an 86-year-old patient who lives alone and is having problems concentrating, loss of memory, crying spells, and fatigue. You recommend a follow-up visit with the primary care physician. The patient is diagnosed with depression and treated with a selective serotonin reuptake inhibitor. Two weeks later, you visit the patient and learn she still has fatigue and now also has loss of appetite and difficulty sleeping.

1. What do you notice in this situation?
2. What patient problems, conditions, or diagnoses are consistent with these findings?
3. What additional information would you collect and why?
4. Discuss the case with a peer and compare interpretations. Decide on next steps to be taken by the home health nurse.

Unfolding Cases

A variation of case method is unfolding cases in which the clinical situation changes, thereby creating a simulation for students to analyze. With an unfolding case, instead of having one scenario, the teacher develops the case to expand the information presented to the student. For example, there might be a change in the patient's condition, clinical situation, or setting similar to what might occur with an actual patient. As the case unfolds, students analyze the new information and make decisions about relevant actions to take.

An example of an unfolding case is:

A patient in extended care is seen by the NP for a cough, wheezing, and short-ness of breath. The patient's symptoms are worse at night.

1. What additional data would you expect to be collected by the NP in the initial assessment? Why?
2. The NP orders spirometry. Explain this test and why it was ordered.

The following day the patient has increased shortness of breath, more frequent coughing, and fatigue. She seems slightly confused.

1. Does this new information change your impression of her problems? Why or why not?
2. List possible problems for this patient with a brief rationale to support each one.
3. What will you report to the NP?

SUMMARY

Cases describe a clinical situation developed around an actual or hypothetical patient for student analysis. In case method, the case is generally shorter and more specific than in case study. Case studies are more comprehensive in nature, thereby presenting a complete picture of the patient and clinical situation. In an unfold-ing case, the clinical situation changes, introducing new information for learners to integrate and analyze.

With these clinical teaching methods, students apply knowledge to practice situ-ations, identify needs and problems, propose varied approaches for solving them considering evidence, decide on courses of action, and evaluate outcomes. As such, cases provide experience for students in thinking through different clinical situa-tions and developing clinical judgment skills.

CNE® EXAMINATION TEST BLUEPRINT CORE COMPETENCIES

1. **Facilitate Learning**
   A. Implement a variety of teaching strategies appropriate to
      5. desired learner outcomes
   B. Use teaching strategies based on
      1. educational theory
      2. evidence-based practices related to education
   G. Model reflective thinking practices, including critical thinking
   H. Create opportunities for learners to develop their own critical thinking skills
   I. Create a positive learning environment that fosters a free exchange of ideas
   N. Use knowledge of evidence-based practice to instruct learners
2. **Facilitate Learner Development and Socialization**
   E. Foster the development of learners in these areas
      1. cognitive domain

CNE®cl EXAMINATION TEST BLUEPRINT CORE COMPETENCIES

1. **Function within the Education and Health Care Environments**
   B. Operationalize the Curriculum
      7. Provide opportunities for learners to develop problem-solving and clinical reasoning skills related to course objectives (e.g., learning outcomes)
2. **Facilitate Learning in the Health Care Environment**
   A. Implement a variety of clinical teaching strategies appropriate to learner needs, desired learner outcomes, content, and context
   B. Ground teaching strategies in educational theory and evidence-based teaching practices
   C. Create opportunities for learners to develop critical thinking and clinical reasoning skills

REFERENCES

Brookhart, S. M., & Nitko, A. J. (2019). *Educational assessment of students* (8th ed.). Pearson.

Foundation for Critical Thinking. (2019). Defining critical thinking. https://www.criticalthinking.org/pages/defining-critical-thinking/766.

National Council of State Boards of Nursing (NCSBN). (2019, winter). Next generation NCLEX news: Clinical judgment measurement model. *NCSBN*. https://www.ncsbn.org/NGN_Winter19.pdf

Noone, T., & Seery, A. (2018). Critical thinking dispositions in undergraduate nursing students: A case study approach. *Nurse Education Today*, *68*, 203–207. https://doi.org/10.1016/j.nedt.2018.06.014

Oermann, M. H., & Gaberson, K. B. (2021). *Evaluation and testing in nursing education* (6th ed.). Springer Publishing Company.

Schön, D. A. (1990). *Educating the reflective practitioner*. Jossey-Bass.

Sommer, S. K., Johnson, J., Clark, C. M., & Mills, C. M. (2021). Assisting learners to understand and incorporate functions of clinical judgment into nursing practice. *Nurse Educator*. [E-pub ahead of print]. https://doi.org/10.1097/NNE.0000000000001020

Tanner, C. A. (2006). Thinking like a nurse: A research-based model of clinical judgment in nursing. *Journal of Nursing Education*, *45*, 204–211. https://doi.org/10.3928/01484834-20060601-04

Von Colln-Appling, C., & Giuliano, D. (2017). A concept analysis of critical thinking: A guide for nurse educators. *Nurse Education Today*, *49*, 106–109. https://doi.org/10.1016/j.nedt.2016.11.007

A robust set of instructor resources designed to supplement this text is located at http://connect.springerpub.com/content/book/978-0-8261-6705-7. Qualifying instructors may request access by emailing textbook@springerpub.com.

Clinical Simulation

Katie Anne Haerling

Simulation refers to any experience where learners participate in a facilitated, interactive scenario or environment that mimics real-life to gain or demonstrate knowledge, skills, or abilities (Lioce et al., 2020). The science of healthcare simulation is rapidly evolving and plays an important role in clinical nursing education. Nursing programs have long faced competition for limited clinical placement sites and restrictions on what students can do within patient-care facilities. More recently, the COVID-19 pandemic required many nursing education programs to completely re-think their approach to clinical teaching and learning. All the while, advances in technology and evidence supporting the use of simulation have made simulation a useful option for nurse educators to provide students with immersive, experiential learning opportunities outside the patient-care environment. This chapter discusses how simulation can be used to enhance clinical teaching to ensure a better prepared nursing workforce. It also discusses the incorporation of best practice standards into clinical simulation activities.

BACKGROUND

The term, *simulation-based experience* (SBE) describes "a broad array of structured activities that represent actual or potential situations in education, practice, and research. These activities allow participants to develop or enhance knowledge, skills, and/or attitudes and provide an opportunity to analyze and respond to realistic situations in a simulated environment" (International Nursing Association for Clinical Simulation and Learning [INACSL] Standards Committee, 2016b, p. S45). While practicing nursing skills on a task-trainer or demonstrating a head-to-toe assessment with a peer may be considered simulation, the principles and practices discussed in this chapter focus specifically on the use of manikin-based, standardized patient (SP), and computer-based (CB) simulation. In manikin-based simulation, manikins are used to represent a patient with heart and lung sounds, pulses, voice interaction and other responses that may be controlled by a simulationist using a computer (Lioce et al., 2020, p. 29). SP simulation refers to a simulation in which the role of the patient is performed by an individual who is trained to portray a real patient (Lioce et al., 2020, p. 43). Finally, while the simulation community does not yet have a unified definition of virtual reality (Kardong-Edgren et al., 2019), this chapter refers to simulations, whether they are screen-based or use more immersive virtual or augmented reality, as CB simulations.

In general, simulations allow students to demonstrate psychomotor skills, clinical reasoning, clinical judgment, problem solving, and critical thinking. Simulation allows teachers to take specific information—such as a patient's personal characteristics; health information; socioeconomic, family, and community components; and physical, mental, and emotional states—and weave it into a real-life scenario that enhances a student's comprehension of the material because it is meaningful (Jeffries, 2021). In the case of clinical nursing scenarios, simulation provides an opportunity to suspend disbelief, engage in a re-creation of reality, and experience a lower-risk, hands-on opportunity to practice a clinical situation involving patient monitoring, management, communication, and multidisciplinary collaboration.

The use of simulation is well-established in industries such as aviation and computer science (Page, 2016) and is quickly becoming standard practice in nursing education. The use of simulation in nursing education has evolved rapidly over the past century: from life-sized dolls used to teach basic nursing skills, to sophisticated, computerized manikins that can mimic human physiology (Aebersold, 2018). In addition to general nursing, specialty areas such as pediatrics, obstetrics, home care, hospice, and palliative care have developed unique opportunities to integrate simulation as part of the clinical experience (Guise & Wiig, 2016; Kunkel et al., 2016; Veltri et al., 2016). Interprofessional education (IPE) has also immerged as a practical application of simulation-based learning (Manning et al., 2016; Pastor et al., 2016). Simulation may never completely replace direct student contact with human patients, but it has the potential to make student and teacher time in clinical settings more valuable and cost-effective while allowing students to explore diverse learning situations that they may not see in clinical settings.

The use of patient simulators has become common practice in many nursing education programs. Using simulation-based pedagogy allows students to integrate psychomotor skill performance, critical thinking, clinical-judgment, and communication skills while gaining self-confidence prior to entering the clinical setting. In addition, simulation offers an opportunity for evaluation and assessment of student skills with options for remediation and continued learning (Jeffries et al., 2022). The active learning component of simulation also appeals to many of today's millennial generation students, helping them to maintain engagement in the learning process, and retain the material learned.

Various organizations have recognized simulation's value as a teaching technique. The Commission on Collegiate Nursing Education (CCNE) accreditation standards encourage the use of innovative teaching methods and the introduction of technology and informatics to improve student learning (CCNE, 2018). The National League for Nursing (NLN) has also provided long-standing leadership and support for simulation in nursing education, conducting a national multisite multimethod study investigating the innovative use of simulation to teach nursing care of ill adults and children (Forneris & Fey, 2016). NLN's leadership continued with the development of the Simulation Innovation Resource Center (SIRC). SIRC provides education and training about simulation while also allowing participants an opportunity to engage in dialogue with colleagues about simulation and providing resources for the development and integration of simulation into the curriculum (NLN, 2021). The NLN Leadership Development Program for Simulation Educators offers an opportunity for experienced simulation nurse educators to examine issues related to research in simulation, curricular integration, and the role of simulation in interprofessional education (NLN, 2020).

Additional organizations, such as INACSL and the interdisciplinary Society for Simulation in Healthcare (SSH) are exclusively dedicated to simulation. Both INACSL and SSH publish journals. *Clinical Simulation in Nursing*, the official journal of INACSL, is a monthly online journal publishing peer-reviewed articles with a mission to "advance the science of simulation in healthcare." (INACSL Journal, 2020b). The Society for Simulation in Healthcare publishes two journals, *Simulation in Healthcare* and *Simulation Technician Operations Resource* magazine, and provides certification and accreditation opportunities (SSH, 2020). These organizations offer a wide variety of webinars, scholarships, and other resources to support both beginning and advanced simulationists. In particular, the INACSL Standards (2021) and SSH Dictionary (Lopreiato et al., 2016) are referenced extensively throughout this chapter.

The National Council of State Boards of Nursing (NCSBN) simulation study provides sound evidence that high-quality simulation experiences can replicate patient situations and allow students to adequately develop their nursing skills. The findings from this national randomized controlled study demonstrated that up to 50% of traditional clinical practice can be replaced with high-quality simulation and produce comparable educational outcomes in prelicensure programs (Hayden et al., 2014). The use of simulation to replace or augment traditional clinical experiences in prelicensure nursing education is growing. A 2019 survey by the National Council of State Boards of Nursing revealed that 75.2% of registered nurse (RN) education programs responded affirmatively to the question: "Does student time in simulation count toward clinical hours?" Of these, 14.3% indicated that on occasion simulation is used as a substitute for clinical practice, and 60.9% indicated that simulation hours were substituted for clinical hours" (Smiley, 2019, p. 56). The evidence informing regulation of simulation in nursing education continues to evolve. For example, Sullivan et al. (2019) and Curl et al. (2016) suggested there is evidence to support counting each hour spent in simulation as two hours of supervised clinical. While nursing experts acknowledge the value of simulation as a teaching–learning approach that mimics reality, experts also emphasize the need for nursing student clinical experiences with real patients, thus encouraging clinical teachers to use all available learning opportunities.

FIDELITY AND SIMULATORS

Depending on the objectives of the simulation-based activity, educators need to incorporate the appropriate level of fidelity into the simulation. Fidelity, "the ability of the simulation to reproduce the reactions, interactions, and responses of the real-world counterpart" (Lioce et al., 2020, p. 18) includes conceptual, physical/environmental, and psychological fidelity. Conceptual fidelity reflects the degree to which the case makes sense (INACSL Standards Committee, 2016b, p. S42). For example, do the respiratory rate, blood pressure, and heart rate of the simulator fluctuate in a way that is congruent with the case? All components of the simulation must fit together appropriately. If the simulation scenario involves a patient having a myocardial infarction, then the subjective and objective data provided to the student should be consistent and reflect the typical activities that would normally occur. Physical/environmental fidelity reflects the degree to which the simulation room, props, equipment, manikin, sounds, and smells represent the environment being simulated (INACSL Standards Committee, 2016b, p. S42). To support physical fidelity, the teacher should consider the sights, sounds, smells, layout, and props used to create a realistic physical environment. Finally, psychological fidelity reflects the degree to which the simulated scenario evokes the feelings and thought processes learners would experience if they were involved in a similar scenario in real life (INACSL Standards Committee, 2016b, p. S42).

Increased fidelity does not necessarily translate to improved learning outcomes. The objectives of the simulation should dictate the level of fidelity. The type of simulator used in a scenario will affect the level of fidelity. However, it is not the only factor to consider. A task-trainer, such as a disembodied pelvis for catheter insertion simulation or a gel pad for intramuscular injection practice, may offer the appropriate level of fidelity for the learning objective such as demonstrating appropriate technique for a specific skill. Similarly, a simple manikin that produces heart and lung sounds, but does not offer the realism of chest movement, is useful for certain scenarios such as completing an assessment that does not require the interactive features of a more sophisticated simulator. Computerized patient simulators produce the most lifelike scenarios. These full-size manikins react to student manipulations in real time and in realistic ways, such as speaking, coughing, and demonstrating chest movements and pulses.

SPs represent another type of simulation used in nursing education. This form of simulation uses live actors with scripts that portray patients and require nursing students to engage in nursing care activities with the SP in an environment that simulates patient care areas (Jeffries et al., 2022). Nursing education programs affiliated with academic health centers may have SPs available to them since SPs are commonly used in medical education. Practice with SPs can provide invaluable learning opportunities for students as they refine their communication skills or practice in sensitive or specialized clinical situations such as oncology, mental health, or end-of-life situations. SPs can offer valuable feedback and insight about the patient perspective to the nursing student (MacLean et al., 2017). Using SPs has also been helpful with health assessment and psychomotor skill development (Ham, 2016; Sarmasoglu et al., 2016; Slater et al., 2016) and can be useful as both a teaching–learning strategy or as an evaluation approach. However, for students who do not have this option available, other well-planned simulation experiences can help to meet their needs. Visual and performing arts students, improvisation group members, nursing alumni, or retired professionals (e.g., actors, physicians, nurses, teachers) may be able to role-play as patients, family members, or interdisciplinary healthcare professionals to enhance simulation realism.

USING SIMULATION AS A TEACHING STRATEGY

Nursing programs are integrating simulation into their curriculum. This integration may be a result of external pressure (visiting prospective students who ask about simulation opportunities), administrators who recognize the need, nurse educators who desire to keep up with the technology-driven millennial generation of students, or teachers seeking alternative learning opportunities for students. Increasingly, compelling evidence about the benefits of simulation is encouraging nurse educators to increase their use of simulation. Well-designed research is necessary to demonstrate how the use of simulation can be optimized to create the desired outcomes in student learning and how knowledge, skills, and abilities learned in simulation can best translate into clinical practice.

The NLN Jeffries Simulation Theory has served as a critical framework to design, implement, and evaluate simulation in nursing (Jeffries, 2016). One component of this theory focuses on simulation design characteristics. Clinical teachers using simulation need to consider the following design characteristics: objectives, fidelity, problem solving, student support, and debriefing. Another component involves outcomes that include measures of participant learning such as skill performance, learner satisfaction, critical thinking, and self-confidence, as well as system and patient level outcomes. Finally, clinical teachers using simulation need to consider the facilitator, the participant, and educational practices when using simulation in clinical education (Jeffries, 2016). Teachers should have adequate training for the development of appropriate clinical scenarios, implementation of the simulation, and evaluation of the pedagogy. Faculty development related to simulation is a critical factor to consider when implementing clinical simulation for teaching–learning purposes to ensure that teachers are adequately prepared to implement simulation appropriately.

Today's nursing students benefit from pedagogy that is based on active participation. By engaging learners directly in the simulation, active learning can occur. Providing constructive feedback during the debriefing session, allowing students to view a recording of their performance, or getting suggestions and critiques from classmates who may be viewing them in a nearby classroom all provide feedback that may enhance student performance (Hallmark et al., 2016). Acknowledging that students learn through many different styles, simulation allows the incorporation of different teaching strategies to appeal to these diverse needs.

PREPARING FOR SIMULATION

To realize the full benefit of clinical simulation, teachers need to ensure that students participating in simulation experiences in clinical nursing laboratories see this as a realistic environment and consider various factors when preparing the clinical scenario for simulation. Specific policies and procedures related to clinical simulation recording and the confidentiality of the recordings need to be developed. Further, students need to be orientated to the manikin and the simulated environment. Presimulation activities include thoughtful scaffolding of content within the curriculum so students have the necessary knowledge, skills, and abilities to meaningfully engage in the scenario (Diaz & Anderson, 2021).

Teachers need to consider many factors and purposively design clinical scenarios that are based on INACSL Standards of Best Practice for simulation (2016a, 2021). The Simulation Design Standard encourages educators to start the simulation design process by completing a needs assessment and developing measurable objectives for the simulation experience (INACSL, 2016a). The Simulation Design Standard emphasizes the need to incorporate an appropriate level of fidelity and include pre- and debriefing activities as well as assessment of not only the participant, but also the simulation experience, environment, and facilitation. The full Simulation Design Standard, along with all of the INACSL Standards of Best Practice: Simulation[SM] is available on the web at the INACSL website: inacsl.org. Program outcomes and course objectives should provide some direction for the type of simulation needed. For example, if a clinical or course objective focuses on client assessment, teachers might decide to create a simulation that has a patient experiencing shortness of breath, decreased oxygen saturation, and abnormal breath sounds. During the simulation, students could use their problem-solving and critical thinking skills to explore the respiratory status of the patient and complete a respiratory assessment.

The level of technology used in clinical simulation depends on several factors. As previously discussed, the primary factor should be the learning objectives. However, teacher familiarity with the technology, the technology available, and support for use of technology also affect which technology is used. Clinical teachers should use the resources and expertise available to provide an optimal simulation experience. Nursing education programs that have access to simulation specialists or information technology (IT) support (ideally, designated IT staff members) may have an easier time incorporating simulation into clinical education. In addition, college or university services that support academic excellence with resources and specialists can assist with faculty development, and other departments can help incorporate components that will make the simulation feel more real. Faculty members in a university department of communication may be able to assist nursing clinical teachers with the dialogue component of scenarios. Performing arts faculty members and students can add to the contextual experience by role-playing anxious family members; nursing education colleagues might apply some of their rich clinical experience by portraying a spouse, parent, or child of the simulated patient.

OTHER PLANNING CONSIDERATIONS

Past simulation and educational experiences, level of student (e.g., first year pre-licensure students vs. advanced practice nurses), and number of clinical students should also be part of the simulation planning considerations. Will all students actively participate in the simulation activities or will a select group of students play an active role serving as the nurse or other healthcare provider in the simulation scenario while others observe? Have the students participated in simulation activities before or are they new to this experience and need a full orientation to the manikins and simulation environment? Does the simulation build on prior knowledge or is it intended to teach new content? Is the simulation an adjunct for clinical learning, an alternate activity in case of an absence from clinical learning activities, or a replacement for activities at a clinical facility? These factors will impact the amount of time and preparation that may be required for the simulation experience.

Another planning consideration is the focus and purpose of the simulation. Is the simulation planned to provide students with practice opportunities, or is the simulation intended to evaluate student performance? Simulated patient experiences are often used for advanced practice nursing students to demonstrate skills needed for practice and are thus used for competency evaluation. Teachers need to consider the high-stakes testing component of simulation as they plan for simulation use. Finally, consider the time for simulation, including lab availability, teacher time, and student time, making sure to include time for introduction, prebriefing, student preparation, simulation implementation, and debriefing. Once these areas have been considered, then further scenario development or selection can occur.

SCENARIO SELECTION

Once some of these preliminary decisions about the simulation have been determined, then teachers can create or select the scenario. Scenario development incorporates evidence and professional standards but is also a creative process.

The use of a simple storyboard template can provide structure without being overwhelming for teachers who are developing their first scenarios. The template typically includes the specific objectives for the simulation activity, simulator settings and other actions, types of cues that the patient and other team members may provide to the students, expected student actions, and suggested debriefing and reflection topics. The use of a storyboard template by teachers as they develop scenarios will increase consistency among teachers across a curriculum and encourage them to start with basic information (e.g., identifying three to five simulation objectives and learning outcomes). It is important to identify essential learning outcomes, taking into consideration social and demographic trends specific to the geographic area, and incorporating cultural sensitivity, spirituality, and ethical considerations.

Similar to other learning activity, it is important to start with the objectives and work backward to develop a simulation scenario that will help learners achieve those objectives. If there are specific specialty areas students are not able to access in the clinical environment, these might be areas to focus on in simulation. Similarly, if existing student outcome data reflect deficits in communication, teamwork, medication administration, or other topics, consider simulation as an opportunity for addressing these deficits. The level of the students, specific course objectives, and teacher clinical expertise all need to be considered when specifying an appropriate learning outcome.

Drawing on common situations seen at clinical sites or relying on past clinical cases will help provide ideas for scenario creation. If you are drawing ideas or information from actual patients, make sure case details are generic and that patient privacy is not compromised by revealing too much personal or identifiable information. Sometimes scenarios are a compilation of many patients seen in clinical practice. Scenarios often incorporate unique aspects of care that can be vividly portrayed in simulations. For example, simulations that use a cluttered, dusty, and insect-infested home during a home health simulation; stressed, arguing parents as part of a pediatric simulation; or a patient experiencing homelessness, low literacy skills, co-morbidities, and limited support systems can effectively portray challenging situations that nurses face in practice. Regardless of the method used to create scenarios, it is important to ensure that they are student-centered, interactive, related to outcomes, and based on best practices.

Many nursing education programs access or purchase existing scenarios from publishers, simulation manufacturers, other nursing education programs, and professional organizations. These already-developed materials aid teachers by providing well-constructed scenarios with the completed template of essential information and support data needed to implement the simulation. When using prepackaged scenarios, it is important to check alignment with course and program outcomes and needs. Sometimes tailoring these scenarios to align with individual course needs may be necessary. Regardless of the origin of the scenario, the scenarios should use lifelike situations that are appropriate for the level of students and clinical course.

OTHER CONSIDERATIONS

Once the scenario is written, teachers should schedule time with lab staff members (equipment managers and IT experts for programming the equipment) for a rehearsal of the simulation on paper and then in real time. Reviewing scenarios for accuracy, current evidence-based practice guidelines, and unnecessary distracters will ensure the quality of the simulation experience for all and help to identify needed resources (e.g., teacher and staff support, props, space, and time). It is necessary to practice the scenario, and it is ideal if students or teachers are present for a practice session prior to implementing the live scenario with the students. Finally, the teacher should prepare the manikin or simulated patient with props and include appropriate moulage or a reproduction of special effects so that students can see, feel, smell, and hear in a lifelike clinical environment.

Because electronic health record (EHR) use and its relationship to patient safety and prevention of adverse events has been documented (Helwig & Lomotan, 2016), teachers should consider use of this technology as part of the simulation. Some nursing programs are using EHRs as a tool to enhance clinical simulation. Students can use the academic EHR to access simulated patient records and document care provided during a simulation, thus giving students an opportunity to develop these essential informatics skills in a safe environment (Hansbrough et al., 2020). Creating a database of mock patient records as part of the EHR that can be accessed and used during simulation will enhance realism while allowing students to access longitudinal patient data and help ensure that students develop the knowledge and skills needed to function in a technology-rich clinical environment. This hands-on approach of using an EHR during simulation will provide additional practice opportunities and help students make the transition to EHR use in the clinical setting.

IMPLEMENTING SIMULATION

Prebriefing is an important component of simulation. It involves planning, briefing, and facilitating (McDermott, 2020). While planning, the teacher should consider the learner. Factors such as type of program, level in the program, previous clinical experience, previous simulation experience, and prior coursework will all influence learning and impact simulation success (Jeffries, 2016; McDermott, 2020). To adequately prepare for the simulation experience, teachers may plan learning activities that require students to complete an assignment prior to the simulation, such as reading relevant background information on pathophysiology or medications that will be used during the simulation, completing preparation worksheets, reviewing and practicing technical skills, viewing Internet resources, or watching a video or online presentation.

Providing students with a brief history of the patient and the diagnosis will then allow students to answer some key questions in preparation for the simulation experience. Exhibit 9.1 provides some sample questions that can be used to prepare for the simulation. Clinical teachers can conduct this presimulation preparation in a variety of ways; students can complete individual written assignments or they can participate in oral discussions with the clinical group. A formal presimulation preparatory group meeting with the students is also an opportunity to review expectations about student performance, remind students about confidentiality of the experience, and obtain signatures for video recording consents.

The simulation should begin with a briefing about the simulation. This is an opportunity for the teacher to assess student preparation for the experience, check on essential student knowledge, review background information about the patient

EXHIBIT 9.1 Sample Preparatory Questions for Simulations

1. What physical assessments should be completed as a priority for this patient?
2. What questions will you ask the patient so you can fully explore and understand the health problem?
3. What data or information do you still need to understand and provide appropriate care for this patient?
4. What lab or diagnostic tests will you review, and what might you expect to find?
5. What are the patient's medications (drug classification, dosage, route, administration, and nursing implications)?
6. What teaching will be necessary?
7. What might be important to discuss with the family or significant others?
8. What other social, emotional, religious, psychological, or environmental issues need to be considered when planning the patient's care?
9. What will be your priority nursing actions?
10. What other healthcare providers should be contacted?
11. What nursing interventions will be necessary?

in the simulation, provide instructions, and assign roles for the simulation. It also is helpful to provide logistical information, set the tone, and clarify expectations before proceeding with the simulation. Teachers should act as facilitators and promote student understanding and answer questions that may arise. Many times, the simulation begins with a report or review of background information about the patient in the form of a handoff or change-of-shift report. It may also include a brief review of the relevant patient health history.

Students begin the scenario and enact the assigned roles, which may include primary nurse, charge nurse, medication nurse, or other supportive staff. Sometimes students or others serve in ancillary or supportive roles that help to enhance the realism of the simulation and add an interprofessional learning opportunity. This is also a chance to collaborate with other disciplines such as students from medicine, speech therapy, respiratory therapy, or dieticians who can serve in their respective roles during the simulation. The teacher, controlling the simulation from a separate room, if feasible, uses the preplanned scenario to respond to student actions during the simulation. Teachers may use either preprogrammed patient vocal responses or spontaneously respond to student questions and actions on behalf of the simulated patient. Teachers should allow students to make mistakes, problem solve throughout the scenario, and find their own way. Many nursing education programs have video recording capabilities that allow for a recording of all events of the scenarios. These recordings can be used for debriefing after the simulation.

Depending on clinical group size, learning goals, and time available, teachers may choose to have some students observe the scenario and provide suggestions and insight during debriefing. Students may experience anxiety when they are performing before others during a simulation (Shearer, 2016). Strategies that may assist in decreasing anxiety during simulation include providing a supportive and respectful learning environment that allows students to make mistakes, ensuring adequate preparation, and validating their feelings (Shearer, 2016). Use of these strategies may help reduce the anxiety during simulation.

DEBRIEFING AND GUIDED REFLECTION

Perhaps most important area of clinical simulation involves debriefing and providing an opportunity for guided reflection on the simulation. Debriefing has been identified as critical for students' learning and satisfaction with their simulation experience; however, it requires adequate time and some preplanning to be effective. Debriefing encourages reflection, self-awareness, and assists in the transfer of knowledge to practice (INACSL Standards Committee, 2016c). Debriefing allows the students to make meaning of the experience, critique performance while reinforcing learning, and figure out how to apply information to practice. Although the importance of debriefing is widely accepted, there are diverse views on best practice approaches to debriefing (Hall & Tori, 2016). The INACSL Standards of Best Practice can provide excellent guidance for clinical teachers using debriefing with simulation.

Because debriefing can be critical for student learning, teachers need to carefully plan and consider the methods, format, and approach used while also ensuring that they can effectively facilitate this activity. The Standards of Best Practice: Simulation^{SM} Debriefing are available on the INACSL website at inacsl.org. Similarly, teachers should identify an accepted method for debriefing. Structured debriefing involves development of prepared questions that can be used to guide the debriefing session. These questions typically arise from simulation objectives and serve as a prompt to focus the debriefing discussion. Teachers should allow enough flexibility so that they can respond to unexpected developments during simulation and incorporate them into the debriefing activities.

Five well-accepted methods for debriefing simulation-based activities include:

- Plus Delta (+/Δ),
- Debriefing for Meaningful Learning©,
- Diffuse, Discover, Deepen (3D Model),
- Gather-Analyze-Summarize (GAS), and
- Promoting Excellence and Reflective Learning in Simulation (PEARLS) (Dreifuerst et al., 2021).

Oral or written format, or a combination of both, may be used to accomplish debriefing. Oral debriefing or discussions about simulation can be done in groups or with individual simulation participants. Group debriefing allows observers, typically other clinical students who observed the simulation, to participate in the debriefing process. Student observers and teachers can provide valuable insight and suggestions after watching the simulation. They may notice actions that the students in the nurse's role may not be aware of and can offer insight from their unique perspective of observer. Sometimes the debriefing process can be sensitive and anxiety-provoking, particularly if the student performance is deficient or problems were encountered, or when video playback of the simulation is reviewed. Teachers may choose to complete private debriefing with only those students playing an active role in the simulation. If group debriefing is used then the teacher should facilitate the use of honest, respectful, and supportive feedback. It is also important to demonstrate regard for the student and the emotional aspect of this experience (INACSL Standards Committee, 2016c).

Regardless of the approach used for oral debriefing, teachers should anticipate and plan for adequate time for debriefing. Time required for debriefing varies based on several factors including the objectives of the simulation, level of simulation participants, actions of simulation participants within the scenario, and practical time constraints (Dreifeurst et al., 2021). Further research in this area is needed, but as a general guideline for planning purposes, teachers should consider spending at least the same amount of time on debriefing as they do with the simulation.

Oral debriefing typically follows immediately at the conclusion of the scenario. This timing for debriefing is helpful in that students can recall recent events and discuss them while they are still current. However, some students may benefit from some additional time to process the simulation events and think about the experience, or they may prefer to privately reflect about the experience in writing rather than orally in a public forum. Journaling activities can be assigned to encourage students to personally reflect on the experience. Electronic activities such as blogging (in a private rather than public format) or threaded electronic discussions can also be used to engage students who are digital natives and promote reflection after simulation. Either structured or unstructured approaches can be used. For example, students can be asked to compose a reflective journal entry that uses a broad prompt, such as, "Write about what you learned from the simulation." Or they can write more specifically about what went well and what could be improved. Structured prompts could direct students to write about specific examples of actions during the simulation. For example, "What were you thinking when the patient complained of shortness of breath during the simulation? What actions did you take and what else could you have done to address this situation?"

Teachers also should consider the use of technology for the debriefing, such as whether and how to incorporate video replay of the simulation. It is important to consider the purpose of the video replay in addition to the risks and benefits of creating and using video recordings of simulation activities. Caution should be exercised to prevent inappropriate distribution of the video and potential violation of student confidentiality. Video review can be required as part of the written journaling activities previously discussed. Limited research is available to provide clear guidance about best uses of video replay; however, use of select video snippets of the simulation may help to remind students of what happened during the simulation and could lead to rich debriefing discussions.

Once decisions about the method, format, and approach to debriefing are complete, the teacher needs to implement activities that will ensure an appropriate climate for debriefing. The instructor's role during debriefing is that of facilitator, coach, or guide—not lecturer and monopolizer of debriefing conversations. At the beginning of a debriefing session, the teacher should orient students to the debriefing process and code of conduct, review the objectives of the simulation, discuss confidentiality, and articulate teacher expectations for students' participation in evaluating themselves and their peers (INACSL Standards Committee, 2016c). Teachers should establish a trusting environment because students may feel vulnerable and anxious, particularly if video playback is used. Sensitive issues need to be openly discussed in a constructive and supportive manner. Once the ground rules of the debriefing session are complete, then discussion about the events and experiences can begin. As students share their impressions and reflections, teachers should listen, redirect discussion as appropriate, and encourage participation.

The use of probing open-ended questions will help to engage students in reflective conversations. Exhibit 9.2 provides some sample questions that can be incorporated into simulation debriefing. The teacher should use what, how, and why questions to promote student discussion and higher-level thinking. Sometimes

EXHIBIT 9.2 Sample Debriefing Questions

Was there anything you missed on report, or was there other information that you needed so you could act more effectively?

What knowledge do you still need to manage the situation more effectively?

What areas require further practice?

What went well?

What would you do differently the next time? Why?

Why do you think the patient responded in the manner that they did?

What were you thinking about during the simulation?

Why did you complete the nursing actions in the order that you did?

How could you have acted differently to meet the patient's needs more effectively and efficiently?

What problems did you identify?

How did you prioritize your care?

teachers may need to clarify inaccuracies or correct misinterpretations in a manner that provides positive feedback and specific examples about performance but also gives students suggestions for areas to strengthen or change. Lastly, the teacher should use verbal and nonverbal responses and engage student observers as well as the simulation participants in the analysis and reflection of the events.

The teacher should conclude the debriefing session with some closing statements about what students identified as effective and efficient, areas they need to work on, and take-away learning messages to summarize the experience. Thanking students for their participation and stating the teacher's appreciation for their attention, efforts in enacting the scenario, and shared reflections provide positive reinforcement and show respect for their efforts. Asking students to identify content that helped them succeed in the scenario and where they received it (classroom, presentations, and scenario preparation) will guide the teacher to further course and curricular improvements.

EVALUATING SIMULATIONS

The final aspect of clinical simulation, evaluating simulations, involves multiple components. As the simulation unfolds, teachers can easily identify areas that are working and areas that are problematic. The dynamic process of the simulation allows for some modification during use, but careful note taking during the scenario, as well as after the debriefing session with students, will document changes necessary to enhance the effectiveness of the simulation for the future. Another method commonly used for simulation evaluation involves asking for student feedback or reactions to the experience. This evaluation can occur in a group debriefing session or individually by each student in a written format. These data, while not directly linked to performance, will provide valuable information about the simulation experience, allowing teachers to consider further revisions and improvements. Reviewing student feedback with teachers and simulation specialists who assisted with the technology component of simulation soon after the scenario is completed provides the best opportunities for change and revision.

There are a variety of ways to assess student performance and determine whether the simulation enabled attainment of the learning objectives. Evaluation methods reflect students' performance and whether they met the objectives and demonstrated the skills and knowledge identified as important outcomes for that scenario. This type of learning can also be assessed with skills checklists, rating scales, or other performance indices. Regardless of the approach used for evaluation, teachers should select instruments with demonstrated reliability and validity evidence and determine if formative or summative evaluations will be completed. Student behaviors can be assessed for items such as level of independence, prompting, accuracy, timeliness, and appropriate sequence of activities. Debriefing is enriched with this information because students are provided with concrete, constructive, and immediate feedback in an objective manner.

Sometimes simulation is used during class time to reinforce content and engage the students, in which case it probably involves more than one student with classmates observing (either live or a recording). In this situation, peer observers can be given an assignment that instructs them to observe for specific actions or activities. Because a simulation can often be complex, assigning students specific areas to observe can allow students to focus more effectively. For example, one student can watch the simulation and note safety measures and another student may watch for communication skills; students can then share their impressions and evaluation about these areas during debriefing. Teachers may find it helpful to agree on and detail the behaviors in a particular scenario that best demonstrate achievement of the defined objectives.

Instruments exist for evaluating multiple aspects of simulation including the facilitator and educational strategies, the participant, simulation design, and simulation outcomes (Haerling, 2021; Jeffries et al., 2015). The INACSL maintains a Repository of Instruments used in Simulation Research on their website at: www.inacsl.org/resources/repository-of-instruments/

Two instruments that have been used extensively in the literature to evaluate simulation participant performance are the Creighton Competency Evaluation Instrument (C-CEI) and the Lasater Clinical Judgment Rubric (LCJR). The C-CEI addresses performance in the areas of Assessment, Communication, Clinical Judgment, and Patient Safety (Creighton, 2020). The developers of the instrument provide extensive resources including access to training and the instrument at their website: nursing.creighton.edu/academics/competency-evaluation-instrument

The LCJR (Lasater, 2007) is based on Tanner's (2006) Model of Clinical Judgment and reflects the four aspects of Clinical Judgment: Noticing, Interpreting, Responding, and Reflecting. Each of the 11 items on the rubric is accompanied by language describing beginning, developing, accomplished, and exemplary performance. This language is useful not only for evaluating performance, but for communicating with simulation participants about their performance and how to improve in the future. Widespread use of both the C-CEI and LCJR contributes valuable reliability and validity evidence about their appropriateness for evaluating student performance. Further research is needed to effectively determine how simulation impacts learning, behavior and, ultimately, patient care.

COMPUTER-BASED SIMULATION

There is no universally accepted terminology related to the use of CB simulation—virtual simulation, virtual reality, and augmented reality—within the simulation literature. Table 9.1 provides descriptions of each of these.

TABLE 9.1	DEFINITIONS OF TYPES OF CB SIMULATION
Term	**Description**
Virtual simulation	"Partially immersive, screen-based experiences"
Virtual reality or virtual-reality simulation	"Fully immersive experience through the use of a headset that covers the eyes"
Augmented reality or augmented-reality simulation	Combination or "overlay of a digital learning environment with real life"

Source: Foronda, C. L., Fernandez-Burgos, M., Nadeau, C., Kelley, C. N., & Henry, M. N. (2020). Virtual simulation in nursing education: A systematic review spanning 1996 to 2018. *Simulation in Healthcare: Journal of the Society for Medical Simulation, 15*(1), 51. https://doi.org/10.1097/SIH.0000000000000411.

CB, Computer-based

While much remains to be learned about the effectiveness of CB simulation in nursing education, a systematic review found that 86% of the 80 reviewed studies found virtual simulation to be associated with positive learning outcomes (Foronda et al., 2020). Since the publication of this review, the COVID-19 pandemic provided a catalyst for closer examination of the use of CB simulation in healthcare education. INACSL and SSH issued a joint Position Statement on Use of Virtual Simulation during the Pandemic in March 2020. In this statement, the organizations indicated that virtual simulation—simulated healthcare experiences on one's computer—has been used successfully for more than a decade and was an effective teaching method that improved learning outcomes (Foronda et al., 2020; Kononowicz et al., 2019). They proposed that regulatory bodies allow the replacement of clinical practice hours in a healthcare setting with virtually simulated experiences during the pandemic (INACSL, 2020a).

Many CB simulations combine multimedia and animation to simulate nursing scenarios that allow students to interact with patients through a branching patient case. Since the simulation is delivered electronically, there may not the usual person, space, cost, or delivery demands found with other types of simulation. These efficiencies, while attractive, may come at a cost. For example, if a facilitator is not actively engaging with learners as they experience the simulation, they may not be able to provide an immediate debriefing session. Much research has gone into best practices for debriefing virtual simulations, and these should be carefully considered when adopting CB simulation pedagogy (Verkuyl, 2020).

Unlike traditional manikin-based and SP-based simulations, CB simulations allow participants to engage with the scenarios at a convenient time and place. Multiple students can complete the simulation and actively participate in the nursing case. Depending on how the CB simulation is designed, the student may receive immediate performance feedback and repeat the simulation. This opportunity to integrate feedback and re-do a simulation can make CB simulations ideal for enhanced learning and remediation activities. CB simulations may offer a cost-effective alternative to clinical site visits and performance evaluations particularly for online or geographically disbursed students. One study comparing manikin-based and CB simulations demonstrated similar learning outcomes between the two types of simulation, but improved cost-utility associated with the CB simulations (Haerling, 2018). As nurse educators continue to adopt CB simulations to augment or replace clinical teaching, and more options for CB simulations become available, these technologies are expected to grow in quality and quantity. A list of virtual simulation resources is provided in Appendix A.3.

CLINICAL SIMULATION INTEGRATION INTO THE CURRICULUM

Simulation activities can be integrated into clinical learning in a variety of ways. First, simulation offers opportunities to prepare students for clinical care by offering practice of psychomotor skills, communication, and problem solving in a simulated environment. By involving a group of clinical students in the simulation activities, students have an opportunity to deliver care, observe performance, reflect on their learning, and critique their practice and that of peers. Simulation also provides a standardized experience for students. It is particularly useful when the clinical teacher would like all students to have practice with a situation that may not be available to everyone due to variability in patient census or setting constraints. Creating a simulation scenario involving a high-risk, life-threatening, or emergency situation allows all students to experience the same scenario without the potential safety concerns to the patient.

Simulation can also be used as a makeup activity to provide additional clinical learning when a student is absent. Or it can be used for additional review and practice to help remediate at-risk students who are having trouble mastering clinical competencies. Students can have repeat practice opportunities with simulation. With video-recording capabilities, simulations can be saved and used for other learning activities such as clinical conferences. Finally, simulation can be used for evaluation purposes as either a way to ensure all students demonstrate satisfactory performance or for competency assessment.

FUTURE IMPLICATIONS

The use of simulation for clinical teaching continues to evolve. The landmark NCSBN study demonstrating up to 50% of traditional clinical practice experiences can be replaced with high-quality simulation further supports simulation use in nursing education. However, further research is indicated, and some suggestions are provided.

- Nurse educators should continue to work with other related professions to conduct interprofessional simulation activities and evaluate their effectiveness.
- Continued research is needed to demonstrate the efficacy of simulation in nursing education and provide sound evidence-based support for simulation activities.
- Teacher support, resources, and curricular integration require administrative support, affordable simulation software and evaluation systems that streamline faculty efforts. As simulation continues to advance, ongoing faculty training on the latest developments is essential to keep teachers up-to-date on simulation advances.
- More research and support are necessary for the use of EHRs and scenario implementation.

■ Simulation research in nursing education needs to move from small-scale, single-site descriptive studies to robust multisite experimental designs using strong methodology, adequate sample sizes, and measurement tools that produce reliable results.

SUMMARY

Clinical simulation plays an increasingly important role in nursing education, and nurse educators will continue to be called on to develop, implement, and evaluate this essential element of clinical nursing education. This chapter discussed the background and evidence related to the use of simulation in clinical nursing education. It provided an overview of essential concepts and educational practices including guidelines for preparing for simulation, choosing a manikin, and creating or selecting a scenario. Prebriefing is an important component of simulation and was discussed in the chapter. The simulation should begin with a briefing about the simulation. This is an opportunity for the teacher to assess student preparation, check on essential student knowledge, review background information about the patient in the simulation, provide instructions, and assign roles for the simulation. Depending on the clinical group size, learning goals, and time available, teachers may choose to have some students observe the scenario and provide suggestions and insight during debriefing.

Perhaps the most important area of clinical simulation involves debriefing and providing an opportunity for guided reflection on the simulation. Debriefing has been identified as critical for students' learning and satisfaction with their simulation experience, and it requires adequate time and some preplanning to be effective. The chapter provided extensive discussion on debriefing with guidelines for implementation.

The final aspect of clinical simulation, evaluating simulations, involves multiple components. As the simulation unfolds, teachers can easily identify areas that are working and areas that are problematic. The dynamic process of the simulation allows for some modification during use, but careful note taking during the scenario and after the debriefing is important to document changes necessary to enhance the effectiveness of the simulation for the future.

Simulation activities can be integrated into clinical learning in a variety of ways, which were described in the chapter. Resources and organizations that can help nurse educators develop and sustain the successful use of simulation were identified throughout the chapter and are also provided in Appendix A. While research to further develop the science of simulation is ongoing, these resources provide guidance for implementing existing best practices.

CNE® EXAMINATION TEST BLUEPRINT CORE COMPETENCIES

1. **Facilitate Learning**
   A. Implement a variety of teaching strategies appropriate to
      1. content
      3. learner needs
      5. desired learner outcomes
      6. method of delivery

B. Use teaching strategies based on
  1. educational theory
  2. evidence-based practices related to education
C. Modify teaching strategies and learning experiences based on consideration of learners
  2. past clinical experiences
  3. past educational and life experiences
D. Use information technologies to support the teaching–learning process
G. Model reflective thinking practices, including critical thinking
H. Create opportunities for learners to develop their own critical thinking skills
I. Create a positive learning environment that fosters a free exchange of ideas
N. Use knowledge of evidence-based practice to instruct learners
O. Demonstrate ability to teach clinical skills
Q. Foster a safe learning environment

2. **Facilitate Learner Development and Socialization**
D. Create learning environments that facilitate learners' self-reflection, personal goal setting, and socialization to the role of the nurse
E. Foster the development of learners in these areas
  1. cognitive domain
  2. psychomotor domain
  3. affective domain
F. Assist learners to engage in thoughtful and constructive self and peer evaluation

3. **Use Assessment and Evaluation Strategies**
C. Use a variety of strategies to assess and evaluate learning in these domains
  1. cognitive
  2. psychomotor
  3. affective
D. Incorporate current research in assessment and evaluation practices
E. Analyze available resources for learning assessment and evaluation
G. Implement evaluation strategies that are appropriate to the learner and learning outcomes
I. Analyze assessment and evaluation data
J. Use assessment and evaluation data to enhance the teaching–learning process
K. Advise learners regarding assessment and evaluation criteria
L. Provide timely, constructive, and thoughtful feedback to learners

6. **Engage in Scholarship, Service, and Leadership**
A. Function as a change agent and leader
  3. Participate in interdisciplinary efforts to address healthcare and education needs
    a. within the institution
    b. locally
    c. regionally
  6. Adapt to changes created by external factors
B. Engage in scholarship of teaching
  1. Exhibit a spirit of inquiry about teaching and learning, student development, and evaluation methods
  2. Use evidence-based resources to improve and support teaching
  3. Participate in research activities related to nursing education

CNE®cl EXAMINATION TEST BLUEPRINT CORE COMPETENCIES

1. **Function within the Education and Health Care Environments**
   A. Function in the Clinical Educator Role
      2. Foster professional growth of learners (e.g., coaching, reflection, and debriefing
      3. Use technologies to enhance clinical teaching and learning
2. **Facilitate Learning in the Health Care Environment**
   B. Ground teaching strategies in educational theory and evidence-based teaching practices
   C. Use technology (e.g., simulation, learning management systems, EHR) skillfully to support the teaching-learning process
   D. Create opportunities for learners to develop critical thinking and clinical reasoning skills
   E. Promote a culture of safety and quality in the healthcare environment
   F. Create a positive and caring learning environment
5. **Facilitate Learner Development and Socialization**
   A. Mentor learners in the development of professional nursing behaviors, standards, and codes of ethics
   B. Promote a learning climate of respect for all
   C. Promote professional integrity and accountability
   F. Assist learners in effective use of self-assessment and professional goal setting for ongoing self- improvement
   H. Assist learners to develop the ability to engage in constructive peer feedback
   I. Inspire creativity and confidence
   K. Act as a role model for self-reflection, self-care, and coping skills
   M. Engage learners in applying best practices and quality improvement processes
6. **Implement Effective Clinical Assessment and Evaluation Strategies**
   A. Use a variety of strategies to determine achievement of learning outcomes
   B. Implement both formative and summative evaluation that is appropriate to the learner and learning outcomes
   D. Maintain integrity in the assessment and evaluation of learners
   E. Provide timely, objective, constructive, and fair feedback to learners

REFERENCES

Aebersold, M. (2018). Simulation-based learning: No longer a novelty in undergraduate education. *The Online Journal of Issues in Nursing, 23*(2). https://doi.org/10.3912/OJIN. Vol23No02PPT39

Commission on Collegiate Nursing Education. (2018). *Standards for accreditation of baccalaureate and graduate degree nursing programs.* https://www.aacnnursing.org/Portals/42/CCNE/PDF/Standards-Final-2018.pdf

Creighton University. (2020). Competency Evaluation Instrument. https://nursing.creighton.edu/academics/competency-evaluation-instrument

Curl, E., Smith, S., Chisholm, L., McGee, L., & Das, K. (2016). Effectiveness of integrated simulation and clinical experiences compared to traditional clinical experiences for nursing students. *Nursing Education Perspectives, 37*(2), 72–77.

Diaz, D. A., & Anderson, M. (2021). Structuring simulation-based education (SBE): From pre-simulation to debriefing. In P. R. Jeffries & National League for Nursing (Eds.), *Simulation in nursing education: From conceptualization to evaluation* (3rd ed., pp. 69–82). National League for Nursing.

Dreifuerst, K. T., Bradley, C. S., & Johnson, B. K. (2021). Debriefing: An essential component for learning in simulation pedagogy. In P. R. Jeffries & National League for Nursing (Eds.), *Simulation in nursing education: From conceptualization to evaluation* (3rd ed., pp. 45–68). National League for Nursing.

Forneris, S. G., & Fey, M. (2016). NLN vision: Teaching with simulation. In P. R. Jeffries (Ed.), *The NLN Jeffries simulation theory*. Wolters Kluwer.

Foronda, C. L., Fernandez-Burgos, M., Nadeau, C., Kelley, C. N., & Henry, M. N. (2020). Virtual simulation in nursing education: A systematic review spanning 1996 to 2018. *Simulation in Healthcare : Journal of the Society for Medical Simulation, 15*(1), 46–54. https://doi.org/10.1097/SIH.0000000000000411

Guise, V., & Wiig, S. (2016). Preparing for organizational change in home healthcare with simulation based training. *Clinical Simulation in Nursing, 12*, 496–503. https://doi.org/10.1016/j.ecns.2016.07.011

Haerling, K. (2018). Cost-utility analysis of virtual and mannequin-based simulation. *Simulation in Healthcare, 13*(1), 33–40. https://doi.org/10.1097/SIH.0000000000000280

Haerling, K. (2021). Simulation evaluation. In P. R. Jeffries & National League for Nursing (Eds.), *Simulation in nursing education: From conceptualization to evaluation* (3rd ed., pp. 83–99). National League for Nursing.

Hall, K., & Tori, K. (2016). Best practice recommendation for debriefing in simulation-based education for Australian undergraduate nursing students: An integrative review. *Clinical Simulation in Nursing, 13*, 39–50. https://doi.org/10.1016/j.ecns.2016.01.006

Hallmark, B. R., Thomas, C. M., & Gantt, L. (2016). The educational practices construct of the NLN/Jeffries simulation framework: State of the science. *Clinical Simulation in Nursing, 10*, 345–352. https://doi.org/10.10166/j.ecns.2013.04.006

Ham, K. (2016). Use of standardized patients to enhance simulation of medication administration. *Nurse Educator, 41*, 166–168. https://doi.org/10.1097/NNE.0000000000000248

Hansbrough, W., Dunker, K. S., Ross, J. G., & Ostendorf, M. (2020). Restrictions on nursing students' electronic health information access. *Nurse Educator, 45*(5), 243–247. https://doi.org/10.1097/NNE.0000000000000786

Hayden, J. K., Smiley, R. A., Alexander, M., Kardong-Edgren, S., & Jeffries, P. (2014). The NCSBN national simulation study: A longitudinal, randomized controlled study replacing clinical hours with simulation in prelicensure nursing education. *Journal of Nursing Regulation, 5*(2), S1–S64. https://doi.org/10.1016/S2155-8256(15)30062-4

Helwig, A., & Lomotan, E. (2016). *Can electronic health records prevent harm to patients?* https://www.ahrq.gov/news/blog/ahrqviews/020916.hmtl

INACSL Standards Committee (2016a). INACSL standards of best practice: Simulation[SM] Simulation design. *Clinical Simulation in Nursing, 12*(S), S5–S12. https://doi.org/10.1016/ j.ecns.2016.09.005

INACSL Standards Committee. (2016b). INACSL standards of best practice: Simulation[SM] Simulation glossary. *Clinical Simulation in Nursing, 12*(S), S39–S47. https://doi.org/10.1016/j.ecns.2016.09.012

INACSL Standards Committee. (2016c). INACSL standards of best practice: Simulation[SM] Debriefing. *Clinical Simulation in Nursing, 12*(S), S21–S25. https://doi.org/10.1016/j.ecns.2016.09.008

International Association for Clinical Simulation and Learning. (2021). *INACSL Standards of Best Practice: Simulation[©]*. https://www.inacsl.org/inacsl-standards-of-best-practice-simulation/

International Nursing Association for Clinical Simulation and Learning. (2020a). *International Nursing Association for Clinical Simulation and Learning and Society for Simulation in Healthcare Position statement on use of virtual simulation during the pandemic.* https://www.inacsl.org/INACSL/document-server/?cfp=INACSL/assets/File/public/covid-19/INACSL_SSH%20Position%20Paper%20FINAL.pdf

International Nursing Association for Clinical Simulation and Learning. (2020b). *Journal.* https://www.inacsl.org/clinical-simulation-in-nursing-journal/

Jeffries, P. R. (2021). *Simulation in nursing education: From conceptualization to evaluation* (3rd ed.). National League for Nursing.

Jeffries, P. R. (2016). *The NLN Jeffries simulation theory*. Wolters Kluwer.

Jeffries, P. R., Dreifuerst, K. T., & Haerling, K. A. (2022). Clinical simulations in nursing education: Overview, essentials, and the evidence. In M. H. Oermann, J. C. De Gagne, & B. C. Phillips (Eds.), *Teaching in nursing and role of the educator: The complete guide to best practice in teaching, evaluation, and curriculum development* (3rd ed., pp. 133–158). Springer Publishing Company.

Jeffries, P. R., Rodgers, B, & Adamson, K. (2015). NLN/ Jeffries Simulation Theory: Brief narrative description. *Nursing Education Perspectives, 36*(5), 292–293. https://doi.org/10.5480/1536-5026-36.5.292

Kardong-Edgren, S. (S.), Farra, S. L., Alinier, G., & Young, H. M. (2019). A call to unify definitions of virtual reality. *Clinical Simulation in Nursing, 31*(C), 28–34. https://doi.org/10.1016/j.ecns.2019.02.006

Kononowicz, A. A., Woodham, L. A., Edelbring, S., Stathakarou, N., Davies, D., Saxena, N., Tudor Car, L., Carlstedt-Duke, J., Car, J., & Zary, N. (2019). Virtual patient simulations in health professions education: Systematic review and meta-analysis by the Digital Health Education Collaboration. *Journal of Medical Internet Research, 21*(7), e14676. https://doi.org/10.2196/14676

Kunkel, C., Kopp, W., & Hanson, M. (2016). A matter of life and death: End-of-life simulation to develop confidence in nursing students. *Nursing Education Perspectives, 37*, 285–286. https://doi.org/10.1097/01.NEP.0000000000000029

Lasater, K. (2007). Clinical judgment development: Using simulation to create an assessment rubric. *Journal of Nursing Education, 46*(11), 496–503. https://doi.org/10.3928/01484834-20071101-04

Lioce L. (Ed.), Downing D., Chang T. P., Robertson J. M., Anderson M., Diaz D. A., & Spain A. E. (Assoc. Eds.) and the Terminology and Concepts Working Group. (2020). *Healthcare simulation dictionary – Second edition*. Agency for Healthcare Research and Quality. AHRQ Publication No. 20-0019. https://doi.org/10.23970/simulationv2

Lopreiato, J. O., Downing, D., Gammon, W., Lioce, L., Sittner, B., Slot, V., Spain, A. E. (Eds.), Terminology and Concepts Working Group. (2016). *Healthcare simulation dictionary*. http://www.ssih.org/dictionary

MacLean, S., Kelly, M., Geddes, F., & Della, P. (2017). Use of simulated patients to develop communication skills in nursing education: An integrative review. *Nurse Education Today, 48*, 90–98. https://doi.org/10.1016/j.nedt.2016.09.018

Manning, S. J., Skiff, D. M., Santiago, L. P., & Irish, A. (2016). Nursing and social work trauma simulation: Exploring an interprofessional approach. *Clinical Simulation in Nursing, 12*, 555–564. https://doi.org/10.1016/j.ecns.2016.07.004

McDermott, D. S. (2020,). Prebriefing: A historical perspective and evolution of a model and strategy (Know: Do: Teach). *Clinical Simulation in Nursing, 49*(C), 40–49. https://doi.org/10.1016/j.ecns.2020.05.005.

National League for Nursing. (2020). *Faculty programs & resources: Leadership development program for simulation educators*. http://www.nln.org/centers-for-nursing-education/nln-center-for-transformational-leadership2/leadership-institute2/leadership-development-program-for-simulation-educators

National League for Nursing. (2021). *Simulation innovation resource center*. http://sirc.nln.org

Page, R. (2016). Lessons from aviation simulation. In R. H. Riley (Ed.), *Manual of simulation in healthcare*. ProQuest Ebook Central. https://ebookcentral.proquest.com

Pastor, D. K., Cunningham, R. P., White, P. H., & Kolomer, S. (2016). We have to talk: Results of an interprofessional clinical simulation in delivering bad health news in palliative care. *Clinical Simulation in Nursing, 12*, 320–327. https://doi.org/10.1016j.ecns.2016.03.005

Sarmasoglu, S., Dinc, L., & Elcin, M. (2016). Using standardized patients in nursing education: Effects on students' psychomotor skill development. *Nurse Educator, 41*, e1–e5. https://doi.org/10.1097/NNE.0000000000000188

Shearer, J. N. (2016). Anxiety, nursing students and simulation: State of the science. *Journal of Nursing Education, 55*, 551–554. https://doi.org/10.3928/01484834-20160914-02

Slater, L. Z., Bryant, K., & Ng, V. (2016). Nursing student perceptions of standardized patient use in health assessment. *Clinical Simulation in Nursing, 12*, 368–376. https://doi.org/10.1016/j.ecns.2016.04.007

Smiley, R. (2019). Survey of simulation use in prelicensure nursing programs: Changes and advancements, 2010–2017. *Journal of Nursing Regulation, 9*(4), 48–61. http://dx.doi.org/10.1016/S2155-8256(19)30016-X

Society for Simulation in Healthcare. (2020). *About SSH*. https://www.ssih.org/About-SSH

Sullivan, N., Swoboda, S. M., Breymier, T., Lucas, L., Sarasnick, J., Rutherford-Hemming, T., Budhathoki, C., & Kardong-Edgren, S. (S.) (2019). Emerging evidence toward a 2:1 clinical to simulation ratio: A study comparing the traditional clinical and simulation settings. *Clinical Simulation in Nursing, 30* (C), 34–41. https://doi.org/10.1016/j.ecns.2019.03.003

Tanner, C. (2006). Thinking like a nurse: A research-based model of clinical judgment in nursing. *Journal of Nursing Education, 45*(6), 204–211. https://doi.org/10.3928/01484834-20060601-04

Veltri, L., Kaakinen, J. R., Shillam, C., Arwood, E., & Bell, K. (2016). Controlled post-partum newborn simulation with objective evaluation exchanged for clinical learning. *Clinical Simulation in Nursing, 12*, 177–186. https://doi.org/10.1016/j.ecns.2016.01.005

Verkuyl, M., Lapum, J. L., St-Amant, O., Hughes, M., Romaniuk, D., & McCulloch, T. (2020, March). Exploring debriefing combinations after a virtual simulation. *Clinical Simulation in Nursing, 40*(C), 36–42. https://doi.org/10.1016/j.ecns.2019.12.002

A robust set of instructor resources designed to supplement this text is located at http://connect.springerpub.com/content/book/978-0-8261-6705-7. Qualifying instructors may request access by emailing textbook@springerpub.com.

Pedagogical Technologies in Clinical Education

Meigan Robb

Practice experiences that occur in the clinical learning environment provide critical opportunities for nursing students to apply theory to practice and demonstrate the essential skills of clinical judgment and clinical reasoning. Advances in technology have permeated the healthcare environment resulting in the need for clinical nurse educators to rethink current practices to best prepare students to meet their future role demands. A national survey of nursing education programs found technology is currently being used for measuring learning outcomes and redesigning learning spaces (Forneris & Tiffany, 2017). Incorporating pedagogical technologies in clinical education should be an ongoing process that reflects best practices while also connecting students to emerging technology that can advance healthcare. Technology should support students and nurses in gathering data and delivering high-quality healthcare (American Association of Colleges of Nursing, 2021). Nursing leaders and educators need to thoughtfully incorporate technology that supports learning complex skills and that develops the competencies demanded of today's healthcare professionals.

This chapter explores technologies for clinical teaching, including simulated electronic health records (EHRs), telepresence, telehealth, electronic escape rooms, and other technology-related approaches. Suggestions are provided for how clinical nurse educators can use these technologies in clinical teaching. This chapter also includes virtual clinical learning experiences and how educators responded with technology use to COVID-19.

TECHNOLOGY USE IN CLINICAL TEACHING

Clinical skills for nursing students have traditionally been cultivated through a combination of laboratory activities and direct observation of skills in actual clinical practice. Over time, nursing students gradually increase their role and responsibility for the care of patients under the supervision of nurse educators and clinical staff. However, current students are accustomed to multimedia environments and expect that educators will integrate technology into the curriculum and not rely on traditional and possibly outdated teaching approaches.

Clinical courses are incorporating more online and other educational technology. However, the range extends from technology as a flashy add-on resource to the incorporation of technology as the major form of instructional delivery and skill practice. Since many nurse educators lack a model of online teaching to follow and may not have the benefit of observation of online instruction, they are frequently creating their own approach to technology integration through trial and error. They learn about new technology and incorporate that into their courses. Or, external forces, such as the COVID-19 pandemic, have forced them to embrace technology for learning. This haphazard approach may lead to fragmented and unsatisfactory learning experiences.

To facilitate effective online educational approaches, nurse educators can benefit from a backward design model. Clinical educators can begin planning for teaching by focusing on the essential learning goals. They should consider the critical elements that students should learn by the end of the clinical course. What should students be able to do by the end of the experience? Then, they can design learning experiences that help students achieve that goal (Darby & Lang, 2019). Successful adoption of technology also requires nurse educators to consider how technology can be utilized to create a holistic learning environment where students are actively engaged in the content being taught (Skiba, 2017). Access to unlimited online resources for learning supports a change in the clinical teacher's role from the direct provider of information to a facilitator and co-learner. Udermann (2017) suggests students require four distinct approaches from educators when facilitating learning with online technology:

1. Create easy to follow design and navigation. Students can become confused when they do not know where to start an activity. Presenting information in a clear and consistent format can provide a comfort level for students, decreasing confusion and apprehension throughout the learning experience.
2. Offer clear expectations and directions. Providing clear instructions that state what is expected of students reduces their confusion and frustration. Having an awareness of performance requirements improves student learning and keeps them engaged in the learning environment.
3. Provide timely responses to questions. Activities in the online environment are usually asynchronous, meaning that students participate independently from each other and the teacher. This physical separation slows communication between the teacher and student and can contribute to a student's frustration when seeking assistance. Stating response times (e.g., within 24 hours of receiving an email) tells students when they can expect to receive answers.
4. Establish online presence. Students may feel isolated from the teacher due to the asynchronous format of the online environment. Engaging in online dialogue with the students by regularly participating in activities, providing feedback, and sending electronic reminders can help improve instructor presence.

Successful adoption of technology in clinical teaching can be enhanced by identifying *technology stewards* or *superusers*. These technology champions help their community of learners choose, organize, and apply technology to meet their needs. It is not unusual that students show leadership in joining the team of technology champions, supporting their peers and teachers in beginning use of technology and in troubleshooting problems. Technology champions need a clear understanding of their learning community so they can respond to both expressed and implied needs. It is helpful if these champions demonstrate technology expertise. Still, even an awareness of possibilities and available products is sufficient to trigger the process of finding others who can help with the selection and installation of more complex programs or equipment. During the adoption of new technology, champions serve the leadership functions of managing the direction and pace of the change. Once a new technology is implemented into practice, these technology stewards or superusers may support upgrading practices and new technology applications in response to emerging needs (Ravert et al., 2020).

Clinical teachers who like to try out new ideas are often natural technology champions, but a team approach supports the successful implementation of more complex systems. Benefits to the clinical teacher of taking on the technology champion role include:

- The satisfaction of moving an initiative forward that does not otherwise have a leader.
- The impact of improving learning or educational practices.
- The opportunity for developing leadership, teaching, and technical skills.
- Enhanced reputation and credibility in both the academic and practice settings.

SELECTING TECHNOLOGY

There are strategies that clinical nurse educators can use to facilitate technology integration into teaching and to promote success with online learning approaches. Educational technology is a tool; finding the right tool or tools for the purpose is vital in selecting pedagogical technology. Clinical teachers who want to incorporate pedagogical technologies into their courses should consider the course objectives and the characteristics of the learners. Start small with easy-to-implement and straightforward strategies rather than a complete course redesign. For example, begin with one electronic post-clinical conference activity using a known technology system rather than switching to an entirely new delivery system and changing activities and technology for an entire course. Test out the planned technology and practice using it before wide-scale implementation. Ask a friend, student, or faculty colleague to try the technology in a practice situation before launching the technology activity with all students. Seek technology training that may be available from product distributors, online support, or campus technology personnel. Select strategies that foster student engagement, stimulate intellectual development, and build rapport (Chunta et al., 2021).

Some technological tools can serve multiple learning support functions and some learning objectives can be supported by more than one tool. For example, simulation and virtual reality–based learning provide experiential learning in contextually rich environments where learners can interact and engage with patients in the virtual environment. They can develop critical thinking and clinical decision making while reflecting and reframing their understanding of clinical practice (Forneris, 2020). Teachers can select virtual environments that reflect real-world best practices while exploring ethical issues and professional boundaries. Environments that support learning activities designed to replicate authentic clinical practice settings should be seen and treated as clinical environments. These environments may support and provide a foundation for learning during future clinical experiences.

Clinical teachers can also choose to use technology that is already familiar to students, such as social networking sites, to facilitate clinical learning. For example, the teacher might establish a Twitter account, separate from their personal account, and use the privacy settings to make tweets visible only to a specific group of students (all of whom must have Twitter accounts). Using this account, the clinical educator can teach followers mini-lessons and update them on relevant topics. The teacher may maximize teachable moments that occur outside of the clinical learning environment, such as sharing a new idea from a conference, alerting students to the publication of a relevant article in a current issue of a professional nursing journal, or suggesting that students view a particular television show that relates to content they are studying. The clinical teacher might send a weekly tweet to students with a question or brainteaser about the competencies they are attempting to master. For students who have clinical learning activities in diverse settings, the clinical teacher may use Twitterchat to conduct post-clinical conferences at a predetermined time. As the moderator, the teacher posts questions (designated as Q1, Q2, and so forth) to prompt responses from students (labeled R1, R2, and so forth) and facilitate discussion among participants. Media dashboard tools such as Hootsuite and Tweetdeck can help the teacher serve as chat host and can also assist in scheduling social media posts and track chat conversations.

Students and clinical instructors may prefer to engage in electronic discussions without the use of social media. Learning management systems provide a venue for interactive discussions among the clinical instructor and students. These discussions can allow students to reflect and comment upon experiences, pose questions, and dialogue with clinical classmates in a secure environment. They may work well for clinical conferencing activities that do not require an immediate response from others. However, sometimes a clinical teacher or student may want quick access to support, ask clarification questions, or dialogue about a clinical situation. In those instances, text messaging services may be an appropriate alternative. Educators should exercise caution with text messaging to ensure compliance with the Health Insurance Portability and Accountability Act (HIPAA). Precautions should take place to guarantee that personal patient information is not messaged. Secure HIPAA compliant text messaging services for healthcare providers such as the free application, Athena text, allow for streamlined, connected, and secure text messaging among clinical students and instructors (Serembus et al., 2020).

Most educational technology is a resource and a means to an end, a tool rather than an intended program outcome. There is no requirement for selecting the most elaborate technology to support clinical learning; expensive and complicated materials and plans may not be a better fit than simple and inexpensive materials and methods for supporting a particular clinical objective. An intensive effort to use specific nonclinical technology to complete a single assignment is generally not worthwhile from the perspective of either the students or the teacher. Clinical teachers should take care that even while striving to support students in using new technology learning tools, the teachers should not trade their responsibility of facilitating learning based on the clinical objectives for a full-time role as the technology support specialist.

Mastering technology that learners will continue to use through their working careers, such as EHRs, may be a worthwhile learning outcome. However, a focus on the specific technology rather than the learning objectives can lead to a misguided instructional effort.

Before choosing technology for clinical teaching, the educator should reflect on the learning objectives and the intended types of interactions to support achieving those objectives. For example, a teacher's plan that learners will create a product such as a patient education pamphlet or an electronic clinical portfolio suggests tools such as design or presentation software. In contrast, a plan to have learners practice clinical decision making might benefit from human patient simulation, virtual reality simulations, or online case study analysis. Table 10.1 provides suggested technology that aligns with the educational intention. Using this table, clinical educators can determine the intention of the learning activity and then select the most appropriate technology approach.

ELECTRONIC HEALTH RECORDS

EHRs are used across most hospitals in the United States and serve as a vital tool for managing patient information and care (Wilbanks & Langford, 2019). Nursing students need to be prepared to use these electronic systems for documentation, to search for information, and to develop essential information technology skills expected of graduates. However, some clinical agencies have policies preventing students and clinical faculty from accessing or entering data in the EHR (Baxter & Andrew, 2018; Sweeney et al., 2019).

Educators have identified several solutions to support nursing students in learning electronic documentation and data review. Nursing schools can lease or purchase simulated EHRs like those found in hospitals and ambulatory health settings; however, simulated EHRs can be costly. An academic institution can develop its own academic electronic health record (AEHR), but this approach requires significant time, technology expertise, and support services (Herbert & Connors, 2016).

Another way to gain healthcare facility EHR access involves the development of a partnership with a specific healthcare organization. These partnering agencies may offer repeated immersive clinical learning experiences for students and may provide in-depth training for EHR use. Orientation to an EHR can sometimes take days of training but partnerships can guarantee that students that receive training will engage in repeated clinical experiences at this agency. Through repeated

TABLE 10.1 SELECTING TECHNOLOGY TO SUPPORT EDUCATIONAL STRATEGIES

Educational Intention	Related Technology
Direct experience	Electronic health records, virtual reality environments, e-learning modules, telepresence, telehealth, multiplayer online role-playing games, electronic escape rooms, virtual case simulations, high-fidelity simulation
Discussion/reflection	Online discussion boards, virtual chat, video conferencing, telepresence, social media sites
Project production	Software or online sites for design and publishing or producing presentations, video recording, posting, and commenting sites
Information access	Websites, mobile applications, online newspapers and journals, pre-recorded or real-time presentations
Drill and practice	Quizzing software, electronic response systems or polling software, online/digital flashcards, knowledge-based games

exposure to the clinical agency and the site-specific EHR system, students begin to develop a familiarity with the operations and the technology used at the clinical site. They gain insight and knowledge about EHR use, thereby making these graduates attractive potential employees as they may require less training upon hiring.

The selection of an AEHR requires significant research and thought to meet the needs of the students, faculty, and the curriculum. The AEHR chosen should provide realism for the students learning to read health documents and allow the students to document a simulated or clinical patient assessment. Faculty should have the opportunity to evaluate the AEHR before a purchase decision. The AEHR selected should provide upgrades and program-specific requests, such as integrating bar-code technology to increase patient safety and decrease medication errors (Baxter & Andrew, 2018).

Educators can plan strategies to help make the implementation of an AEHR successful and meaningful for the faculty and the students. An AEHR can be integrated across all curriculum levels to complete assignments such as planning care or developing written situation, background, assessment, recommendation (SBAR) reports. Clinical faculty can begin to implement EHRs in nursing programs by having students review the health records developed for simulation patients in the school's AEHR. Students can search the records for the information needed to provide safe patient care; for example, allergies, diagnostic test results, and medications. They also can document the simulation assessment and any interventions performed during the simulation in the AEHR.

The use of an AEHR as a teaching strategy across various learning environments (e.g., classroom, skills lab, simulation lab) exposes students to different situations that will improve their professional role readiness (Badowski et al., 2018). Incorporating repetitive practice opportunities with EHRs is necessary for nursing students to become competent in utilizing these systems within the clinical environment (Badowski et al., 2018). Sweeney et al. (2019) suggest creating shared content by integrating simulated EHR patients across multiple courses in a single semester. This approach reinforces essential content and allows students to become more familiar and competent with electronic documentation.

Several barriers exist to using AEHRs for clinical teaching in nursing education. Frequently identified barriers include limited access to funding for AEHR integration and the associated costs of AEHR purchases. Faculty may resist the change and/or may not have adequate faculty training, limited to no release time for learning, and insufficient ongoing support for use. Shifting from traditional learning activities to meaningful AEHR activities requires significant time and effort for faculty. Additionally, technology issues such as Internet connectivity, inadequate backup systems, and software incompatibility create further implementation challenges (Mollart et al., 2020).

It is important to have a strategic plan to address the barriers before implementing an AEHR. Involving faculty in planning and implementation while providing ongoing support and training will help engage faculty in AEHR use. Successful implementation requires strong administrative support and access to funding for AEHR implementation costs (Herbert & Connors, 2016). Nursing programs that successfully use EHRs often have a program champion who has positive attitudes toward technology and can serve as a change leader and an early adopter. These program champions are faculty or staff members familiar with the program and can provide initial training and refresher courses while also serving as a resource to both faculty and students.

VIRTUAL LEARNING

Virtual learning, a learning experience that is enhanced by computers and/or Internet use, creates opportunities for students to gain clinical experiences outside of the traditional face-to-face clinical setting (MacRae et al., 2021). These learning experiences span a continuum from a simple case study delivered in an online format to more elaborate and technologically sophisticated learning involving video-based interactive simulated learning experiences. One advantage of these virtual learning experiences is they can be structured for flexibility and self-direction. Instructors can allow students to complete virtual clinical activities at their own pace and permit students to engage in repeated practice and mastery of the virtual learning activity.

One virtual learning approach that clinical teachers can use involves creating an e-learning module contained in a learning management system. These e-learning modules address one or two topics and use various teaching tools (e.g., videos, web-links, narratives, games), self-directed activities, and assessment approaches that students complete independently. The clinical teacher can use e-learning modules to prepare students for pre- and post-conference activities or other learning experiences. As an example, a module can be created that addresses the topic of cardiovascular disease. Students complete the module before starting their scheduled clinical day. Embedded web links and videos presenting lifestyle modifications, medications, and diet will further reinforce course content. In a virtual discussion, the clinical teacher can ask probing questions that require student engagement and demonstration of clinical judgment and clinical reasoning. Using these online discussions will facilitate the interleaving of classroom and clinical learning experiences and assist in applying theory to practice. Students' answers to provided discussion questions can serve as a starting point for critical dialogue during a post-conference session. E-learning modules would be applicable for all student levels and across all clinical areas. Logan et al. (2021) described using virtual e-learning modules as a self-paced supplemental resource to enhance student engagement with content, and better prepare them for simulated pediatric scenarios.

Virtual learning opportunities also solve some of the limitations associated with limited clinical learning spaces. For example, students can access virtual activities without the time and cost of traveling to clinical sites. The virtual environment also allows students to have experiences that may not exist during an actual clinical rotation. For example, students may not have an opportunity to engage in neonatal intensive care unit activities, but the development and use of a virtual reality learning activity that simulates high-risk neonatal infection allow students to repetitively practice these needed clinical and problem-solving skills (Yu & Mann, 2021). Implementing such learning with simulated patients in a virtual environment allows each student to have a similar experience at a predetermined level of complexity.

Telepresence

Clinical learning experiences can present challenges when the virtual activity requires students to interact synchronously from different locations. Telepresence is a modality that can extend the nuances and presence of face-to-face clinical interactions to a virtual learning experience. Telepresence technology allows remote students to feel as if they are physically present with their peers without distance being a barrier. Rudolph et al. (2017) described telepresence as an effective method to promote engagement, satisfaction, and self-confidence when completing clinical learning activities. Telepresence is most commonly incorporated using a robot in simulated clinical learning experiences when students are participating both in-person and remotely (Mudd et al., 2020; Rudolph et al., 2017). A telepresence robot is a roaming remote-controlled wheeled device with a screen that allows for face-to-face real-time interactions among the teacher, in-person students, and remote students (Mudd et al., 2020). This pedagogical technology requires remote students to use a computer with a webcam and Internet connection to control the robot and participate in the clinical activity.

There are many benefits of using telepresence technology as a clinical teaching strategy. Incorporating telepresence creates an immersive opportunity that moves remote students from being observers to engaged learners. Remote students who participate in simulated activities via telepresence versus cloud-based audio-video communications report feeling more present and engaged in the virtual learning activity (Dang et al., 2019). Telepresence also creates unique learning opportunities for students that support their development of effective communication and collaborative problem-solving skills. Rudolph et al. (2017) suggested using telepresence technologies to develop interprofessional learning opportunities for undergraduate prelicensure students and nurse practitioner students for simulated activities. Providing exposure to telepresence technologies during clinical learning equips students with knowledge and experience to function in the complex healthcare environment.

Telehealth

Like telepresence, telehealth is an emerging technology gaining a routine presence in healthcare. In nursing, telehealth involves the remote monitoring of patients, the delivery of patient education, and the facilitation of consultations through audio and video communications (Mataxen & Webb, 2019). Face-to-face clinical encounters can be supplemented or enhanced with virtual and electronic experiences. Wynn (2019) described the incorporation of telehealth technologies into a psychiatric mental health nursing clinical course as an innovative way for students to gain psychosocial interviewing and assessment skills with clients at remote locations. Although faced with some technology challenges of security settings and firewalls, students positively evaluated their learning and improved understanding of health informatics. Other research on telehealth use for clinical nursing education supports positive learning outcomes. For example, participating in a telehealth simulation of a homebound geriatric client improved students' self-reported confidence, competency in screening, assessment, and patient education (Lister et al., 2018).

Many clinical education settings provide culturally limited environments. Virtual encounters may offer an opportunity to prepare learners for actual encounters with patients and colleagues in real clinical settings. Educators can infuse diversity and inclusion learning concepts into telehealth experiences to aid in the training and developing of culturally competent healthcare providers (Hilty et al., 2021). Exposure to different cultural backgrounds in the virtual setting helps nursing students learn how to interact in new and often uncomfortable contexts. For example, a clinical teacher could utilize interactive video conferencing technology to create a simulated telehealth environment using standardized patients. Students can explore the nurse's role in providing end-of-life care and practice therapeutic communication skills. Or virtual learning activities could be structured with different cultural groups or clients with different social beliefs.

Experiences in virtual or other technological environments with the potential to evoke strong emotional responses should include both thoughtful preparation activities and guided debriefing/reflection sessions. Preparation for what to expect and how to behave in a virtual environment reduces student anxiety and focuses on the intended outcomes. Facilitated reflection on the virtual telehealth experience may help students develop understanding and skills related to culture, diversity, and sensitive topics that they can bring to the clinical practicum setting. Debriefing after the experience helps ensure that students and teachers meet targeted learning objectives and encourages further reflection.

VIRTUAL GAME-BASED LEARNING

The current generation of nursing students—digital natives—expects technology to be incorporated in learning activities and prefers individualized, engaging, and technologically enhanced experiences (Chicca & Shellenbarger, 2018). Virtual game-based learning represents a clinical teaching tool capable of engaging students through interaction based on narratives, decision-making processes, rewards, and consequences. Virtual games are often used in conjunction with simulation. An integrative review of game elements used for assessing students' experiences in learning clinical reasoning with simulation games revealed that the mechanics (space, time, feedback, and action), story, aesthetics (immersive, realistic, and authentic), and technology format are essential to game element considerations. Most of the reviewed simulated games involved students assuming the nurse's role and collecting information or addressing a clinical problem. However, few of the reviewed games contained all essential game elements. Clinical educators are encouraged to select gaming approaches that provide realistic and authentic storylines that offer appropriate learning opportunities and serve a purpose beyond entertainment (Havola et al., 2020).

Narratives provide valuable cues in virtual game-based learning to direct student performance in the virtual world. The teacher can think of the narrative as the background information provided to students during a virtual game-based learning experience. However, instead of the teacher simply providing the patient's history by reading it aloud to students, the virtual scenario unfolds based on the students' interaction with the environment. Storylines also provide spaces for reflection on the consequences of one's decisions. The virtual world can offer different narrative endings from multiple perspectives based on learners' ongoing interactions with their environments. In this way, students can engage in deliberate decision making that will produce varying scenario outcomes. Learners can be encouraged to see the consequences of action or inaction from multiple perspectives.

When students care for patients in a clinical setting, they do not have the luxury of revisiting the same clinical encounter to make a better or different decision. Virtual game-based learning environments allow students to take responsibility for their choices in a situated and safe context. Teachers can monitor students' progress as they adjust their behavior and decision making to negotiate more acceptable outcomes. For students engaged in virtual game-based learning, an error simply becomes an opportunity for reflection, learning, and potential behavior change.

Electronic Escape Rooms

The use of escape rooms in education has gained popularity since being introduced in Japan in 2007 (Garwood, 2020) and are viewed as a helpful learning tool (Gutiérrez-Puertas et al., 2020). Traditionally, when used in nursing education, escape rooms are structured around a face-to-face simulated learning activity. Students are provided with a clinically based storyline and determine answers to immersive problems and challenges to find clues that can unlock a series of boxes. Students can use mobile devices to retrieve web-based resources to support the application of evidence-based practice for solving scenarios related to assessment skills, medication administration, and topic-specific nursing interventions. Escape rooms, when developed appropriately, support specific learning outcomes (Garwood, 2020), facilitate teamwork and collaboration (Haley & Palmer, 2020), and serve as a method for formative evaluation (Oermann & Gaberson, 2021).

The clinical teacher can apply the design principles of a traditional escape room to support a virtual learning experience. Electronic escape rooms are developed using web-page survey administration software. Students' progression through the electronic escape room is managed by skip-logic pathways that serve as locks (Dobbs, n.d.). For example, an escape room challenge might require students to select three medications from a list of drugs appropriate to treat a patient exhibiting symptoms of peptic ulcer disease. The first letter of each correct medication serves as the code to unlock the virtual box. When the code is entered correctly, skip logic directs the students to the next challenge. If the code is entered incorrectly, skip logic will direct the students back to repeat the challenge. The clinical teacher can review the results and determine what content areas need further instruction and more clinical practica. Electronic escape rooms can be incorporated into asynchronous or synchronous virtual learning experiences. For example, using an electronic escape room in an e-learning module as an asynchronous learning activity can be a helpful tool to reinforce specific learner competencies. Or forming small groups of students who use video conference break-out rooms to solve escape room challenges may support synchronous learning and the development of communication, teamwork, and collaborative practice skills.

RESPONSE TO COVID-19

Clinical education quickly changed with the emergence of COVID-19. The educational impact of the global pandemic required educators to swiftly transition in-person clinical learning experiences to exclusively virtual environments. Clinical teachers were forced to quickly select innovative methods and use technology to offer appropriate learning experiences outside of traditional care settings. The lack of available clinical sites resulted in many educators selecting virtual learning platforms from textbook publishers or other companies to facilitate the demonstration of required clinical competencies (Mariani et al., 2020). Virtual clinical education using modalities such as telehealth and faculty skills instruction using video conferencing technology provided an alternative for some programs (Shea & Rovera, 2021). Other approaches used to develop critical clinical competencies included unfolding cases and video teleconferencing to support immersive experiences and dialogue between the clinical teacher and students (Oermann, 2020). Clinical teachers used interactive video technology such as Zoom™ for Socratic questioning and engagement with students in live discussions about clinical learning topics (Konrad et al., 2021).

Dewart et al. (2020) and Yancey (2020) suggest nursing programs reflect on lessons learned from these clinical teaching transitions to best plan for future learning experiences. Clinical teachers should consider new ways of extending traditional learning as part of the preparation of nurses. During the pandemic, the experiences of clinical educators highlighted the need for teachers to become aware of and comfortable integrating various pedagogical technologies in clinical education. As clinical educators look to future technology trends, they should consider advances such as biometric sensors and wearable technology, technology-enhanced patient engagement, cloud computing, and big data (Risling, 2017). Nurse educators should consider current and emerging technology and how they can be integrated into clinical education to prepare students and graduates to face anticipated clinical issues and challenges.

SUMMARY

Advances in technology require clinical nurse educators to rethink current practices to best prepare students to meet their future role demands. Today's learners are accustomed to multimedia environments and expect technology integration into their curricula. Clinical teachers can serve as technology stewards in adopting effective tools for teaching and learning. Careful curricular integration and ongoing evaluation of technology-supported activities help promote positive learning outcomes. Using pedagogical technologies that incorporate virtual learning, such as telepresence, telehealth, and virtual game-based learning in clinical education, can enhance clinical virtual learning opportunities. Technology supported learning activities can expand boundaries beyond cultures, professions, and locations and help cultivate needed critical thinking and clinical-judgment skills. The COVID-19 pandemic accelerated the use of virtual learning and provided educators with issues to consider for future clinical teaching.

CNE® EXAMINATION TEST BLUEPRINT CORE COMPETENCIES

1. **Facilitate Learning**
   A. Implement a variety of teaching strategies appropriate to
      1. content
      2. setting
      3. learner needs
      4. learning style
      5. desired learner outcomes
   B. Use teaching strategies based on
      1. educational theory
      2. evidence-based practices related to education
   C. Modify teaching strategies and learning experiences based on consideration of learners'
      2. past clinical experiences
      3. past educational and life experiences
      4. generational groups (i.e., age)

    D. Use information technologies to support the teaching–learning process

    N. Use knowledge of evidence-based practice to instruct learners

2. **Facilitate Learner Development and Socialization**

    B. Provide resources for diverse learners to meet their individual learning needs

    D. Create learning environments that facilitate learners' self-reflection, personal goal-setting, and socialization to the role of the nurse

    E. Foster the development of learners in these areas

        1. cognitive domain

        2. psychomotor domain

        3. affective domain

6. **Engage in Scholarship, Service, and Leadership**

    A. Function as a change agent and leader

        4. Implement strategies for change within the nursing program

        6. Adapt to changes created by external factors

CNE®cl EXAMIANTION TEST BLUEPRINT CORE COMPETENCIES

1. **Function within the Education and Health Care Environments**

    A. Function in the Clinical Educator Role

        3. Use technologies to enhance clinical teaching and learning

    B. Operationalize the Curriculum

        2. Plan meaningful and relevant clinical learning assignments and activities

        4. Prepare learners for clinical experiences (e.g., facility, clinical expectations, equipment, and technology-based resources)

        7. Provide opportunities for learners to develop problem-solving and clinical reasoning skills related to course objectives (e.g., learning outcomes)

2. **Facilitate Learning in the Health Care Environment**

    C. Use technology (e.g., simulation, learning management systems, electronic health records) skillfully to support the teaching-learning process

4. **Apply Clinical Expertise in the Health Care Environment**

    H. Demonstrate competence with a range of technologies available in the clinical learning environment

5. **Facilitate Learner Development and Socialization**

    G. Create learning environments that are focused on socialization to the role of the nurse

6. **Implement Effective Clinical and Assessment Evaluation Strategies**

    A. Use a variety of strategies to determine achievement of learning outcomes

    B. Implement both formative and summative evaluation that is appropriate to the learner and learning outcomes

    F. Use learner data to enhance the teaching-learning process in the clinical learning environment

    K. Evaluate the quality of the clinical learning experiences and environment

REFERENCES

American Association of Colleges of Nursing. (2021). *The essentials: Core competencies for professional nursing education.* https://www.aacnnursing.org/Portals/42/AcademicNursing/pdf/Essentials-2021.pdf

Badowski, D., Horsley, T. L., Rossler, K. L., Mariani, B., & Gonzalez, L. (2018). Electronic charting during simulation: A descriptive study. *CIN: Computers, Informatics, Nursing, 36*(9), 430–437. https://doi.org/10.1097/CIN.0000000000000457

Baxter, P. M., & Andrew, L. A. (2018). Successful integration of an academic electronic health records into the curriculum of an associate degree nursing program. *Nursing Education Perspectives, 39*(4), 250–251. https://doi.org/10.1097.01.NEP.0000000000000255

Chicca, J., & Shellenbarger, T. (2018). Connecting with Generation Z: Approaches in nursing education. *Teaching and Learning in Nursing, 13*(3), 180–184. https://doi.org/10.1016/j.teln.2018.03.008

Chunta, K., Shellenbarger, T., & Chicca, J. (2021). Generation Z students in the online environment: Strategies for nurse educators. *Nurse Educator, 46*(2), 87–91. https://doi.org/10.1097/NNE.0000000000000872

Dang, B. K., O'Leary-Kelley, C., Palicte, J. S., Badheka, S., & Vuppalapati, C. (2019). Comparing virtual reality telepresence and traditional simulation methods: A pilot study. *Nursing Education Perspectives, 41*(2), 119–121. https://doi.org/10.1097/01.NEP.0000000000000496

Darby, F., & Lang, J. M. (2019). *Small teaching online: Applying learning science in online classes.* Jossey-Bass.

Dewart, G., Corcoran, L., Thirsk, L., & Petrovic, K. (2020). Nursing education in a pandemic: Academic challenges in response to COVID-19. *Nurse Education Today, 92,* 104471. https://doi.org/10.1016/j.nedt.2020.104471

Dobbs, M. (n.d.). How to build a digital escape room using Google Forms. *Bespoke ELA.* https://www.bespokeclassroom.com/blog/2019/10/4/how-to-build-a-digital-escape-room-using-google-forms

Forneris, S. (2020). Teaching and learning using simulation. In D. M. Billings & J. A. Halstead (Eds.), *Teaching in nursing: A guide for faculty* (6th ed., pp. 353–373). Elsevier.

Forneris, S., & Tiffany, J. (2017). Future of technology in nursing education part 2: How nursing education programs are currently using educational technology. *NLN Nursing Edge.* https://www.wolterskluwer.com/en/expert-insights/future-of-technology-in-nursing-education-part-2-how-nursing-education-programs-are-currently-using?utm_landingPage=https://www.wolterskluwer.com/en/expert-insights/future-of-technology-in-nursing-education-part-2-how-nursing-education-programs-are-currently-using

Garwood, J. (2020). Escape to learn! An innovative approach to engage students in learning. *Journal of Nursing Education, 59*(5), 278–282. https://doi.org/10.3928/01484834-20200422-08

Gutiérrez-Puertas, L., Márquez-Hernández, V. V., Román-López, P., Rodríquez-Arrastia, M. J., Ropero-Padilla, C., & Molina-Torres, G. (2020). Escape rooms as a clinical evaluation method for nursing students. *Clinical Simulation in Nursing, 49*(2020), 73–80. https://doi.org/10.1016/j.ecns.2020.05.010

Haley, B., & Palmer, J. (2020). Escape tasks: An innovative approach in nursing education. *Journal of Nursing Education, 59*(1), 655–657. https://doi.org/10.3928/01484834-20201020-11

Havola, S., Koivisto, J., Mäkinen, H., & Haavisto, E. (2020). Game elements and instruments for assessing nursing students' experiences in learning clinical reasoning by using simulation games: An integrative review. *Clinical Simulation in Nursing, 46*(2020), 1–14. https://doi.org/10/1016/j.ecns.2020.04.003

Herbert, V. M., & Connors, H. (2016). Integrating an academic electronic health record: Challenges and success strategies. *Computers, Informatics, Nursing, 34*(8), 345–354. https://doi.org/10.1097/CIN.0000000000000264

Hilty, D. M., Crawford, A., Teshima, J., Nasatir-Hilty, S. E., Luo, J., Chisler, L. S. M., Gutierrez Hilty, Y. S. M., Servis, M. E., Godbout, R., Lim, R. F., & Lu, F. G. (2021). Mobile health and cultural competencies as a foundation for telehealthcare: Scoping review. *Journal of Technology in Behavioral Science, 6,* 197–230. https://doi.org/10.1007/s41347-020-00180-5

Konrad, S., Fitzgerald, A., & Deckers, C. (2021). Nursing fundamentals—Supporting clinical competency online during the COVID-19 pandemic. *Teaching and Learning in Nursing, 16*(1), 53–56. https://doi.org.10.1016/j.teln.2020.07.005

Lister, M., Vaughn, J., Brennan-Cook, J., Molloy, M., Kuszajewski, M., & Shaw, R. J. (2018). Telehealth and telenursing using simulation for pre-licensure USA students. *Nurse Education in Practice, 29*(1), 59–63. https://doi.org/10.1016/j.nepr.2017.10.031

Logan, R. M., Johnson, C. E., & Worsham, J. W. (2021). Development of an e-learning module to facilitate student learning and outcomes. *Teaching and Learning in Nursing, 16*(2), 139–142. https://doi.org/10.1016/j.teln.2020.10.007

MacRae, D., Jara, M. R., Tyerman, J., & Luctkar-Flude, M. (2021). Investing in engagement: Integrating learning experiences across an undergraduate nursing program. *Clinical Simulation in Nursing, 52,* 17–32. https://doi.org/10.1016/j.ecns.2020.12.005

Mariani, B., Havens, D. S., & Metz, S. (2020). A college of nursing's upward spiral during a global pandemic. *Journal of Nursing Education, 59*(12), 675–682. https://doi.org/10.3928/01484834-20201118-04

Mataxen, P. A., & Webb, L. D. (2019). Telehealth nursing: More than just a phone call. *Nursing, 49*(4), 11–13. https://doi.org/10.1097/01.NURSE.0000553272.16933.4b

Mollart, L., Newell, R., Geale, S. K., Noble, D., Norton, C., & O'Brien, A. P. (2020). Introduction of patient electronic medical records (EMR) into undergraduate nursing education: An integrated literature review. *Nurse Education Today, 94*(2020), 1–13. https://doi.org/10.1016/j.nedt.2020.104517

Mudd, S. S., McIltrot, K. S., & Brown, K. M. (2020). Utilizing telepresence robots for multiple patient scenarios in an online nurse practitioner program. *Nursing Education Perspectives, 41*(4), 260–262. https://doi.org/10.1097/01.NEP.0000000000000590

Oermann, M. (2020). COVID-19 disruptions to clinical education: Nurse educators rise to the challenges. *Nurse Educator, 46*(1), 1. https://doi.org/10.1097/NNE.0000000000000947

Oermann, M., & Gaberson, K. (2021). *Evaluation and testing in nursing education* (6th ed.). Springer Publishing Company.

Ravert, P., Whipple, K., & Hunsaker, S. (2020). Academic health record implementation: Tips for success. *Clinical Simulation in Nursing, 41,* 9–13. https://doi.org/10.1016/j.ecns.2019.12.008

Risling, T. (2017). Educating the nurses of 2025: Technology trends of the next decade. *Nurse Education in Practice, 22*(2017), 89–92. https://doi.org/10.1016/j.nepr.2016.12.007

Rudolph, A., Vaughn, J., Crego, N., Hueckel, R., Kuszajewski, M., Molloy, M., Brisson, R., & Shaw, R. (2017). Integrating telepresence robots into nursing simulation. *Nurse Educator, 42*(2), E1–E4. https://doi.org/10.1097/NNE.0000000000000329

Serembus, J. F., Hunt-Kada, P., Lenahan, K., & Lydon, A. (2020). Internet, apps, and tweets: Enhancing clinical learning through just-in-time training. *Nursing Education Perspectives, 41*(5), E33–E34. https://doi.org/10.1097.01/NEP.0000000000000486

Shea, K. L., & Rovera, E. J. (2021). Preparing for the COVID-19 pandemic and its impact on a nursing simulation curriculum. *Journal of Nursing Education, 60*(1), 52–55. https://doi.org/10.3928/01484834-20201217-12

Skiba, D. (2017). Horizon report: Knowledge obsolescence, artificial intelligence, and rethinking the educator role. *Nursing Education Perspectives, 38*(3), 165–167. https://doi.org/10.1097/01.NEP.0000000000000154

Sweeney, A. B., Morse, C. Y., & Carofiglio, C. (2019). Integrating simulated electronic health record patients across multiple nursing courses. *Journal of Nursing Education, 58*(8), 495–496. https://doi.org/10.3928/01484834-20190719-14

Udermann, B. (2017). What do students really want from online instructors? *The Teaching Professor.* https://www.teachingprofessor.com/topics/online-learning/teaching-strategies-techniques/students-really-want-online-instructors/

Wilbanks, B. A., & Langford, P. A. (2019). Using clinical simulation to design and evaluate electronic health records. *Journal of Informatics Nursing, 4*(2), 6–11. www.ania.org

Wynn, S. T. (2019). Limited mental health clinical sites: Telehealth is the answer. *Journal of Nursing Education, 58*(3), 187. https://doi.org/10.3928/01484834-20190221-14

Yancey, N. R. (2020). Disrupting rhythms: Nurse education and a pandemic. *Nursing Science Quarterly, 33*(4), 299–302. https://doi.org/10.1177/0894318420946493

Yu, M., & Mann, J. S. (2021). Development of virtual reality simulation program for high-risk neonatal infection control education. *Clinical Simulation in Nursing, 50*(2021), 19–26. https://doi.org/10.1016/j.ecns.2020.10.006

A robust set of instructor resources designed to supplement this text is located at http://connect.springerpub.com/content/book/978-0-8261-6705-7. Qualifying instructors may request access by emailing textbook@springerpub.com.

Preceptors as Clinical Teachers

In Chapter 5, the preceptor teaching model was introduced is an alternative to the traditional clinical teaching model. In the preceptor model, an experienced nurse, known as a preceptor, directs student learning in a clinical setting. This approach, drawing upon apprenticeship theory, allows students to be immersed in clinical learning with an expert as the coach and primary teacher. The preceptor guides the student and provides opportunities for the student to gain clinical nursing knowledge and skills and facilitates opportunities to translate theory into practice. Additionally, the preceptor helps socialize the student in understanding the role of the nurse.

Preceptorships have been used with prelicensure nursing students, graduate students preparing for advanced practice roles, and new staff nurse orientees (Ulrich, 2019). These preceptor experiences may be known by other names such as practicums, internships, immersion experiences, clinical partnerships, coaching models, capstone experiences, or externships (Oermann & Shellenbarger, 2020). Regardless of the name used, this approach allows students an opportunity to work one-to-one in a clinical setting with an expert who facilitates and supervises clinical learning. This chapter discusses the effective use of preceptors as clinical teachers and coaches. The advantages and disadvantages of preceptorships are examined, and suggestions are made for selecting, preparing, implementing, evaluating, and rewarding preceptors.

PRECEPTORSHIP MODEL OF CLINICAL TEACHING

A preceptorship involves a time-limited, one-to-one relationship between a learner and an experienced nurse who is employed in a healthcare setting in which the learning activities take place. The academic clinical teacher may not be physically present during the learning activities; the preceptor provides intensive, individualized learning opportunities that improve the learner's clinical competence, confidence, and clinical reasoning. Regardless of learners' levels of education and experience, preceptorships provide opportunities for socialization into professional nursing roles. They also enhance the personal and professional development of the preceptors and allow preceptors to contribute to the growth of the profession (Amirehsani et al., 2019).

The preceptor model is collaborative. The teacher is a faculty member who has overall responsibility for the quality of the clinical teaching and learning. The teacher provides the link between the educational program and the practice setting by selecting and preparing preceptors, assigning students to preceptors, providing guidance for the selection of appropriate learning activities, serving as a resource to the preceptor–student pair, and evaluating student and preceptor performance. The preceptor functions as a role model and provides individualized clinical instruction, coaching, support, and socialization for the learner. The preceptor also provides input into the evaluation of learner performance, although the teacher has ultimate responsibility for summative evaluation decisions (American Association of Colleges of Nursing [AACN], 2021; L'Ecuyer et al., 2018).

USE OF PRECEPTORSHIPS IN NURSING EDUCATION

In academic programs that prepare nurses for initial entry into practice, preceptorships are usually used for students in their final year of study. The decision to use preceptors for clinical teaching should be based on the perceived benefits to students, the educational program and focus, student learning needs, clinical sites and staff available, and accreditation and practice requirements.

Preceptorships are frequently used in graduate programs that prepare nurses for advanced clinical practice, administration, and education roles. At this level, a preceptorship involves well-defined learning objectives based on the student's education and experience. The student participates in learning activities that demonstrate functional role components, allowing rehearsal of role behaviors in a safe setting before assuming the advanced practice role. Depending upon the focus of the graduate program, these learning experiences can involve 500 or more clinical hours with preceptors (Doherty et al., 2020). The preceptor for graduate students must be an expert practitioner who can model the advanced practice role functions including decision making, problem solving, clinical reasoning, and leadership.

ADVANTAGES AND DISADVANTAGES OF USING PRECEPTORS

The use of preceptors in clinical teaching has both advantages and disadvantages for the involved parties. Effective collaboration and adequate preparation of students and preceptors are required to minimize the drawbacks and achieve advantages for the educational programs, clinical agencies, teachers, preceptors, and students.

Preceptorships hold many potential advantages for preceptors and the clinical agencies that employ them. The presence of students in the clinical environment tends to enhance the professional development, leadership, professional growth, and teaching skills of preceptors (Amirehsani et al., 2019). While preceptors enjoy sharing their clinical knowledge and skill, they also appreciate the stimulation of working with students who challenge the status quo and raise questions about clinical practice. Preceptors also report increased job and career satisfaction (Ciocco, 2021). The interest and enthusiasm of students are often rewarding to nurses who take on the additional responsibilities of the preceptor role. In agencies that use a clinical ladder, serving as a preceptor may be a means of advancing professionally within the system or developing essential leadership and teaching skills. Additionally, working with students may be counted toward specialty recertification requirements. For the clinical site, the preceptorship model also produces opportunities to recruit potential staff members for the agency from among students who work with preceptors.

Typically, one of the greatest drawbacks of preceptorships to agencies and preceptors is the expected time commitment. Some clinical agencies may not agree to provide preceptors because of increased patient acuity and staffing concerns. Or potential preceptors may decline to participate because of the perception that guiding and evaluating a student would add to their workloads and be time intensive (Gatewood & De Gagne, 2019; Luimes, 2020). An added consideration involves changes resulting from the Affordable Care Act that have led to competition for clinical sites. Now medical schools that provided clinical training for residents in their clinics no longer receive Medicare and Medicaid reimbursement. As a result, medical resident training has shifted to other community placements, thus creating competition for the same clinical sites as advanced practice nursing students (Hawkins, 2019). Other factors such as compliance requirements, preceptor fatigue, institutional constraints, lack of incentives and preceptor support, limited resources, and poor preparation for teaching are some of the reasons contributing to the difficulty in securing clinical sites and preceptors to work with students (Doherty et al., 2020; Gatewood & De Gagne, 2019; Hawkins, 2019).

Students who participate in preceptorships enjoy several benefits. They have the advantage of working one-on-one with experts who can coach them to increased clinical competence and performance. Preceptorships also provide opportunities for students to experience the realities of clinical practice, including scheduling learning activities on evening and night shifts and weekends to follow their preceptors' schedules. However, following their preceptors' schedules often creates conflicts with students' academic, work, and family commitments. Additionally, a preceptor's clinical assignment may not always be appropriate or align with the student's clinical learning objectives.

Preceptorships offer many advantages for the educational program in which they are used. The use of preceptors provides rich educational experiences for students and more intensive, individualized guidance of students' learning activities. Working collaboratively with preceptors also helps teachers to stay informed about the current realities of practice; up-to-date clinical information benefits ongoing curriculum development.

Several disadvantages related to the use of preceptors may affect educational programs. Contrary to a common belief, teachers' responsibilities do not decrease when students work with preceptors. Initial identification of appropriate clinical sites, selection of preceptors, preparation of preceptors and students, and ongoing collaboration and communication with preceptors and students require as much time or more as the traditional clinical teaching model. The preceptorship model requires considerable indirect teaching time for the development of relationships with agencies and preceptors and the evaluation of preceptors and students. When preceptors are used as clinical teachers, faculty members may be responsible for more students in several clinical agencies and feel uncertain whether student learning aligns with course objectives. Additionally, with the growth of online graduate programs, clinical sites may not be easily accessible, yet site visits may be expected by staff and students. Conducting a traditional in-person site visit may require substantial time and financial expenditures, especially in remote or geographically distant areas. Lastly, educators report that it may be difficult to secure preceptors in specialty areas. Baccalaureate programs face challenges locating preceptors in pediatric, acute care, obstetric, and mental health sites. In graduate program, preceptors are difficult to find in select advanced practice specialities such as pediatric primary care, women's health, and family practice/primary care (AACN and the American Organization for Nursing Leadership [AONL], 2020; Carelli et al., 2019).

SELECTING PRECEPTORS

The success of preceptorships largely depends on the selection of appropriate preceptors; such selection is one of the teacher's most important responsibilities. Most faculty members consider the experience and educational preparation of the preceptor to be important. Most academic programs require the preceptor to have at least the degree for which the student is preparing, although insistence on this level of educational preparation does not guarantee that learners will be exposed only to professional role models. Nursing accreditors may also provide specific guidelines for preceptor selection. The Commission on Collegiate Nursing Education (CCNE, 2018) requires that preceptors be academically and experientially qualified for their role and have the expertise to support student achievement of expected outcomes. Similarly, the Accreditation Commission for Education in Nursing (ACEN, 2020) also indicates that preceptors be academically and experientially qualified but add they should be oriented, mentored, and monitored and have clearly documented roles and responsibilities. The accreditation standards for nursing programs provided by the National League for Nursing Commission for Nursing Education Accreditation (NLN CNEA, 2016) provides a quality indicator for preceptors suggesting that they are qualified and prepared for their role and responsibilities. They provide further interpretive guidelines and allow the nursing program to define the academic and experience qualifications ensuring that they align with regulatory agency rules and standards.

There is little standardization of regulations for nurse preceptors across the United States. The state board of nursing within each state regulates qualifications, preparation, training, and role responsibilities for preceptors, yet there is little uniformity from state to state (L'Ecuyer et al., 2018). Nine U.S. states do not mention preceptors in their regulations, and those states that do mention preceptors vary in their definition. Twenty-nine states indicate that the preceptors need to have a professional license in the state. Surprisingly, four states indicate that the preceptor can be a nonnurse. Years of experience is also a consideration for preceptor selection. The amount of clinical experience expected of preceptors varies, but some states require between 1- and 3-year's experience as a nurse. Educational preparation of the preceptor also varies. For prelicensure programs, some states require a baccalaureate degree in nursing, other states only prefer a baccalaureate degree, while some regulations just suggest that preceptors have a comparable degree or more education than the students (L'Ecuyer et al., 2018). Other considerations for preceptor selection involve the amount of clinical time students engage in the preceptorship experience and the level of student permitted in the preceptorship experience. There is also variability in the regulations regarding preceptor orientation and teacher expectations. State boards of nursing may provide guidance about the preceptor-to-student ratio. Most recommendations suggest a ratio of one preceptor to either one or two students. Lastly, faculty-to-student ratios may be specified with maximums ranging from one faculty for up to 24 students, as is found in Texas (L'Ecuyer et al., 2018).

Regardless of the state mandated regulations, the desire to teach and willingness to serve as a preceptor are important qualities of potential preceptors. Nurses who feel obligated to enact this role may not make enthusiastic, effective preceptors. Additional attributes of effective preceptors, according to Ciocco (2021), include:

▪ *Clinical expertise or proficiency, depending on the level of the learner:* Preceptors should be able to demonstrate expert psychomotor, problem-solving, critical thinking, clinical reasoning, and decision-making skills in their clinical practice. Prelicensure nursing students need preceptors who are proficient clinicians; graduate students need preceptors who are expert clinicians.
▪ *Leadership abilities:* Good preceptors are change agents in the healthcare organizations in which they are employed. They demonstrate effective communication skills and are trusted and respected by their peers. Additionally, they are team players and work well with others.
▪ *Teaching interest and skill:* Preceptors must understand and use principles of adult learning. They should be able to communicate ideas effectively to learners and give descriptive positive and negative feedback.
▪ *Professional role behaviors and attitudes:* Because preceptors act as role models for learners, they must demonstrate behaviors that represent important professional values. They are accountable for their actions and accept responsibility for their decisions. Good preceptors demonstrate maturity and self-confidence; their approach to learners is nonthreatening and nonjudgmental. They need effective communication skills and should welcome questions from learners. They should not interpret the questions as criticisms or judgments about the practice setting or care approach. Flexibility, accessibility, and approachability are also important considerations for preceptors (Chicca & Shellenbarger, 2020). Additionally, having preceptors who are open-minded, enthusiastic about working with students, demonstrate a positive attitude, are willing to work with a diverse population of learners, and exhibit a sense of humor are additional desirable attributes of effective preceptors.

The selection of preceptor and setting should also take into account the learner's interest in a specific clinical specialty, as well as the need for development of particular skills. The teacher may collaborate with nurse managers to select appropriate preceptors. It may be unwise to choose preceptors from newly established practice areas or those with recent high staff turnover.

Potential preceptors for nursing students may be found in any clinical setting that meets the requirements of the nursing education program. There are variable approaches to the identification and selection of nurse preceptors. Doherty et al. (2020) report findings from a recent national survey of nurse practitioner (NP) programs regarding the student clinical placement process. They identified the process for securing preceptors varied across programs. Thirty-one percent of respondents to the survey indicated that most preceptors are arranged by the school with some effort by the student. This was followed closely by the school securing all preceptors (29%). Another method used by 26% of nursing programs require the student to locate the preceptor but having some assistance from the school. Lastly, only 14% of NP students needed to find their own preceptor. This arrangement may be in direct conflict with legal statutes in certain states so it may not be appropriate in all programs. Some states, such as Kentucky, have statutes preventing advanced practice nursing students from finding their own preceptors (Hawkins, 2019).

Therefore, prior to mandating students to independently self-identify preceptors, it is important for the educational institution to check state regulations to ensure compliance with legal statutes. Regardless of the selection process, it appears that many schools and faculty are involved in the preceptor selection process.

Clinical teachers should carefully screen and select preceptors to ensure that the preceptor complies with program requirements and state board of nursing regulations. Graduate programs need to confirm that preceptors have the appropriate advanced nursing experience and qualifications. To facilitate preceptor identification and the matching process, some schools are using electronic modalities and algorithms for matching students with preceptors (Doherty et al., 2020). Independent companies are now also emerging that offer, for a fee, a preceptor matching service and help to broker clinical placements (Delaney et al., 2019; Gardenier et al., 2019). Since these are relatively new services, students, teachers, and nursing programs should carefully investigate the services offered, costs, and the appropriateness of the match.

When trying to locate appropriate nurse preceptors within a healthcare agency, the staff development or education department is a good first contact. Some agencies ask that all requests for preceptors for nursing students be directed to a specified staff member who serves as a gatekeeper and can suggest appropriate matches. If appropriate, students may be able to suggest good potential preceptors from their work experience or from their contacts with nursing staff members in their previous clinical learning experiences. Alumni of the nursing program are a rich source of potential preceptors; many of them would like to give back to their alma mater and are flattered to be asked to serve as a preceptor for students. These potential preceptors can be recruited at alumni association gatherings, by telephone or email, via professional social media groups, or through an alumni newsletter.

Another trend emerging, in part because of the difficulty in securing clinical preceptors, especially in hard to place advanced practice areas, involves paying preceptors. In the past many nursing programs provided nonmonetary incentives for preceptors, but that may no longer be sufficient in acknowledging the work of the preceptor. The literature suggests that many preceptors believe that they should receive payment for their precepting efforts due to lost productivity and as compensation for their time working with students (Delaney et al., 2019). Preceptors who are paid report higher satisfaction with this role (Gardenier et al., 2019).

The preceptor payment trend is occurring in other health-related fields, with approximately 21% of physician assistant programs paying preceptors. The shift in compensation for preceptors in other related disciplines will generate increasing discussion in nursing education and should be carefully monitored to assess the impact upon students, preceptors, and nursing programs. At present, most schools report not paying for clinical preceptors; however, there are some program and regional differences (AACN & AONL, 2020). Graduate programs are more likely to pay for preceptors than baccalaureate programs. Additionally, baccalaureate programs in the North Atlantic region and graduate schools in the South and Midwest are more likely to pay clinical preceptors (AACN & AONL, 2020).

Funding to support preceptor payment is emerging in various ways. Some schools are charging students additional fees for clinical courses, while other schools allocate students a designated honorarium to distribute to all preceptors. Preceptor compensation is also being tackled at the state level, with states such as Colorado, Georgia, Maine, Maryland, South Carolina, and Texas offering an income tax incentive credit program to APRN preceptors in support of APRN training (AACN &

AONL, 2020; Delaney et al., 2019). Other states have unsuccessfully attempted to pass similar tax credit legislation. Regardless of the source of the compensation or credit, this preceptor payment approach deserves careful monitoring as it may seriously impact nursing programs, thereby creating financial pressure for the institution and competition among programs.

In addition to payment issues, nursing programs face additional challenges when offering nursing education through distance delivery modalities. Nursing programs are now reaching previously untapped student populations in remote settings through innovative delivery methods. However, these programs and students face added challenges when planning preceptor experiences. Online programs may need to work with boards of nursing and regulatory bodies to ensure compliance with appropriate approval processes. When students are working with preceptors at remote or distant sites, the board of nursing in those states will need to be aware of clinical experiences occurring in their jurisdiction and the program must comply with any approval regulations or state authorization requirements. Clinical teachers or clinical coordinators are advised to contact the appropriate state board of nursing as other requirements may vary from state to state. Additionally, to streamline distance education program delivery and ensure quality, nursing programs may also wish to explore the National Council for State Authorization Reciprocity Agreements (NC-SARA) at www.nc-sara.org. It is important to identify possible clinical sites and preceptors early in the planning process so that appropriate screening can occur, and programs can ensure compliance with all regulations is complete before the clinical experience begins.

Working with preceptors at clinical sites, particularly those at distant locations or involving advanced practice programs, can be challenging. Developing partnerships with preceptors may be an effective approach to ensure that qualified and adequately prepared preceptors are available for students. Clinical teachers can work closely with the clinical site preceptors to understand the unique aspects of the clinical site, the populations served, the clinical role, and to ensure that clinical placements align with program and student needs.

PREPARING THE PARTICIPANTS

Thorough preparation of preceptors and students for their roles is key to the success of preceptorships. Teachers are responsible for initial orientation and continuing support of all participants; preparation can be formal or informal.

Preceptor Preparation

Preparation of preceptors may begin with a general orientation, possibly for groups of potential preceptors at the selected clinical site or for all preceptors working with students from one nursing education program. Or, with the rapid rise in remote preceptorship experiences and restricted faculty and preceptor time, educators may develop and implement an electronic orientation for preceptors. A preceptorship preparation program acknowledges the need for and commitment to collaboration in nursing education and helps to decrease feelings of isolation, anxiety, or uncertainty associated with the preceptor role. This preparation supports the learning needs of preceptors enabling them to enact their role effectively and confidently and it may also help to prevent problems.

Content of a preceptorship preparation program may include the following information:

- Benefits and challenges of precepting
- Characteristics of a good preceptor
- Facilitating learning
- Principles of adult learning
- Assessment of learner needs
- Communication and conflict resolution
- Clinical teaching methods, including motivating and challenging learners, dealing with difficult learning situations, and when to use coaching techniques
- Evaluation of learning, including how to give effective feedback and use of clinical evaluation tools
- Preceptor's role in developing and implementing an individualized learning contract, if used
- Course and faculty expectations
- Academic program curriculum structure, framework, and goals (Amirehsani et al., 2019; Pearson & Hensley, 2019; Pitts et al., 2019)

After preceptors have been selected, they need a specific orientation to their responsibilities. This orientation may take the form of a face-to-face, telephone, or videoconference meeting. Technology-supported orientation programs using online learning modules or websites offer flexibility, especially for preceptors that are geographically separated from the nursing school (Luimes, 2020). Written guidelines may also be used. Exhibit 11.1 is an example of written guidelines for preceptors of graduate nursing students. The conference and written materials may include information such as:

- *The educational level and previous experience of the student*: Preceptors will find it helpful to understand what courses and content students previously completed so the preceptor can develop realistic performance expectations and select appropriate learning experiences.
  Beginning students may not have developed the knowledge and skill to participate in all of the preceptor's activities. Graduate students need learning activities that build on their previous learning and experience to produce advanced practice outcomes.
- *Structure of the course:* Information about the course including the number of hours required for the experience.
- *How to choose specific learning activities based on learning objectives:* The teacher may share samples of learning contracts or lists of learning activities to guide the preceptor's selection of appropriate activities for the student.
- *Scheduling of clinical learning activities*: A common feature of preceptorships is the scheduling of the student's learning activities according to the preceptor's work schedule. Preceptors should be advised of dates that students and teachers may not be available because of school holidays, examinations, and other course requirements.
- *Contacts:* How and under what circumstances to contact the course faculty member.

EXHIBIT 11.1 Sample Guidelines for a Preceptor of a Graduate Nursing Student

The preceptor is expected to:

Facilitate the student's entry into the healthcare organization

Provide the student with an orientation to the organization

After receiving the student's learning goals for the precepted experience, provide suggestions for how these goals can be accomplished

Assist the student to identify activities that are consistent with organizational needs and the student's interests, abilities, and learning needs

Meet with the student at regular intervals to discuss progress and achievement of individual and course objectives

Provide the student with regular feedback regarding their performance

Communicate regularly with the faculty member regarding the student's progress

Serve as a role model and facilitate learning opportunities

At the end of the preceptorship, provide a written evaluation of the student's performance related to goal achievement, clinical knowledge and skill, problem-solving and decision-making skills, communication, and interpersonal skills

New preceptors have learning needs much like those of students and new staff nurses; supportive role models and coaching are essential to success.

Student Preparation

Learners also need to understand the purposes and processes of the preceptorship. They need an orientation to the process of planning individual learning activities, an explanation of teacher and preceptor roles, and a review of policies specific to student practice. At the beginning of the preceptorship, teachers should clarify evaluation responsibilities and expectations such as dates for learning contract approval, site visits frequency and format, and conferences with faculty members.

IMPLEMENTATION

Successful implementation of preceptorships depends on mutual understanding of the roles and responsibilities of the participants. The teacher, student, and preceptor collaborate to plan and implement learning activities that will facilitate the student's goal attainment. Key to these processes is frequent, clear, effective communication among the participants.

Roles and Responsibilities of Participants

PRECEPTORS

Preceptors are responsible for patient care delivery in addition to clinical teaching of the student. The preceptor is expected to be a positive role model and a resource person for the student. The clinical teaching responsibilities of the preceptor include creating a positive learning climate, including the student in activities that relate to learning goals, and providing feedback to the student and teacher. The Preceptor Expectation Checklist, developed by the National Organization of Nurse Practitioner Faculties (NONPF) and the American Association of Nurse Practitioners (AANP), provides a guide that faculty can use to ensure clear preceptor expectations.

Role model behaviors important for preceptors to demonstrate can be classified into four categories:

- **Technical and Technology Skills**: Demonstrates nursing care procedures; operation of equipment unique to that clinical setting; use of the electronic health record, and evidence-based, current nursing practices.
- **Interpersonal Skills**: Uses effective communication techniques with patients and family members; interacts with members of the interdisciplinary healthcare team in a collegial, confident manner; displays appropriate use of humor; demonstrates caring attitude toward patients; gives constructive feedback; uses questioning techniques.
- **Clinical Reasoning and Clinical Judgment**: Listens carefully during reporting and asks pertinent questions about patients' conditions; demonstrates proficient problem solving, critical thinking, and clinical reasoning; and incorporates skills of noticing, interpreting, responding, and reflecting as part of clinical decision making (Caputi, 2019).
- **Professional Role Behaviors**: Keeps patient information confidential; encourages discussion of ethical issues; demonstrates enthusiasm about nursing; demonstrates accountability for own actions.

Sometimes preceptors experience conflict between the educator and evaluator roles. Preceptors play a key role as professional gatekeepers ensuring the delivery of safe and competent care. Although preceptors may lack experience and confidence with the evaluator role and be hesitant to suggest that a student is failing, they must seek faculty support and devise approaches for offering feedback and communicating with students who are unable to meet competency requirements (Nugent et al., 2020). If the learner is unable to perform according to expectations, the faculty member must be notified so that a plan for correcting the deficiencies may be established.

When preceptors perceive that a student is unable to perform nursing care appropriately, they are often tempted to step in and take over the care. This inclination may be due to the preceptor's concurrent responsibility to the patient and a genuine desire to share clinical knowledge and skill with the student. However, doing so interferes with the learning experience and is a missed opportunity for student development.

To support students as they learn their nursing role, preceptors should use a coaching process. In sports, coaches stand on the sidelines; they do not participate in or interfere with the game unless there is a risk of injury (e.g., the soccer coach who sees lightening on the horizon interrupts the game by getting the referee's attention to stop play and clear the field). A good preceptor, using coaching techniques, allows the learner to be in control of the patient situation and stands nearby, monitoring the unfolding situation, offering verbal cues when needed, asking questions to guide the student's problem solving and clinical reasoning, offering encouragement (e.g., "that's right," "keep going"), and then giving immediate feedback for the student to reflect on (Shellenbarger & Robb, 2016). The coach's expression of belief in the student's capacity to succeed helps the student develop self-efficacy and self-confidence. Thus, effective coaching can help students feel more confident in their clinical abilities and see themselves as authentic care providers. However, if a student "freezes" because of overwhelming anxiety, an error, inadequate preparation, or an unexpected occurrence, the preceptor may need to intervene if this places the patient at risk. The preceptor may need to temporarily assume responsibility for the nursing responsibilities the student was attempting to perform, beginning or taking the next step of the task, and then encouraging the student to continue while continuing to coach from the sidelines.

STUDENTS

The student is expected to actively participate in planning their own learning activities. Planning may take the form of a learning contract that specifies individualized objectives and clinical learning activities. Because the teacher is not always present during learning activities, the student must communicate frequently with the teacher. Communication may take many forms, such as a written assignment like a reflective journal or an electronic discussion. Graduate students will be expected to track their clinical hours and experiences. Some nursing programs use electronic data tracking systems to record clinical time logs, assignments, portfolio documents, and evaluations. Written assignments allow students to share experiences with the teacher on a regular basis throughout the semester. The pervasiveness and accessibility of mobile technology allows immediate access to faculty during clinical time.

The student must notify the teacher immediately of any problems encountered in the implementation of the preceptorship. Students may experience problems or conflict during their preceptor experiences yet may not report conflict for several reasons. They perceive that they are expected to fit in to the practice setting with minimal disruption, or they feel powerless and dependent upon the preceptor's evaluation to complete the clinical practicum successfully. The student's responsibilities also include self-evaluation and evaluation of the preceptor's teaching effectiveness, as will be discussed later in this chapter.

TEACHERS

As previously discussed, the teacher is responsible for making preceptor selections, pairing students with preceptors, and orienting preceptors and students. Gathering information about the site, either through a site visit or a conversation with the staff, prior to students beginning their experience, may be helpful for teachers to learn about the population served. These discussions can also help establish a relationship with the nursing staff. The teacher can use this time to provide an overview and/or orientation to the program and explain clinical expectations. The teacher is an important resource to preceptors and students and can assist in problem solving as issues arise. The teacher must be alert to any sign of conflict in the student–preceptor relationship and promptly take a proactive role in resolving it. If a conflict cannot be resolved to the satisfaction of student, preceptor, and faculty member, the student's well-being should take precedence, and, if necessary, the student should be reassigned.

Teacher availability is particularly important if a problem arises at the clinical site and the preceptor and student cannot resolve the issue independently. The teacher must plan for consultation via telephone, email, text messaging, or electronic conferencing. The teacher also arranges individual and group conferences with students and preceptors and visits the clinical sites as needed or requested by any of the participants. During a clinical site visit, the teacher may observe student performance and ask questions of both the preceptor and the student. If problems are identified, the teacher may need to work collaboratively to strategize resolutions. However, teachers may need to initiate remediation plans if potentially unsafe practices are identified (Oermann & Gaberson, 2021). Close monitoring by the preceptor and/or faculty may be necessary to ensure patient and student safety is maintained. Teachers have the responsibility to gather input from the preceptor about the student performance and use that as part of the overall evaluation of learner performance. Faculty should also gather input from the student about the effectiveness of the preceptor and the opportunities for learning at the clinical site.

Planning and Implementing Learning Activities

A common strategy for planning and implementing students' learning activities in the preceptorship model of clinical teaching is the use of an individualized learning contract. A learning contract is an explicit agreement between a teacher and student that clarifies expectations of each participant in the teaching–learning process. It specifies the learning goals that have been established, the learning activities selected to meet the objectives, and the expected outcomes and criteria by which they will be evaluated. In a preceptorship experience, the learning contract is negotiated among the teacher, student, and preceptor and guides the planning and implementation of the student's learning activities. Even though the learning contract is individualized to meet student and agency needs, it needs to be consistent with course learning outcomes. Exhibit 11.2 is an example of a learning contract that could be adapted for any level of learner.

As discussed previously, effective communication among the preceptor, student, and teacher is critical to the success of the preceptorship. Communication between teacher and student may be facilitated by the student keeping a reflective journal and sharing it with the teacher on a regular basis. In the journal, the student describes and analyzes learning activities that relate to the objectives, reflecting on the meaning and value of the experiences. Journals provide an opportunity for students to review and record their thoughts, impressions, and reactions. They can also assist students to understand and clarify clinical situations, link clinical learning to theory, and examine their thinking and actions while helping to keep the teacher informed of the learning experiences. The journal entries may be recorded in a computer file, on paper, on audiotape, or posted to an online discussion board. Additionally, the student and teacher have telephone, email, or face-to-face contact as necessary for the teacher to give consultation and guidance. Similarly, the teacher and preceptor should have regular contact by telephone, email, text messaging, or face-to-face meetings so that the teacher receives feedback about learner performance and offers guidance and consultation as needed.

EXHIBIT 11.2 Learning Contract Template

Student Information
　　Name and credentials:
　　Address:
　　Home phone number:
　　Mobile phone number:
　　Email address:
Teacher Information
　　Name and credentials:
　　Address:
　　Office phone number:
　　Mobile phone number:
　　Email address:
Preceptor Information
　　Name and credentials:
　　Address:
　　Office phone number:
　　Mobile phone number:
　　Email address:

Clinical Learning Objectives	Learning Activities and Resources	Evaluation Evidence, Responsibility, and Time Frame

　　Start date: _____　　Completion date: _____
Student Signature _____　　Date _____
Preceptor Signature _____　　Date _____
Teacher Signature _____　　Date _____

One way to ensure regular contact with the student and preceptor is to conduct site visits. Both students and preceptors report that site visits are valuable and worthwhile as they enhance connection with the faculty and program, provide real-time opportunities for feedback, and enhance student confidence (Pericak et al., 2017). It is recommended that faculty make site visit expectations clear and then spend adequate time with the student and preceptor during the visit to ensure mentoring and communication of progress and needs. NP research suggests that the site visits are best after the student has an opportunity to get comfortable in the setting, thus scheduling the visit after mid semester may be best. NP preceptors recommend at least one site visit per semester while NP students prefer that several site visits occur (Amirehsani et al., 2019; Pericak et al., 2017).

A growing trend, particularly with the growth of online program delivery, is the use of virtual site visits. Given the cost and faculty time needed for conducting in-person site visits, virtual visits are becoming more popular. These remote visits can be conducted using interactive videos that enable the teacher to observe student performance at the clinical site, provide real time interaction, and enable the delivery of feedback to all parties. Exhibit 11.3 offers some suggestions for how

EXHIBIT 11.3 Virtual Site Visits

Secure approval from the clinical site for a virtual site visit

Select a secure interactive video platform that ensures privacy, provides password protection, offers encryption, and complies with the Health Insurance Portability and Accountability Act (HIPAA)

Train faculty and students for device use

Test the video platform prior to using to guarantee a quality transmission

Seek permission from all parties including patients, family (if appropriate), and preceptors

Position device, such as a laptop, iPad, or phone, so that the student and their actions can be observed

Consider use of an adjustable technology stand, such as gooseneck holders, that allow for manipulation and movement of the recording device during an exam

Provide adequate lighting and avoid positioning directly in front of windows that may create shadows or glare

Arrange for technology support to assist with problem troubleshooting

preceptors, teachers, and students can work together to ensure that the virtual visit is successful (Alton et al., 2018; Harris et al., 2020).

The realities of clinical and academic cultures present challenges to effective communication among teacher, preceptor, and student. Preceptors often work a variety of shifts, students often have complex academic, personal, and work demands, and teachers have multiple responsibilities in addition to clinical teaching. Flexibility and commitment to establishing and maintaining communication are essential to overcome these challenges.

EVALUATING THE OUTCOMES

Students, teachers, and preceptors share responsibility for monitoring the progress of learning and for evaluating outcomes of the preceptorship. Student performance may be evaluated according to the terms specified in the learning contract or through the clinical evaluation methods used by the educational program. Throughout the clinical experiences, students should be encouraged to self-assess their performance to identify strengths and areas needing ongoing improvement (Oermann & Gaberson, 2021). If a learning contract is used, student self-evaluation is usually an important strategy for assessing outcomes. As discussed earlier, preceptors are expected to give feedback to the learner and to the teacher, but the teacher has the responsibility for the summative evaluation of learner performance (L'Ecuyer et al., 2018).

An important aspect of evaluation concerns the teaching effectiveness of preceptors. Students are an important source of information about the quality of their preceptors' clinical teaching, but the teacher should also assess the degree to which preceptors were able to effectively guide the students' learning. A modified form of a teaching effectiveness tool used to evaluate clinical teachers may be used to collect data from students regarding their preceptors. Exhibit 11.4 is an example of a form for student evaluation of preceptor teaching effectiveness. Because each preceptor may be assigned to only one student at a time, it is usually impossible to maintain anonymity of student evaluations. Therefore, teachers may wish to share a summary of the student's evaluation, instead of the raw data, with the preceptor.

EXHIBIT 11.4 Sample Tool For Student Evaluation of Preceptor Teaching Effectiveness

Directions: Rate the extent to which each statement describes your preceptor's teaching behaviors by circling a number following each item, using the following scale:

     4 = to a large extent
     3 = to a moderate extent
     2 = to a small extent
     1 = not at all

1. The preceptor was an excellent professional role model.   4   3   2   1

2. The preceptor guided my clinical problem solving.   4   3   2   1

3. The preceptor helped me to apply theory to clinical practice.   4   3   2   1

4. The preceptor was responsive to my individual learning needs.   4   3   2   1

5. The preceptor provided constructive feedback about my performance.   4   3   2   1

6. The preceptor communicated clearly and effectively.   4   3   2   1

7. The preceptor encouraged my independence.   4   3   2   1

8. The preceptor was flexible and open-minded.   4   3   2   1

9. Overall, the preceptor was an excellent clinical teacher.   4   3   2   1

10. I would recommend this preceptor for other students.   4   3   2   1

REWARDING PRECEPTORS

Preceptors make valuable contributions to nursing education programs, and they should receive appropriate rewards and incentives for their participation. At minimum, every preceptor should receive an individualized thank-you letter, specifying some of the benefits that the student received from the preceptorship. A copy of the letter may be sent to the preceptor's supervisor or manager to be used as evidence of clinical excellence. Some preceptors prefer nonmaterial rewards such as lighter workloads and support from managers and teachers; however, teachers may not be able to provide all these things as a reward and may use other methods of demonstrating appreciation.

Other formal and informal ways of acknowledging the contributions of preceptors for nursing students are:

- A name badge or pin that identifies the nurse as a preceptor
- A certificate of appreciation, signed by the administrator of the nursing education program
- An annual preceptor recognition event, including refreshments and an inspirational speaker
- Free or reduced-price registration for continuing education programs offered by the nursing education program or clinical facility (Amirehsani et al., 2019; Delaney et al., 2019)

- Documentation of hours for certification renewals (Doherty et al., 2020; Drayton-Brooks et al., 2017)
- Free or reduced-rate tuition for one or more academic courses or the opportunity to audit a nursing course
- A free meal
- Campus guest privileges such as library access
- Adjunct or affiliate faculty appointment
- Differential pay or adjustment of work schedule (e.g., exemption from weekend shifts)
- Nomination of preceptors for awards, providing letters of reference, and collaborating on research projects
- A small gift such as a fruit basket, plant, or gift certificate

SUMMARY

The use of preceptors is an alternative to the traditional clinical teaching model based on the assumption that a consistent relationship between an experienced nurse and a nursing student is an effective way to provide individualized guidance in clinical learning and professional socialization. Preceptorships have been used extensively with prelicensure as well as graduate nursing students preparing for advanced practice roles.

A preceptorship is a time-limited, one-to-one relationship between a learner and an experienced nurse. The teacher may not be physically present during the learning activities; the preceptor provides intensive, individualized learning opportunities that improve the learner's clinical competence and confidence. The teacher has overall responsibility for the quality of the clinical teaching and learning and provides the link between the educational program and the practice setting. The preceptor functions as a role model and provides individualized clinical instruction, coaching, support, and socialization for the learner.

Preceptorships are frequently used for students in their last semester of academic preparation for entry into practice and for graduate students preparing for advanced clinical practice, administration, and education roles.

The use of preceptors in clinical teaching has both advantages and disadvantages for the educational program, clinical agency, teachers, preceptors, and students. Benefits for preceptors and their employers include the stimulation of working with learners who raise questions about clinical practice, rewards through a clinical ladder system for participation as a preceptor, and opportunities to recruit potential staff members for the agency from among students who work with preceptors. The greatest drawback of preceptorships to agencies and preceptors is usually the expected time commitment.

Students experience the benefits of working one-on-one with clinical experts who can coach them to improved performance as well as opportunities to experience the realities of clinical practice. However, following their preceptors' schedules often creates conflicts with students' academic, work, and family commitments.

Preceptorships offer many advantages to teachers and educational programs. The use of preceptors provides more clinical teachers for students and thus more intensive guidance of students' learning activities. Working collaboratively with preceptors also helps teachers to stay informed about the current realities of practice. Disadvantages include the amount of indirect teaching time required to select, prepare, and communicate with preceptors and students.

Selection of appropriate preceptors is important to the success of preceptorships. Most academic programs require the preceptor to have at least the degree for which the student is preparing. Desire to teach and willingness to serve as a preceptor are very important qualities of potential preceptors. Additional attributes of effective preceptors include clinical expertise or proficiency, leadership abilities, teaching skill, and professional role behaviors and attitudes.

Teachers are responsible for the initial orientation and continuing support of all participants; preparation can be formal or informal. A general orientation for potential preceptors may include information about benefits and challenges of precepting, characteristics of a good preceptor, principles of adult learning, clinical teaching and coaching techniques, evaluation methods, and the structure and goals of the nursing education program. After preceptors have been selected, they need a specific orientation to their responsibilities, including information about the student's educational level and previous experience, choosing specific learning activities based on learning objectives, and scheduling of clinical learning activities. Learners also need an orientation that includes information about the purposes of the preceptorship, the process of planning individual learning activities, and an explanation of teacher and preceptor roles.

Successful implementation of preceptorships depends on mutual understanding of the roles and responsibilities of the participants. The preceptor is expected to be a positive role model and a resource person for the student. The responsibilities of the preceptor include creating a positive learning climate, including the student in activities that relate to learning goals, and providing feedback to the student and teacher. The student usually arranges the schedule of clinical learning activities to coincide with the preceptor's work schedule and is expected to participate actively in planning learning activities. Because the teacher is not always present during learning activities, the student must keep the teacher informed about progress through frequent communication. In addition to making preceptor selections and orienting preceptors and students, the teacher is an important resource to preceptors and students to assist in problem-solving. Teachers must make adequate arrangements for communication with participants.

A common strategy for planning and implementing students' learning activities is the use of an individualized learning contract—an explicit agreement between the teacher, student, and preceptor that specifies the learning goals, learning activities selected to meet the objectives, and the expected outcomes and criteria by which they will be evaluated. The learning contract guides the planning and implementation of the student's learning activities.

Students, teachers, and preceptors share responsibility for monitoring the progress of learning and for evaluating outcomes of the preceptorship. Student performance is assessed according to the terms specified in the learning contract or through the clinical evaluation methods used by the educational program, through self-evaluation, and through feedback from preceptors. The teacher is responsible for the summative evaluation of learner performance. Students are an important source of information about their preceptors' clinical teaching effectiveness, but the teacher should also assess the degree to which preceptors were able to effectively guide students' learning.

Preceptors should receive appropriate rewards and incentives for the contributions they make to the educational program. At minimum, every preceptor should receive an individualized thank-you letter, specifying some of the benefits that the student received from the preceptorship. Other formal and informal ways of acknowledging the contributions of preceptors were discussed.

CNE® EXAMINATION TEST BLUEPRINT CORE COMPETENCIES

1. **Facilitate Learning**
   A. Implement a variety of teaching strategies appropriate to
      1. content
      2. setting
      3. learner needs
      4. desired learner outcomes
   B. Use teaching strategies based on
      1. educational theory
      2. evidence-based practices related to education
   E. Practice skilled oral and written (including electronic) communication that reflects an awareness of self and relationships with learners (e.g., evaluation, mentorship, and supervision)
   F. Communicate effectively orally and in writing with an ability to convey ideas in a variety of contexts
   H. Create opportunities for learners to develop their own critical thinking skills
   I. Create a positive learning environment that fosters a free exchange of ideas
   N. Use knowledge of evidence-based practice to instruct learners
2. **Facilitate Learner Development and Socialization**
   E. Foster the development of learners in these areas
      1. cognitive domain
      2. psychomotor domain
      3. affective domain
   F. Assist learners to engage in thoughtful and constructive self and peer evaluation
3. **Use Assessment and Evaluation Strategies**
   C. Use a variety of strategies to assess and evaluate learning in these domains
      1. cognitive
      2. psychomotor
      3. affective
   J. Use assessment and evaluation data to enhance the teaching–learning process
   K. Advise learners regarding assessment and evaluation criteria
   L. Provide timely, constructive, and thoughtful feedback

CNE®cl EXAMINATION TEST BLUEPRINT CORE COMPETENCIES

1. **Function within the Education and Health Care Environments**
   A. Function in the Clinical Educator Role
      1. Bridge the gap between theory and practice by helping learners to apply classroom learning to the clinical setting
      2. Foster professional growth of learners (e.g., coaching, reflection, and debriefing)
      3. Use technologies to enhance clinical teaching and learning
   B. Operationalize the Curriculum
      1. Assess congruence of the clinical agency to curriculum, course goals, and learner needs when evaluating clinical sites
      2. Plan meaningful and relevant clinical learning assignments and activities
      3. Identify learner's goals and outcomes
      4. Prepare learners for clinical experiences (e.g., facility, clinical expectations, equipment, and technology-based resources)

    5. Structure learner experiences within the learning environment to promote optimal learning

    7. Provide opportunities for learners to develop problem-solving and clinical reasoning skills related to course objectives (e.g., learning outcomes)

    8. Implement assigned models for clinical teaching (e.g., traditional, preceptor, simulation, dedicated education units)

  C. Abide by Legal Requirements, Ethical Guidelines, Agency Policies, and Guiding Framework

    1. Apply ethical and legal principles to create a safe clinical learning environment

    2. Assess learner abilities and needs prior to clinical learning experiences

    4. Inform others of program and clinical agency policies, procedures, and practices

    5. Adhere to program and clinical agency policies, procedures, and practices when implementing clinical experiences

2. **Facilitate Learning in the Health Care Environment**

  D. Create opportunities for learners to develop critical thinking and clinical reasoning skills

  F. Create a positive and caring learning environment

  G. Develop collegial working relationships with learners, faculty colleagues, and clinical agency personnel

3. **Demonstrate Effective Interpersonal Communication and Collaborative Interprofessional Relationships**

  B. Foster a shared learning community and cooperate with other members of the healthcare team

  C. Create multiple opportunities to collaborate and cooperate with other members of the healthcare team

  D. Support an environment of frequent, respectful, civil, and open communication with all members of the healthcare team

  E. Act as a role model showing respect for all members of the healthcare team, professional colleagues, clients, family members, as well as learner

  F. Use clear and effective communication in all interactions (e.g., written, electronic, verbal, non-verbal)

  N. Communicate performance expectations to learners and agency staff

5. **Facilitate Learner Development and Socialization**

  B. Promote a learning climate of respect for all

  C. Promote professional integrity and accountability

  F. Assist learners in effective use of self-assessment and professional goal setting for ongoing self-improvement

  G. Create learning environments that are focused on socialization to the role of the nurse

6. **Implement Effective Clinical and Assessment Evaluation Strategies**

  A. Use a variety of strategies to determine achievement of learning outcomes

  B. Implement both formative and summative evaluation that is appropriate to the learner and learning outcomes

  D. Maintain integrity in the assessment and evaluation of learners

  E. Provide timely, objective, constructive, and fair feedback to learners

  H. Assess and evaluate learner achievement of clinical performance expectations

  J. Document learner clinical performance, feedback, and progression

  K. Evaluate the quality of the clinical learning experiences and environment

REFERENCES

Accreditation Commission for Education in Nursing. (2020). *ACEN accreditation manual.* https://www.acenursing.org/acen-accreditation-manual/

Alton, S., Luke, S. A., & Wilder, M. (2018). Cost-effective virtual clinical site visits for nurse practitioner students. *Journal of Nursing Education, 57*(5), 308–311. https://doi.org/10.3928/01484834-20180420-11

American Association of Colleges of Nursing. (2021). *APRN clinical preceptor resources guide.* https://www.aacnnursing.org/Education-Resources/APRN-Education/APRN-Clinical-Preceptor-Resources-Guide

American Association of Colleges of Nursing and the American Organization for Nursing Leadership. (2020). *AACN-AONL clinical preceptor survey summary report.* https://www.aacnnursing.org/Portals/42/Data/AACN-AONL-Clinical-Preceptor-Survey-May-2020.pdf

Amirehsani, K. A., Kennedy-Malone, L., & Alam, M. T. (2019). Supporting preceptors and strengthening academic-practice partnerships: Preceptors' perceptions. *The Journal for Nurse Practitioners, 15*(8), e151–e156. https://doi.org/10.1016/j.nurpra.2019.04.011

Caputi, L. J. (2019). Reflections on the next generation NCLEX with implications for nursing programs. *Nursing Education Perspectives, 40*(1), 2–3. https://doi.org/10.1097/01.NEP.0000000000000439

Carelli, K. V., Gatiba, P. N., & Thompson, L. S. (2019). Tax incentives for preceptors of nurse practitioner students in Massachusetts: A potential solution. *Journal of the American Association of Nurse Practitioners, 31*(8), 462–467. https://doi.org/10.1097/JXX.0000000000000257

Chicca, J., & Shellenbarger, T. (2020). Implementing successful clinical nursing preceptorships. *Nurse Educator, 45*(4), E41–E42. https://doi.org/10.1097/NNE.0000000000000750

Ciocco, M. (2021). *Fast facts for the nurse preceptor* (2nd ed.). Springer Publishing Company.

Commission on Collegiate Nursing Education. (2018). *Standards for accreditation of baccalaureate and graduate nursing programs.* https://www.aacnnursing.org/Portals/42/CCNE/PDF/Standards-Final-2018.pdf

Delaney, K. R., Swartwout, K., Livesay, S. L, & Bavis, M. P. (2019). Establishing nurse practitioner clinical practicums: Addressing fiscal realities. *Journal of the American Nurse Practitioners, 31*(11), 657–662. https://doi.org/10.1097/JXX.0000000000000333

Doherty, C. L., Fogg, L., Bigley, M. B., Todd, B., & O'Sullivan, A. L. (2020). Nurse practitioner student clinical placement processes: A national survey of nurse practitioner programs. *Nursing Outlook, 68*(1), 55–61. https://doi.org/10.1016/j.outlook.2019.07.005

Drayton-Brooks, S. M., Gray, P. A., Turner, N. P., & Newland, J. A. (2017). Building clinical education training capacity in nurse practitioner programs. *Journal of Professional Nursing, 33*(2017), 422–428. https://doi.org/10.1016/j.profnurs.2017.02.002

Gardenier, D., Arends, R., & Selway, J. (2019). Should preceptors be paid? *The Journal for Nurse Practitioners, 15*(8), 542–543. https://doi.org/10.1016/j.nurpra.2019.06.007

Gatewood, E., & De Gagne, J. C. (2019). The one-minute preceptor model: A systematic review. *Journal of the American Association of Nurse Practitioners, 31*(1), 46–57. https://doi.org/10.1097/JXX.0000000000000099

Harris, M., Rhoads, S. J., Rooker, J. S., Kelly, M. A., Lefler, L., Lubin, S., Martel, I. L., & Beverly, C. J. (2020). Using virtual site visits in the clinical evaluation of nurse practitioner students: Student and faculty perspectives. *Nurse Educator, 45*(1), 17–20. https://doi.org/10.1097/NNE.0000000000000693

Hawkins, M. D. (2019). Barriers to preceptor placement for nurse practitioner students. *Journal of Christian Nursing, 36*(1), 48–53. https://doi.org/10.1097/CNJ.0000000000000519

L'Ecuyer, K. M., von der Lancken, S., Malloy, D., Meyer, G., & Hyde, M. J. (2018). Review of state boards of nursing rules and regulations for nurse preceptors. *Journal of Nursing Education, 57*(3), 134–141. https://doi.org/10.3928/01484834-20180221-02

Luimes, J. (2020). Supporting preceptors of distance nurse practitioner students. *Teaching and Learning in Nursing*, 1–7. Advance online publication. https://doi.org/10.1016/j.teln.2020.10.005

National League for Nursing Commission for Nursing Education Accreditation. (2016). *Accreditation standards for nursing programs.* https://cnea.nln.org/standards-of-accreditation

Nugent, O., Lydon, C., Part, S., Dennehy, C., Fenn, H., Keane, L., Prizeman, G., & Timmins, F. (2020). Who is failing who? A survey exploration of the barriers and enablers to accurate decision making when nursing students' competence is below required standards. *Nurse Education in Practice, 45*(2020), 102791. https://doi.org/10.1016/j.nepr.2020.102791

Oermann, M. H., & Gaberson, K. B. (2021). *Evaluation and testing in nursing education* (6th ed.). Springer Publishing Company.

Oermann, M. H., & Shellenbarger, T. (2020). Clinical education in nursing: Current practices and trends. In D. Nestel, G. Reedy, L. McKenna, & S. Gough (Eds.), *Clinical education for the health professions: Theory and practice* (pp. 1–20). Springer Nature. https://doi.org/10.1007/978-981-13-6106-7_10-1

Pearson, T., & Hensley, T. (2019). Positive precepting: Identifying NP student learning levels and needs. *Journal of the American Association of Nurse Practitioners, 31*(2), 124–130. https://doi.org/10/1097/JXX.0000000000000106

Pericak, A., Graziano, M., & McNelis, A. M. (2017). Faculty clinical site visits in nurse practitioner education. *Nurse Educator, 42*(4), E1–E3. https://doi.org/10.1097/NNE.0000000000000362

Pitts, C., Padden, D., Knestrick, J., & Bigley, M. B. (2019). A checklist for faculty and preceptor to enhance nurse practitioner student clinical experiences. *Journal of the American Association of Nurse Practitioners, 31*(10), 591–597. https://doi.org/10/1097/JXX.0000000000000310

Shellenbarger, T., & Robb, M. (2016). Effective mentoring in the clinical setting. *American Journal of Nursing, 116*(4), 64–68.

Ulrich, B. (2019). *Mastering precepting: A nurse's handbook for success* (2nd ed.). Sigma Theta Tau.

Evaluation Strategies in Clinical Teaching

Clinical Evaluation and Grading

Nursing practice requires the development of clinical judgment and higher level thinking skills, psychomotor and technological skills, attitudes and values, and other competencies for care of patients across settings. Through clinical evaluation, the teacher arrives at judgments about students' competencies—their performance in practice. After establishing a framework for evaluating students in clinical practice and exploring one's own values, attitudes, and biases that may influence evaluation, the teacher identifies a variety of methods for collecting data on student performance. Clinical evaluation methods are strategies for assessing learning outcomes in clinical practice. Some evaluation methods are most appropriate for use by faculty members or preceptors who are on-site with students and can observe their performance; other evaluation methods assess students' knowledge, cognitive skills, and other competencies but do not involve direct observation of their performance. This chapter describes the process of clinical evaluation in nursing, methods for evaluating clinical performance, and how to grade students in clinical courses.

CONCEPT OF CLINICAL EVALUATION

Clinical evaluation is a process by which judgments are made about learners' competencies in practice. This practice may involve care of patients, families, and communities; other types of learning activities in the clinical setting; simulation activities; performance of varied skills in learning laboratories; or activities using multimedia and technologies. Most frequently, clinical evaluation involves observing performance and arriving at judgments about the student's competence. Judgments influence the data collected—that is, the specific types of observations made to evaluate the student's performance—and the inferences and conclusions drawn from the data about the quality of that performance. Teachers may collect different data to evaluate the same outcomes, and when presented with a series of observations about a student's performance in clinical practice, there may be minimal consistency in their judgments about how well that student performed.

Clinical evaluation is not an objective process; it involves subjective judgments by the educator and others involved in the process. This is most apparent in judging clinical performance, where the nurse educator's values may influence the observations made of students and the judgments about the quality of performance. Thus, it is important for nurse educators and other involved in teaching to be aware of their own values that might bias their judgments of students. For example, if the teacher prefers students who initiate discussions and participate actively in conferences, this value should not influence the assessment of students' competencies in other areas. Or, if the teacher is used to the fast pace of most acute care settings, when working with beginning students or someone who moves slowly, the teacher should be cautious not to let this prior experience influence expectations of performance. Clinical nurse educators and preceptors should examine their values, attitudes, and beliefs so that they are aware of them as they teach and assess students' performance in practice settings.

Clinical Evaluation Versus Grading

Clinical evaluation is not the same as grading. In evaluation, the teacher makes observations of performance and collects other types of data, then compares this information to a set of standards to arrive at a judgment. From this assessment, a quantitative symbol or grade may be applied to reflect the evaluation data and judgments made about performance. The clinical grade, such as pass–fail or A through F, is the symbol to represent the evaluation. Clinical performance may be evaluated and not graded, such as with formative evaluation or feedback to the learner, or it may be graded. Grades, however, should not be assigned without sufficient data about clinical performance. Grades are important to students at all educational levels in nursing (Poorman & Mastorovich, 2019).

Formative and Summative Clinical Evaluation

Clinical evaluation may be formative or summative. Formative evaluation in clinical practice provides feedback to learners about their progress in developing the clinical competencies and meeting the outcomes of the clinical course or practicum. The purposes of formative evaluation are to enable students to develop further their clinical knowledge, skills, and values; indicate areas in which learning and practice are needed; and provide a basis for suggesting additional instruction to improve performance. With this type of evaluation, after identifying the learning needs, instruction is provided to move students forward in their learning. Feedback is critical to learning in the clinical setting: The teacher provides specific information that fills in gaps in learning and helps students improve their performance. Formative evaluation, therefore, is diagnostic; it should not be graded (Brookhart & Nitko, 2019). For example, the clinical nurse educator or preceptor might observe a student perform wound care and give feedback on changes to make with the technique. The goal of this assessment is to improve subsequent performance, not to grade how well the student carried out the procedure.

Summative clinical evaluation, however, is designed for determining clinical grades because it summarizes competencies the student has developed in clinical practice. Summative evaluation is done at the end of a period of time—for example, at midterm or at the end of the clinical practicum—to assess the extent to which learners have achieved the clinical competencies. Summative evaluation is not diagnostic; it summarizes the performance of students at a particular point in time. For much of clinical practice in a nursing education program, summative evaluation comes too late for students to have an opportunity to improve performance. At the end of a course involving care of children, for instance, there may be behaviors the student would not have an opportunity to practice in subsequent courses.

Any protocol for clinical evaluation should include extensive formative evaluation and periodic summative evaluation. Formative evaluation is essential to provide feedback to improve performance while practice experiences are still available.

Fairness in Clinical Evaluation

The goal is for evaluation to be fair. This means that:

1. Clinical educators should identify their own values and biases that may influence the evaluation process. These can affect both the observations made about students and judgments about whether the competencies were met.
2. Clinical evaluation should be based on the competencies to be achieved. The competencies should be the focus of the evaluation.
3. The clinical nurse educator, preceptor, and others in the clinical setting should develop a supportive learning environment where students are comfortable asking questions about care and seeking their guidance. A supportive environment is critical for effective assessment because students need to recognize that the teacher's feedback is intended to help them improve performance.

FEEDBACK IN CLINICAL EVALUATION

For clinical evaluation to be effective, the teacher should provide continuous feedback to students about their performance and how they can improve it. Feedback is the communication of information to students, based on an assessment, that enables students to reflect on their performance, identify continued learning needs, and decide how to meet them (Altmiller, 2016; Bonnel, 2008). Feedback may be verbal, by describing observations of performance and explaining what to do differently, or visual, by demonstrating correct performance. Feedback should be accompanied by further instruction from the teacher or by working with students to identify appropriate learning activities.

The ultimate goal is for students to progress to a point at which they can judge their own performance, identify resources for their learning, and use those resources to further develop competencies. Students must have an underlying knowledge base and beginning skills to judge their own performance. Sometimes students are not able to perform at the expected level because they lack the prerequisite knowledge and skills for developing the new competencies. As such, it is important to begin the clinical instruction by assessing whether students have learned the necessary concepts and skills and, if not, to start there.

Principles of Providing Feedback as Part of Clinical Evaluation

There are five principles for providing feedback to students as part of the clinical evaluation process. First, the feedback should be precise and specific. General information about performance, such as, "You need to work on your assessment" or "You need more practice in the simulation laboratory," does not indicate what behaviors need improvement or how to develop them. Instead of using general statements, the teacher should indicate what specific areas of knowledge are lacking, where there are problems in clinical judgments, and what particular competencies need more development. Rather than saying to a student, "You need to work on your assessment," the student would be better served if the teacher identified the specific areas of data collection omitted and the physical examination techniques that need improvement. Specific feedback is more valuable to learners than a general description of their behavior.

Second, for procedures and any psychomotor skills, the teacher should provide both verbal and visual feedback to students. This means that the teacher should explain first, either orally or in writing, where the errors were made in performance and then demonstrate the correct procedure or skill. This should be followed by deliberate practice: repetitive practice of a skill with assessment of performance and instruction to guide performance (Johnson et al., 2020; Kardong-Edgren et al., 2019). This practice is essential to retain skills and develop proficiency in them.

Third, feedback about performance should be given to students at the time of learning or immediately following it. Providing prompt and rich feedback is equally important when teaching nurses and other learners. The longer the period of time between performance and feedback from the teacher, the less effective is the feedback. As time passes, neither student nor teacher may remember specific areas of clinical practice to be improved. This principle holds true whether the performance relates to cognitive learning, a procedure or clinical skill, or an attitude or value expressed by the student, among other areas.

Whether working with a group of students in a clinical setting, communicating with preceptors about students, or teaching an online course, the teacher needs to develop a strategy for giving focused and immediate feedback to students and following up with further discussion as needed. Recording short notes about observations of students' performance for later discussion with individual students helps the teacher remember important points about performance.

Fourth, students need different amounts of feedback and positive reinforcement. In beginning practice and with clinical situations that are new to learners, most students will need frequent and extensive feedback. As students' progress through the program and become more competent, they should be able to assess their own performance and identify personal learning needs. Some students will require more feedback and direction from the teacher than others.

One final principle is that feedback should be diagnostic. After identifying areas in which further learning is needed, the teacher's responsibility is to guide students so that they can improve their performance. The process is cyclical—the teacher observes and assesses performance, gives students feedback about that performance, and then guides their learning and practice so they can become more competent.

RELATIONSHIP OF EVALUATION TO CLINICAL COMPETENCIES

The clinical competencies provide the basis for clinical evaluation. Competencies are the knowledge, skills, and attitudes that students need to develop in clinical practice; they are the basis for the evaluation (American Association of Colleges of Nursing, 2020). In some nursing programs, outcomes or objectives to be met in clinical practice may be specified for clinical learning. For example, each course might have an outcome on communication. In a beginning clinical course, the outcome might be, "Identifies verbal and nonverbal techniques for communicating with patients." In a later course, the communication outcome might be, "Collaborates with other healthcare providers in care of patients." Outcomes can be stated specifically, or they can be stated more broadly with specific behaviors students should demonstrate to meet those outcomes in a particular course. For example, the outcome on communication might be stated as, "Communicates effectively with patients and others in the health system." Examples of behaviors that indicate achievement of this outcome in a course on care of children include, "Uses appropriate verbal and nonverbal communication based on the child's age, developmental status, and patient condition" and "Interacts effectively with parents, caregivers, and others."

Regardless of how these are stated in a nursing program, the clinical competencies represent *what* is evaluated in clinical practice. For nurses in practice, these competencies reflect the expected level of performance to care for patients in the healthcare setting. Competencies for nurses are assessed as part of the initial employment and orientation to the healthcare setting and on an ongoing basis.

Caution should be exercised in developing clinical competencies to avoid having too many for evaluation, considering the number of learners for whom the teacher is responsible, types of clinical learning opportunities available, and time allotted for clinical learning. In preparing competencies for a clinical course, teachers should keep in mind that they need to collect sufficient data about students' performance of each competency specified for that course. The clinical competencies need to reflect safe and effective practice, be realistic, and be useful for guiding the assessment.

CLINICAL EVALUATION METHODS

There are many evaluation methods for use in nursing education. Some methods, such as journals, are most appropriate for formative evaluation, while others are useful for either formative or summative evaluation.

Selecting Clinical Evaluation Methods

There are several factors to consider when selecting clinical evaluation methods to use in a course. First, the evaluation methods should provide information on student performance of the clinical competencies associated with the course. With the evaluation methods, the teacher collects data on performance to judge whether students are developing the clinical competencies or have achieved them by the end of the course.

Second, for many competencies, different strategies can be used, thereby providing flexibility in choosing methods for evaluation. Varying the methods maintains student interest and takes into account learners' individual needs, abilities, and characteristics. Some students may be more proficient in methods that depend on writing, while others prefer strategies such as conferences and other discussions. Using multiple evaluation methods in clinical practice takes into consideration these differences among students. It also avoids relying on one method, such as a rating scale, for determining the entire clinical grade.

Third, the teacher should select evaluation methods that are realistic considering the number of students to be evaluated, available practice or simulation activities, and constraints such as the teacher's or preceptor's time. Planning for an evaluation method that depends on patients with specific health problems or particular clinical situations is not realistic considering the types of experiences with actual or simulated patients available to students. Some methods are not appropriate because of the number of students who would need to use them within the time frame of the course. Others may be too time consuming for educators to provide feedback to students. Discussions with students one-to-one or in small groups, cases analyzed by students in postclinical conferences, group writing activities, and similar methods might replace strategies that require more teacher time for assessment and accomplish the same purposes.

Fourth, evaluation methods can be used for formative or summative evaluation. In the process of deciding how to evaluate students' clinical performance, the teacher should identify whether the methods will be used to provide feedback to learners (formative) or for grading (summative). In clinical practice, students should know ahead of time whether the assessment by the teacher is for formative or summative purposes. Some of the methods designed for clinical evaluation provide feedback to students on areas for improvement and should not be graded. Other methods, such as rating scales and written assignments, can be used for summative purposes and can be included as part of the clinical grade.

Fifth, before finalizing the plan for how students will be evaluated in a course, the teacher should review the purpose and number required of each assignment completed by students. What are the purposes of these assignments, and how many are needed to demonstrate competency? In some clinical courses, students complete an excessive number of written assignments. Students benefit from continuous feedback from the teacher, not from repetitive assignments that contribute little to their development of clinical knowledge and skills.

Observation

The main strategy for evaluating clinical performance is observing students in clinical practice, simulation and learning laboratories, and other settings. Although observation is widely used, there are threats to its validity and reliability. First, observations of students may be influenced by the teacher's values and biases, as discussed earlier. There may also be overreliance on first impressions, which might change as the teacher or preceptor observes the student over a period of time and in different situations. Altmiller (2016) emphasized that feedback about performance should be an unbiased reflection of observations and events. In any performance evaluation, there needs to be a series of observations made before drawing conclusions about performance. Every observation in the clinical setting reflects only a sampling of the learner's performance. An observation of the same student at another time may reveal a different level of performance.

Second, in clinical practice, there are many aspects of performance on which the educator may focus attention. For example, while observing a student change a surgical wound dressing, the teacher may focus mainly on the technique and not how the student interacts with the patient, while another educator observing this same student may zero in on the interaction. The competencies should guide the teacher on what to observe, but all observations about performance should be shared with the students.

Third, the teacher may arrive at incorrect judgments about the observation, such as inferring that a student is inattentive during conference when, in fact, the student is thinking about the comments made by others in the group. It is important to discuss observations with students, obtain their perceptions of their performance, and be willing to modify one's own judgments when new data are presented.

Fourth, it is difficult, if not impossible, to remember the observations made of each student for each clinical activity. For this reason, clinical educators need some type of notes that describe the observations made of students. The notes can include a description of the observations only or the observations with a statement about how well the student performed. Notes about the student's performance should be recorded as close to the time of the observation as possible and should be shared frequently with students. Considering that many factors may influence observations of performance, educators should discuss their observations with students and be willing to incorporate students' impressions of their performance. These notes are also useful in conferences with students—for example, at midterm and at the end of the practicum—for reviewing a pattern of performance over time. Notes can be handwritten or recorded using some technology.

Checklists

A checklist contains specific behaviors or activities to be observed with a place for marking whether they were present during the performance (Brookhart & Nitko, 2019). A checklist often lists the steps to be followed in performing a procedure or demonstrating a skill. Checklists guide the teacher's observation of procedures performed by students and nurses and also provide a way for learners to assess their own performance.

For common procedures, teachers can often find checklists already prepared that can be used for evaluation. When these resources are not available, teachers can develop their own checklists but should avoid including every possible step, which makes the checklist too cumbersome and prescriptive. Instead, the focus should be on critical behaviors for safe performance of the procedure or skill.

Rating Scales

Rating scales, also referred to as clinical evaluation tools, forms, or instruments, provide a means of recording judgments about the observed performance of students in clinical practice. A rating scale has two parts: (a) a list of competencies (or outcomes and behaviors) the student is to demonstrate in clinical practice and (b) a scale for rating their performance of them. Rating scales are most useful for summative evaluation of performance. After observing students over a period of time, the teacher determines if the competencies were achieved and, for tools with multiple levels, rates the quality of the performance. A few examples of evaluation tools are provided in Appendix B. The Quality and Safety Innovation Center, at the College of New Jersey, provides access to content-validated Quality and Safety Education for Nurses (QSEN)-based Clinical Evaluation tools. There are instruments for use in nursing courses in prelicensure and nurse practitioner programs. These tools are available at https://qsicenter.tcnj.edu/resources/.

The same rating scale can be used for multiple purposes. Exhibit 12.1 shows sample competencies from a rating scale that is used midway through a course and at the end as for the final summative rating.

TYPES OF RATING SCALES

Many types of rating scales are used for evaluating clinical performance. The scales may have multiple levels for rating performance, such as 1 to 5 or exceptional to

EXHIBIT 12.1 Sample Competencies From Rating Scale

COMPETENCIES	Midterm			Final	
	S	NI	U	S	U
1. Provides patient-centered care for patients with chronic health problems across the life span					
A. Completes a comprehensive assessment using multiple sources of data					
B. Develops an individualized plan of care reflecting patient values, preferences, and needs					
C. Implements nursing interventions based on evidence					
D. Evaluates the outcomes of care					
E. Demonstrates caring behaviors					
2. Collaborates with nurses, the interprofessional team, and others in the healthcare system and community					
A. Demonstrates effective communication skills (with patients, families/caregivers, nurses, and other healthcare providers)					
B. Communicates relevant information about the patient and clinical situation using SBAR (Situation-Background-Assessment-Recommendation)					
C. Collaborates with members of intra- and interprofessional teams					
D. Identifies resources for patients and caregivers for discharge and transitions of care					
3. ...					

Student Name _____ Faculty Name _____
Date _____

S, satisfactory; NI, needs improvement; U, Unsatisfactory

Source: Oermann, M. H., & Gaberson, K. B. (2021). *Evaluation and testing in nursing education* (6th ed.). Springer Publishing Company. p. 274. Reprinted by permission, 2021.

below average, or have two levels, such as pass–fail. Types of scales with multiple levels for rating performance include:

- Letters: A, B, C, D, E or A, B, C, D, F
- Numbers: 1, 2, 3, 4, 5
- Qualitative labels: Excellent, very good, good, fair, poor; exceptional, above average, average, below average
- Frequency labels: Always, usually, frequently, sometimes, never
- Combinations of these scales

A short description included with the letters, numbers, and labels for each of the competencies rated improves objectivity and consistency (Brookhart & Nitko, 2019). For example, with a scale based on numbers, short descriptions of each level in the scale could be written to clarify the expected performance. For the competency "Collects relevant data from patients," the descriptors might be:

4. Differentiates relevant from irrelevant data, analyzes multiple sources of data, collects comprehensive data, identifies data needed for evaluating possible patient problems.
3. Collects significant data from patients, uses multiple sources of data as part of assessment, identifies possible patient problems based on the data.
2. Collects significant data from patients, uses data to develop main patient problems.
1. Does not collect significant data and misses important cues in data; unable to explain relevance of data for patient problems.

However, even with descriptors the level of performance is often not clear cut, and there may be inconsistency in clinical nurse educator and preceptor interpretations of the quality of performance. What is the difference between a 2, 3, or 4 level of performance? Do all clinical educators in the course agree? Scales based on frequency labels are often difficult to implement because of limited experiences for students to practice and demonstrate a level of skill rated as "always, usually, frequently, sometimes, and never." How should teachers rate students' performance in situations in which they practiced the skill perhaps once or twice? With rating scales that have two levels, such as pass–fail, satisfactory–unsatisfactory, and met–did not meet the competency, there is less variability in the judgments to be made by educators, but even two-dimensional scales present room for variability. It is critical that everyone involved in the evaluation has an opportunity to discuss each of the competencies on a tool, what they mean, the expected performance, and the rating for that performance level, and come to an agreement.

RATING ERRORS

Brookhart and Nitko (2019) identified common errors that can occur with rating scales applicable to rating clinical performance. The first three errors can occur with tools that have multiple points on the scale for rating performance, such as 1 to 5 or below average to exceptional. The other errors can occur with any type of clinical performance rating scale.

1. Leniency error results when the teacher tends to rate all students toward the high end of the scale.
2. Severity error is the opposite of leniency, tending to rate all students toward the low end of the scale.
3. Central tendency error is hesitancy to mark either end of the rating scale and instead use only the midpoint of the scale.
4. Halo effect is a judgment based on a general impression of the student. With this error, the teacher lets an overall impression of the student influence the ratings of specific aspects of the student's performance. The halo may be positive, giving the student a higher rating than is deserved, or negative, letting a general negative impression of the student result in lower ratings of performance.
5. Personal bias occurs when the teacher's biases influence ratings.
6. Logical error results when similar ratings are given for items on the scale that are logically related to one another. This is a problem with rating scales that are too long and often too detailed. For example, there may be multiple competencies on communication to be rated. The teacher observes some of these but not all of them. In completing the clinical evaluation form, the teacher gives the same rating to all competencies related to communication on the tool. When this occurs, some of the items on the rating scale can often be combined.
7. Rater drift occurs when the clinical nurse educators and others involved in the evaluation redefine the competencies to be observed and assessed. Initially, in developing a clinical evaluation form, all agree on the competencies to be rated and the scale to be used. However, over time, the competencies may be interpreted differently, drifting away from the original intent. For this reason, discussion of the tool is critical at the beginning and mid-point of a course.
8. Reliability decay is a similar issue. Brookhart and Nitko (2019) indicated that immediately following training on using a rating tool, educators tend to use the tool consistently across students and with each other. As the course continues, though, educators may become less consistent in their ratings. Discussion of the tool among evaluators, as indicated earlier, may improve consistency in its use.

Although there are issues with rating scales, they allow clinical educators, preceptors, and others to rate performance over time and to assess patterns of performance. Exhibit 12.2 provides guidelines for using rating scales for clinical evaluation in nursing.

EXHIBIT 12.2 Guidelines for Using Rating Scales for Clinical Evaluation

1. Be alert to the possible influence of your own values, attitudes, and biases in observing performance and drawing conclusions about it.
2. Use the clinical competencies to focus your observations. Give students feedback on your observations.
3. Collect sufficient data on students' performance before rating it summatively. Students should be observed more than one time. Rating scales, when used for clinical evaluation, are intended for assessing performance over a period of time.
4. Do not rely on first impressions; they may not be accurate.

(continued)

EXHIBIT 12.2 Guidelines for Using Rating Scales for Clinical Evaluation (*continued*)

5. Always discuss observations with students, obtain their perceptions of performance, and be willing to modify judgments and ratings when new data are presented.
6. Avoid using rating scales as the only source of data about a student's performance—use multiple evaluation methods for clinical practice.
7. Rate each competency individually based on the observations made of performance. If you have insufficient information about achievement of a particular competency, do not rate it—leave it blank.
8. If the rating form is not useful for judging student performance, then revise and re-evaluate it. Consider these questions: Does the form yield data that can be used to make valid decisions about students' competence? Does the form yield reliable, stable data? Is it easy to use? Is it appropriate considering the types of learning activities that students have in their clinical settings or can obtain in simulation or skills laboratory?
9. Discuss as a group (with other educators, preceptors, and others involved in the evaluation) each competency on the rating scale. Come to agreement about the meaning of the competencies and what a student's performance would look like at each rating level in the tool. Share examples of performance, how you would rate them, and your rationale. As a group exercise, observe a video clip or other simulation of a student's performance, rate it with the tool, and come to agreement about the rating. Such exercises and discussions should be held before the course begins and periodically during it to ensure reliability across teachers and settings.

Simulations for Clinical Evaluation

Simulations are not only effective for instruction in nursing, but they are also useful for clinical evaluation. Students can demonstrate skills, conduct assessments, analyze scenarios and make decisions about problems and actions to take, carry out nursing interventions, and evaluate the effects of their decisions. Many nursing education programs have simulation laboratories with human patient simulators, manikins and models for skill practice and assessment, areas for standardized patients, clinically equipped examination rooms, and a wide range of multimedia that can be used to facilitate performance evaluations. Video conferencing and other technology can be used to conduct clinical evaluations of students in settings at a distance from the nursing education program, effectively replacing on-site performance evaluations by faculty members.

The same principles for evaluating student performance in the clinical setting apply to using simulations. The first task is to identify which clinical competencies will be assessed with a simulation. It is important to remember when deciding on evaluation methods that assessment can be done for feedback to students and thus remain ungraded, or it can be used for grading purposes. If the evaluation using simulation is for high-stakes decisions, where students need to pass the assessment to progress in the course or program, more than one evaluator should observe and rate performance; evaluators should be trained and use a valid and reliable tool; they need to practice to be comfortable with the tool and observation of performance; and evaluators should not know the students being evaluated (Oermann & Gaberson, 2021; Oermann, Kardong-Edgren, & Rizzolo, 2016).

Standardized Patients

One type of simulation for clinical evaluation uses standardized patients—individuals who have been trained to accurately portray the role of a patient with a specific diagnosis or condition. With simulations using standardized patients, students can be evaluated on a history and physical examination, related skills and procedures, and communication techniques, among other competencies. Champlin et al. (2020) noted that standardized patients might provide feedback to students about their professionalism and bedside manner, but this would not count toward the students' score or grade. Standardized patients are effective for evaluation because the actors are trained to re-create the same patient condition and clinical situation each time they are with a student, providing for consistency in the performance evaluation.

When standardized patients are used for formative evaluation, they provide feedback to the students on their performance, an important aid to their learning. Ballman et al. (2016) developed interactive case studies using technology to allow students in a distance education program to interact with standardized patients.

Objective Structured Clinical Examination

An objective structured clinical examination (OSCE) provides a means of evaluating performance in a simulation laboratory rather than in the clinical setting. In an OSCE, students rotate through a series of stations; at each station, they complete an activity or perform a task, which is then evaluated. Some stations assess the student's ability to take a patient's history, perform a physical examination, and implement other interventions while being observed by the teacher or an examiner. The student's performance can then be rated using a rating scale or checklist. At other stations, students might be tested on their knowledge and clinical judgment—they might be asked to analyze data, identify patient problems, select interventions and treatments, and manage the patient's condition. There may also be post-encounter stations to facilitate the evaluation of cognitive skills such as interpreting lab results and other data, developing management plans, and making other types of judgments and decisions about patient care. In a scoping review of 204 studies, Goh et al. (2019) found that OSCEs were valid, reliable, and an acceptable method for evaluating performance in nursing. OSCEs were used across various nursing specialties in 33 countries. OSCEs are typically used for summative clinical evaluation but can also be used formatively to assess performance and provide feedback to students.

Written Assignments

Written assignments accompanying the clinical practicum are effective methods for assessing students' higher-level learning, understanding of concepts and content relevant to clinical practice, and ability to express ideas in writing. Many types of written assignments for clinical courses were described in Chapter 7. Written assignments can be included as part of the clinical evaluation.

EVALUATING WRITTEN ASSIGNMENTS

Written assignments may be evaluated formatively or summatively. Periodic assessment of drafts of papers and work in progress is formative in nature and is not intended for arriving at a grade. For written assignments that are not graded, the teacher's role is to give prompt and sufficient feedback for students to learn from the assignment. If the assignment will be graded at a later time (summative evaluation), then criteria for grading and the rubric to be used should be shared with students. Some writing assignments, such as journals, do not lend themselves to grading and instead are best used for formative evaluation only.

To improve writing, drafts of papers should be submitted for feedback on writing and content. Students need specific suggestions about revisions, not general statements such as "unclear introduction." Instead, tell students exactly what needs to be changed; for example, "The introduction is about noise reduction strategies rather than the problem on the unit with noise. Revise the introduction to explain the problem with noise on the unit, supporting data on noise levels, and why we need strategies to reduce noise for both patients and staff." Feedback is typically provided in written form but can also be given using various technology tools. Madson (2017) described used screencasts, a digital audiovisual technology that records what is displayed on the teacher's computer screen, for giving writing feedback to students.

CRITERIA FOR EVALUATION

The criteria for evaluation of a paper should relate to the learning outcomes to be met. For example, if students write a short paper to meet the objective, "Compare interventions for nausea associated with chemotherapy," criteria should relate to the appropriateness and evidence for the interventions selected for critique, how effectively the student compared them, the rationale developed for the analysis, and the like. General criteria for evaluating written assignments in clinical courses are presented in Exhibit 12.3. For assignments that are graded, students should have the criteria for evaluation and rubric (scoring guide) before they begin writing so they know what will be assessed.

GRADING ASSIGNMENTS

In grading written assignments, a rubric, which is a scoring guide, should be developed based on the criteria established for evaluation. The rubric includes the areas to be evaluated and points allotted for each one and keeps the evaluation focused on the criteria, not some other standard. Some teachers tend to be more lenient, and others tend to be more critical in their review of papers. Rubrics lead to more consistent and transparent scoring (Fulbright, 2018; Minnich et al., 2018).

There are different types of rubrics. With a holistic rubric, the teacher scores the paper as a whole without assessing individual parts. An analytic rubric guides the assessment of separate parts of the paper and then sums them for a total score. Exhibit 12.4 is an example of a rubric that was developed using the general criteria in Exhibit 12.3.

PRINCIPLES FOR ASSESSING WRITTEN ASSIGNMENTS

Written assignments that are graded should be read anonymously if at all possible. This is sometimes difficult with small groups of students. There is a tendency in evaluating papers and other written assignments, similar to essay items, for the teacher to be influenced by a general impression of the student. This is called the

EXHIBIT 12.3 General Criteria for Evaluating Papers in Clinical Courses

Content
    Content is relevant to patient or clinical situation.
    Content is accurate.
    Significant information is presented.
    Concepts and theories are used appropriately for analysis.
    Content is comprehensive.
    Content reflects current research and evidence.
    Hypotheses, conclusions, and decisions are supported.

Organization
    Content is organized logically.
    Ideas are presented in logical sequence.
    Paragraph structure is appropriate.
    Headings are used appropriately to indicate new content areas.

Process
    Process used to arrive at approaches, decisions, judgments, and so forth is adequate.
    Consequences of decisions are considered.
    Sound rationale is provided.
    For papers analyzing issues, rationale supports position taken.
    Multiple perspectives and new approaches are considered.

Writing Style
    Ideas are described clearly.
    Sentence structure is clear.
    There are no grammatical errors.
    There are no spelling errors.
    Appropriate punctuation is used.
    Writing does not reveal bias.
    Length of paper is consistent with requirements.
    Literature used in paper is up to date (within the past 3–5 years)
    References are cited appropriately throughout paper.
    References are accurate and prepared according to required format.

halo effect. The teacher may have positive or negative feelings about the student or other biases that may influence evaluating and grading the assignment.

Another reason to read papers anonymously is to avoid a carryover effect, in which the teacher carries an impression of the quality of one written assignment to the next one that the student completes. If the student develops an outstanding paper, the teacher may be influenced to score subsequent written assignments at a similarly high level; the same situation may occur with a poor paper. The impression of the student is carried from one written assignment to the next (Oermann & Gaberson, 2021).

Papers and other types of written assignments should be read in random order. After the first reading, educators can shuffle the papers so they are read in a random order the second time. Papers read early may be scored higher than those read near

EXHIBIT 12.4 Sample Scoring Rubric for Papers in Clinical Courses

Content		
Content relevant to patient or clinical situation, comprehensive, and in-depth 5	Content relevant to patient or clinical situation with critical information included 4–3	Some content not relevant to patient or clinical situation, critical information missing, lacks depth 2–1
Content accurate 5	Most of content accurate 4–3	Major errors in content 2–1
Sound background developed from peer-reviewed articles and wide range of information sources 5	Textbook and websites are predominant sources of information for developing background 4–3	Background not developed, limited support for ideas 2–1
Current research and evidence synthesized and integrated effectively 10–7	Current research and evidence summarized 6–4	Limited research and evidence in paper, not used to support ideas 3–1
Organization		
Purpose of paper well developed and clearly stated 3	Purpose apparent but not developed sufficiently 2	Purpose poorly developed, not clear 1
Content well organized and logically presented, organization supports arguments and development of ideas 10–7	Clear organization of main points and ideas 6–4	Poorly organized, content not developed adequately 3–1
Effective conclusions based on analysis 3	Conclusions based on summary of content, limited analysis 2	Poor conclusions, not based on content in paper 1

(continued)

EXHIBIT 12.4 Sample Scoring Rubric for Papers in Clinical Courses *(continued)*

Writing Style and Format		
Sentence structure clear, smooth transitions, correct grammar and punctuation, no spelling errors **10–7**	Adequate sentence structure and transitions; few grammar, punctuation, and spelling errors **6–4**	Poor sentence structure and transitions; errors in grammar, punctuation, and spelling **3–1**
Writing Style and Format		
Professional appearance of paper, all parts included, length consistent with requirements **3**	Paper legible, some parts missing or too short or too long considering requirements **2**	Unprofessional appearance, missing sections, paper too short or too long considering requirements **1**
References used appropriately, references current, no errors in references, correct use of APA style **6–5**	References used appropriately but limited, most references current, some citations or references with errors or some errors in APA style **4–3**	Few references and limited breadth, old references (not classic), errors in references, errors in APA style **2–1**
Total score _____ (sum points for total score; maximum score 60)		

the end (Oermann & Gaberson, 2021). Teacher fatigue may also set in and influence the grading of papers. Although this section was on grading written assignments, many writing assignments are for learning and are not graded.

JOURNALS

Journals allow students to describe experiences in clinical practice and reflect on them. With journals, students can think aloud and share their feelings with the educator. Journals are not intended to develop students' writing skills. Instead, they provide a means of expressing feelings and reflections on clinical practice, engaging in a dialogue with the teacher about clinical experiences, developing clinical judgment, and assessing own learning needs (Bussard, 2015, 2018; Fernandez-Pena et al., 2016; Hwang et al., 2018). Students need to be clear about the objectives of the journal. For example, a journal intended for reflection would require different entries than one for documenting activities done in clinical practice as a means of communicating them to faculty.

Cases

Cases for clinical learning were described in Chapter 8. Cases can be completed by students individually or as a group activity. They are effective methods for group discussion and peer review in postclinical conferences and for online discussions. In an online course, the case scenario can be presented with open-ended questions, and, based on student responses, other questions can be introduced for discussion. Using this approach, cases are effective for encouraging higher level thinking. By discussing cases as a clinical group, students are exposed to other possible approaches and perspectives they may not have identified themselves. With this method, the teacher can provide feedback on the content and thought process used by students to arrive at their answers. One advantage of cases is they can be done for instructional purposes and not graded, or they can be graded as part of the clinical evaluation grade.

Electronic Portfolio

An electronic portfolio (e-portfolio) is a collection of projects and materials (also referred to as artifacts) developed by the student that documents achievement of the outcomes of the clinical course. With a portfolio, students can demonstrate what they have learned in clinical practica and the competencies they have developed. Portfolios are valuable for clinical evaluation because students provide evidence in their portfolios to confirm their clinical competencies and document new learning and skills acquired in a course. Most portfolios are developed electronically, which facilitates updating and revising entries, as compared with portfolios that include hard copies of materials.

E-portfolios are used increasingly in doctor of nursing practice programs to provide documentation of student achievement of competencies and program outcomes (Anderson et al., 2017; Melander et al., 2018; Willmarth-Stec & Beery, 2015). They also are used in prelicensure, RN-to-BSN, and master's programs. Portfolios can be evaluated and graded by faculty members or clinical educators or used for students' self-assessment of their progress in meeting personal and professional goals and not be evaluated by the teacher.

Brookhart and Nitko (2019) identified two types of portfolios: best work and growth. Best-work portfolios contain the students' best final products. These provide evidence that the students have demonstrated certain competencies and met the outcomes of the course, and thus are appropriate for summative evaluation. Growth portfolios are designed for monitoring students' progress and providing feedback, and for self-reflection on learning (Brookhart & Nitko, 2019).

The contents of the portfolio depend on the outcomes of the clinical practicum and competencies to be developed, but any documents that communicate what students have learned would be appropriate. The key is for students to choose materials and products they have developed that demonstrate their learning. Steps for planning an e-portfolio for clinical evaluation are in Exhibit 12.5.

Conferences

The ability to present ideas orally is an important outcome of clinical practice. Sharing information about a patient, leading others in discussions about clinical practice, presenting ideas in a group format, and giving presentations are skills

EXHIBIT 12.5 Steps for Planning an Electronic Portfolio for a Clinical Practicum

1. Identify the purpose of the portfolio. (Provide evidence of students' best work in clinical practice, their learning over a period of time, or both? Used for formative or summative evaluation, or both? Provide assessment data for a clinical course or for program evaluation and accreditation?)
2. Identify the type of documents and content to be included in the e-portfolio. (Required types of documents? Minimum number required? How to organize?)
3. Decide on the evaluation of the e-portfolio including criteria for evaluation. (How will the e-portfolio be integrated within the grade, if at all? Develop rubric for scoring the e-portfolio and/or individual documents.)

Source: Brookhart, S. M., & Nitko, A. J. (2019). *Educational assessment of students* (6th ed.). Pearson.

that students need to develop in a nursing program. Working with nursing staff members and the interprofessional team requires the ability to communicate effectively. Conferences provide a method for developing oral communication skills and for evaluating competency in this area. Discussions also can lead to higher level thinking if questions are open ended and used as prompts for clinical judgment.

Criteria for assessing conferences include the ability of students to:

- Present ideas clearly and in a logical sequence to the group
- Participate actively in the group discussion
- Offer ideas relevant to the topic
- Demonstrate knowledge of the content discussed in the conference
- Offer different perspectives on the topic, engaging the group in critical thinking
- Assume a leadership role, if relevant, in promoting group discussion and arriving at group decisions

Most conferences are evaluated for formative purposes, with the teacher giving feedback to students as a group or to the individual who led the group discussion. When conferences are evaluated as a portion of the clinical or course grade, the teacher should have specific criteria to guide the evaluation and should use a scoring rubric. Exhibit 12.6 provides a sample form that can be used to evaluate how well a student leads a clinical conference or to assess student participation in a conference.

Group Projects

Most of the clinical evaluation methods presented in this chapter focus on individual student performance, but group projects also can be assessed as part of the clinical evaluation in a course. Some group work is short term—only for the time it takes to develop a product, such as a teaching plan or group presentation. Other groups may be formed for the purpose of cooperative learning, with students working in small groups or teams in clinical practice over a longer period of time. With any of these group formats, both the products developed by the group and the ability of the students to work cooperatively can be assessed.

There are different approaches for grading group projects. The same grade can be given to every student in the group (i.e., a group grade), although this does not take into consideration individual student effort and contribution to the group product.

EXHIBIT 12.6 Evaluation of Participation in a Clinical Conference

Student's name _____

Conference topic _____

Date _____

Rate the behaviors listed here by circling the appropriate number. Some behaviors will not be applicable depending on the student's role in the conference; mark those as not applicable (na).

Behaviors	Rating					
	Poor				Excellent	
States goals of conference	1	2	3	4	5	na
Leads group in discussion	1	2	3	4	5	na
Asks thought-provoking questions	1	2	3	4	5	na
Uses strategies that encourage all students to participate	1	2	3	4	5	na
Participates actively in discussion	1	2	3	4	5	na
Includes important content	1	2	3	4	5	na
Includes evidence for practice	1	2	3	4	5	na
Offers new perspectives to group	1	2	3	4	5	na
Considers different points of view	1	2	3	4	5	na
Assists group members in recognizing biases and values	1	2	3	4	5	na
Is enthusiastic about topic	1	2	3	4	5	na
Is well prepared for discussion	1	2	3	4	5	na
If leading group, monitors time	1	2	3	4	5	na
Develops quality materials to support discussion	1	2	3	4	5	na
Summarizes major points at end of conference	1	2	3	4	5	na

Another approach is for the students to indicate in the finished product the parts to which they contributed, providing a way of assigning individual student grades, with or without a group grade. Students can also provide a self-assessment of how much they contributed to the group project, which can then be integrated into their grade. Alternatively, students can prepare both a group and an individual product.

Rubrics should be used for assessing group projects and should be geared specifically to the project. To assess students' participation and collaboration in the group, the rubric also needs to reflect the goals of group work. With small groups, the teacher can observe and rate individual student cooperation and contributions to the group. However, this is often difficult because the teacher is not a member of the group, and the group dynamics change when the teacher is present. As another approach, students can assess the participation and cooperation of their peers. These peer evaluations can be used for the students' own development and shared among peers but not with the teacher, or they can be incorporated by the teacher in the grade for the group project. Students can also be asked to assess their own participation in the group.

Self-Assessment

Self-assessment is the ability of students to assess their own clinical competencies and identify where further learning is needed. Self-evaluation begins with the first clinical course and develops throughout the nursing program, continuing into professional practice. Through self-evaluation, students examine their clinical performance and identify both strengths and areas for improvement. Using students' own assessments, teachers can develop plans to assist students in gaining the knowledge and skills they need to meet the outcomes of the course. Self-evaluation is appropriate only for formative evaluation and should never be graded.

CLINICAL EVALUATION IN DISTANCE EDUCATION

Nursing programs use different strategies for offering the clinical component of distance education courses. In one strategy, widely used in advanced practice nursing programs, schools in collaboration with students arrange clinical sites and preceptors to work one-to-one with students to guide their learning and evaluate performance. If cohorts of students are available in an area, adjunct or part-time faculty members might be hired to teach a small group of students in the clinical setting. In other programs, students independently complete clinical learning activities to gain the clinical knowledge and competencies of a course. Regardless of how the clinical component is structured, the course syllabus, competencies to be developed, rating forms, guidelines for clinical practice, and other materials associated with the clinical course need to be available to whomever is providing the instruction and evaluating student learning. Course management systems facilitate communication among students, preceptors, course faculty, and others involved in the students' clinical activities.

The clinical evaluation methods presented in this chapter can be used for distance education. The critical decision for the teacher is to identify which clinical competencies and skills, if any, need to be observed and the performance rated, because that decision suggests different evaluation methods than if the focus of the evaluation is on the cognitive outcomes of the clinical course. In programs in which preceptors or adjunct nurse educators are on-site, any of the clinical evaluation methods presented in this chapter can be used as long as they are congruent with the competencies and clinical practicum outcomes. There should be consistency, though, in how the evaluation is done across preceptors and clinical sites.

Even in clinical courses involving preceptors, faculty members may decide to evaluate some of the clinical competencies themselves by reviewing digital recordings of performance or observing students through video conferencing and other technology. Digitally recording performance is valuable to assess competencies during (for feedback) and at the end of a clinical practicum and for review by students for self-assessment. Some schools are using telehealth and related technology to conduct virtual site visits for evaluating the performance of nurse practitioner and other advanced practice nursing students at a distance (Bice & Parker, 2019; Harris et al., 2020).

Simulations and standardized patients are other strategies useful in assessing clinical performance in distance education. Performance with standardized patients can be recorded, and students can submit their patient histories and other written documentation that would commonly be done in practice in that situation. Students can also complete case analyses related to the standardized patient encounter for assessing their knowledge base and rationale for their decisions. Further discussion about evaluating students in online nursing courses is provided in Chapter 13.

GRADING CLINICAL PRACTICE

Grading systems for clinical practice are often two-dimensional, such as pass–fail, satisfactory–unsatisfactory, and met or did not meet the clinical competencies. Some nursing programs add a third category, honors, to acknowledge performance that exceeds the level required. Other grading systems are multidimensional—for example, using letter grades A through F; integers 1 through 5; and percentages. With any of these grading systems, it is not always easy to summarize the multiple types of evaluation data collected about the student's performance into a symbol representing a grade. This is true even in a pass–fail system; it may be difficult to arrive at a judgment to pass or fail based on the evaluation data and the circumstances associated with the student's clinical and simulated practice.

Regardless of the grading system for clinical practice, there are two criteria to be met: (a) the evaluation methods for collecting data about student performance should reflect the clinical competencies for which a grade will be assigned, and (b) students need to understand how their clinical practica will be evaluated and graded. In planning the course, the faculty decides which of the evaluation methods should be incorporated in the clinical grade. Some of these methods are for summative evaluation, thereby providing a source of information for including in the clinical grade. Other methods, though, are used in clinical practice for feedback only and are not incorporated in the grade.

Categories for grading clinical practice such as pass–fail have advantages over a system with multiple levels, although there are some disadvantages as well. Pass–fail places greater emphasis on giving feedback to the learner because only two categories of performance need to be determined. With a pass–fail grading system, clinical nurse educators may be more inclined to provide continual feedback to learners because they do not have to ultimately differentiate performance according to four or five levels of proficiency such as with a multidimensional system.

A pass–fail system requires only two types of judgment about clinical performance. Do the evaluation data indicate that the student has demonstrated satisfactory performance of the competencies to indicate a pass? Or do the data suggest that the performance of those competencies is not at a satisfactory level? Deciding whether the learner has passed or failed is often easier for the teacher than using the same evaluation information for deciding on multiple levels of performance.

A letter system for grading clinical practice, however, acknowledges the differ-ent levels of clinical proficiency students may have demonstrated in their clinical practica.

A disadvantage of pass–fail for grading clinical practice is the inability to include a clinical grade into the course grade. One strategy is to separate nursing courses into two components for grading: one for theory and the second for clinical practice (designated as pass–fail). Typically, guidelines for the course indicate that the students must pass the clinical component to pass the course. A second mecha-nism is to offer two separate courses with the clinical course graded on a pass–fail basis.

Methods for Assigning the Clinical Grade

Once the grading system is determined, there are varied ways of using it to arrive at the clinical grade. The grade can be assigned based on the competencies achieved by the student. To use this method, faculty can designate some of the competencies as critical for achievement in the course. For example, an A might be assigned if all of the clinical competencies were met; a B might be assigned if all of the competen-cies designated by the faculty as critical behaviors and at least half of the others were met. For pass–fail grading, the faculty might indicate that all of the compe-tencies must be met to pass the course or can designate critical ones required for passing the course. For both of these grading systems, the clinical evaluation meth-ods provide the data for determining whether the student's performance reflects achievement of the competencies. These evaluation methods may or may not be graded separately as part of the course grade.

Another way of arriving at the clinical grade is to base it on the clinical evalu-ation methods. In this system, the clinical grade is computed based on the evalu-ation methods. The rating on the clinical evaluation tool is only a portion of the clinical grade (Table 12.1). An advantage of this approach is that it incorporates into the grade the summative evaluation methods completed by students. If pass–fail is used for grading clinical practice, the grade might be computed as shown in Table 12.2.

TABLE 12.1 EXAMPLE OF CLINICAL GRADE BASED ON EVALUATION METHODS WITH PERFORMANCE GRADED

Assignment	Percent of Grade
Paper on analysis of clinical practice issue	10
Analysis of clinical case	5
Online conference presentation	15
Community resource paper	5
Electronic portfolio	25
Rating scale (of performance)	40
Total	100

TABLE 12.2 EXAMPLE OF CLINICAL GRADE BASED ON EVALUATION METHODS WITH PASS-FAIL GRADING

Assignment	Percent of Grade
Paper on analysis of clinical practice issue	10
Analysis of clinical case	5
Online conference presentation	15
Community resource paper	5
Electronic portfolio	25
OSCE	40
Rating scale (of performance)	Pass required
Total	100

OSCE, Objective Structured Clinical Examination.

FAILING CLINICAL PRACTICE

Clinical nurse educators and preceptors may be faced with students not demonstrating sufficient competence to pass the clinical course. There are principles that should be followed in evaluating and grading clinical practicum, which are critical if a student fails a clinical practicum or course or has the potential for failing it.

Communicate Evaluation and Grading Methods in Writing

The evaluation methods used in a clinical course; how each will be graded, if at all; and how the clinical grade will be assigned should be in writing and communicated to the students. The teacher's practices in evaluating and grading clinical performance must reflect this written information. In courses with adjunct faculty, part-time clinical nurse educators, and preceptors, it is critical that they understand the clinical competencies and outcomes of the course, the evaluation methods, how to observe and rate performance, and responsibilities when students are not performing adequately. Preceptors are reluctant to assign failing grades to students whose competence is questionable (Anthony & Wickman, 2015).

Identify Effect of Failing Clinical Practicum on Course Grade

If failing clinical practice, whether in a pass–fail or a letter system, means failing the nursing course, this should be stated clearly in the course syllabus and policies. By stating it in the syllabus, which all students receive, they have it in writing before clinical learning activities begin. A sample policy statement for pass–fail clinical grading is:

> The clinical component of NUR XXX is evaluated with a pass or fail. A failing grade in the clinical component results in failure of the course, even if the theory grade is 75% or higher.

In a letter grade system, the policy should include the letter grade representing a failure in clinical practice—for example, below a C grade. A sample policy statement is:

> Students must pass the clinical component of NUR XXX with the grade of C or higher. A grade lower than a C in the clinical component of the course results in failure of the course, even if the theory grade is 75% or higher.

Ask Students to Sign Rating Forms and Evaluation Summaries

Students should sign any written clinical evaluation documents—rating forms (of clinical practicum, clinical examinations, and performance in simulations), notes and any other narrative comments about the student's performance, and summaries of conferences in which performance was discussed. Their signatures do not mean they agree with the ratings or comments, only that they have read them. Students should have an opportunity to write in their own comments. These materials are important because they document the student's performance and indicate that the teacher provided feedback and shared concerns about that performance. This is critical in situations in which students may be failing the clinical course because of performance problems.

Identify Performance Problems Early and Develop Learning Plans

Students need continuous feedback on their clinical performance. Observations made by the teacher, the preceptor, and others, and evaluation data from other sources, should be shared with the student. Together they should discuss these. Students may have different perceptions of their performance and, in some cases, may provide new information that influences the teacher's judgment about clinical competencies.

When the clinical nurse educator or preceptor identifies performance problems and clinical deficiencies that may affect passing the course, conferences should be held with the student to discuss these areas of concern and develop a plan for remediation. It is critical that these conferences focus on problems in performance combined with specific learning activities for addressing them. The conferences should not be the teacher telling the student everything that is wrong with clinical performance: The student needs an opportunity to respond to these concerns and identify how to address them.

One of the goals of the conference is to develop a plan with learning activities for the student to correct deficiencies and develop competencies further. The plan should indicate that (a) completing the remedial learning activities does not guarantee that the student will pass the course, (b) one satisfactory performance of the competencies will not constitute a pass clinical grade (the improvement must be sustained), and (c) the student must demonstrate satisfactory performance of the competencies by the end of the course. A template is provided in Exhibit 12.7 that can be used to develop a learning plan for students. It is important to remember that students have until the end of the clinical practicum (the course) to improve their performance unless they are unsafe in the clinical setting. In that case, the student may be removed from the clinical course depending on the policies of the nursing program, which every clinical educator, preceptor, and student should understand.

EXHIBIT 12.7 Template of a Learning Plan

1. List of clinical competencies and areas of performance to be improved.
2. For each of the competencies/areas, identify specific learning activities to be completed by the student with due dates.
3. List the process to be used for evaluating the student's progress and performance. Include dates for achieving competencies and specific meeting times for feedback on progress.

Any discussions with students at risk of failing clinical practice should focus on the student's inability to meet the clinical objectives and perform the specified competencies, not on the teacher's perceptions of the student's intelligence and overall ability. In addition, opinions about the student's ability in general should not be discussed with others.

Conferences should be held in private, and a summary of the discussion should be prepared. The summary should include the date and time of the conference, who participated, areas of concern about clinical performance, and the learning plan with a time frame for completion. The summary should be signed by the teacher, the student, and other participants. All clinical teachers should review related policies of the nursing education program because they might specify other requirements.

Students who are at risk of failing clinical practice may have other problems affecting their performance. Teachers should refer students to counselling and other support services and not attempt to provide these resources themselves. Attempting to counsel the student and help the student cope with other problems may bias the clinical educator and influence judgment of the student's clinical performance.

Document Performance

As the clinical practicum progresses, the teacher should give feedback to the student about performance and continue to guide learning. It is important to document the observations made, other types of evaluation data collected, and the learning activities completed by the student. The documentation should be shared routinely with students, discussions about performance should be summarized, and students should sign these summaries to confirm that they read them.

The teacher cannot observe and document the performance of only the student at risk of failing the course. The students at risk for failure can be observed more closely than is necessary for the majority of students in the clinical group but not to the extent that the student perceives that they were treated differently than others. One strategy is to plan a general number of observations of performance and documentation to be made for all students in the clinical group (in the traditional model) to avoid focusing only on the student with performance problems.

Follow Policy on Unsafe Clinical Performance

There should be a policy in the nursing program about actions to be taken if a student is unsafe in clinical practice. Students who have problems performing some of the competencies can continue in the clinical practicum as long as they demonstrate safe care. This is because the clinical competencies and outcomes of a course are identified for achievement at the end of the course, not during it.

If the student demonstrates performance that is potentially unsafe, however, the teacher can remove the student from the clinical site, following the policy of the nursing program. Specific learning activities outside of the clinical setting need to be offered for students to develop the knowledge and skills they lack; practice in the skills laboratory and in simulation may be valuable in these situations. A learning plan should be prepared and implemented as described earlier.

In all cases, the teacher must follow the policies of the nursing program. If the student fails the clinical course, the student must be notified of the failure and its consequences as indicated in these policies. In some nursing programs, students are allowed to repeat only one clinical course, and there may be other requirements to be met. If the student will be dismissed from the program because of the failure, the student must be informed of this in writing. Generally, there is a specific time frame for each step in the process, which must be adhered to by the faculty, administrators, and students.

SUMMARY

Through clinical evaluation, a teacher arrives at judgments about students' performance in clinical practice. The teacher's observations of performance should focus on the competencies to be developed or outcomes to be met in the clinical practicum. These provide the framework for learning and the basis for evaluating performance. Clinical nurse educators, preceptors, and other clinicians involved in teaching students need to examine their own values, attitudes, and biases that may affect evaluation.

Many clinical evaluation methods are available for assessing student competencies in clinical practice. The teacher should choose evaluation methods that provide information on how well students are performing the clinical competencies. The teacher also decides whether the evaluation method is intended for formative (feedback to students) or summative (grading) evaluation.

The predominant method for clinical evaluation is in observing the performance of students in clinical practice. Although observation is widely used, there are threats to its validity and reliability. In observing clinical performance, there are many aspects of that performance on which the teacher may focus attention. Every observation reflects only a sampling of the student's performance during a clinical learning activity. Such issues point to the need for a series of observations before drawing conclusions about performance. There are several ways of recording observations of students, including notes about performance, checklists, and rating scales. Other methods for clinical evaluation are simulations, standardized patients, OSCEs, written assignments, cases, electronic portfolios, conferences, group projects, and self-evaluation. Some methods are appropriate only for formative evaluation and providing feedback to students. Other methods can be used for both formative and summative evaluation.

Important guidelines for grading clinical practice and working with students who are at risk for failing a clinical course were discussed in the chapter. These guidelines give direction to teachers in establishing sound grading practices and following them when working with students in clinical practice.

Note: This chapter included content from *Evaluation and Testing in Nursing Education*, 6th ed. (Chapters 13, 14, and 17), by M. H. Oermann and K. B. Gaberson, 2021, Springer Publishing Company. Copyright ©2021 by Springer Publishing Company. Adapted with permission.

CNE® EXAMINATION TEST BLUEPRINT CORE COMPETENCIES

1. **Use Assessment and Evaluation Strategies**
   A. Provide input for the development of nursing program standards and policies regarding progression
   B. Enforce nursing program standards related to progression
   C. Use a variety of strategies to assess and evaluate learning in these domains
      1. cognitive
      2. psychomotor
      3. affective
   D. Incorporate current research in assessment and evaluation practices
   E. Analyze available resources for learner assessment and evaluation
   F. Create assessment instruments to evaluate outcomes
   G. Use assessment instruments to evaluate outcomes
   H. Implement evaluation strategies that are appropriate to the learner and learning outcomes
   I. Analyze assessment and evaluation data
   J. Use assessment and evaluation data to enhance the teaching–learning process
   K. Advise learners regarding assessment and evaluation criteria
   L. Provide timely, constructive, and thoughtful feedback to learners

CNE®cl EXAMINATION TEST BLUEPRINT CORE COMPETENCIES

6. **Implement Effective Clinical Assessment and Evaluation Strategies**
   A. Use a variety of strategies to determine achievement of learning outcomes
   B. Implement both formative and summative evaluation that is appropriate to the learner and learning outcomes
   C. Engage in timely communication with course faculty regarding learner clinical performance
   D. Maintain integrity in the assessment and evaluation of learners
   E. Provide timely, objective, constructive, and fair feedback to learners
   F. Use learner data to enhance the teaching-learning process in the clinical learning environment
   G. Demonstrate skill in the use of best practices in the assessment and evaluation of clinical performance
   H. Assess and evaluate learner achievement of clinical performance expectations
   I. Use performance standards to determine learner strengths and weaknesses in the clinical learning environment
   J. Document learner clinical performance, feedback, and progression
   K. Evaluate the quality of the clinical learning experiences and environment

REFERENCES

Altmiller, G. (2016). Strategies for providing constructive feedback to students. *Nurse Educator, 41*(3), 118–119. https://doi.org/10.1097/nne.0000000000000227
American Association of Colleges of Nursing. (2020, November 5). *DRAFT: The Essentials: Core competencies of professional nursing education.* https://www.aacnnursing.org/Portals/42/Downloads/Essentials/Essentials-Draft-Document-10-20.pdf
Anderson, K. M., DesLauriers, P., Horvath, C. H., Slota, M., & Farley, J. N. (2017). From metacognition to practice cognition: The DNP e-portfolio to promote

integrated learning. *Journal of Nursing Education, 56*(8), 497–500. https://doi. org/10.3928/01484834-20170712-09

Anthony, M. L., & Wickman, M. (2015). Precepting challenges: The unsafe student. *Nurse Educator, 40*(3), 113–114. https://doi.org/10.1097/nne.0000000000000118

Ballman, K., Garritano, N., & Beery, T. (2016). Broadening the reach of standardized patients in nurse practitioner education to include the distance learner. *Nurse Educator, 41*(5), 230–233. https://doi.org/10.1097/nne.0000000000000260

Bice, A. A., & Parker, D. L. (2019). Piloting virtual clinical site visits in a family nurse practitioner program. *Journal of Nursing Education, 58*(3), 160–164. https://doi. org/10.3928/01484834-20190221-06

Bonnel, W. (2008). Improving feedback to students in online courses. *Nursing Education Perspectives, 29*, 290–294.

Brookhart, S. M., & Nitko, A. J. (2019). *Educational assessment of students* (6th ed.). Pearson.

Bussard, M. E. (2015). Clinical judgment in reflective journals of prelicensure nursing students. *Journal of Nursing Education, 54*(1), 36–40. https://doi. org/10.3928/01484834-20141224-05

Bussard, M. E. (2018). Evaluation of clinical judgment in prelicensure nursing students. *Nurse Educator, 43*(2), 106–108. https://doi.org/10.1097/nne.0000000000000432

Champlin, A. M., Roberts, L. R., Pueschel, R. D., Saunders, J. S. D., Huerta, G. M., & Yang, J. (2020). Using objective structured clinical examination as a teaching tool in a hybrid advanced health assessment course. *Nurse Educator, 46*(2), 101–105. https://doi. org/10.1097/nne.0000000000000849

Fernandez-Pena, R., Fuentes-Pumarola, C., Malagon-Aguilera, M. C., Bonmati-Tomas, A., Bosch-Farre, C., & Ballester-Ferrando, D. (2016). The evaluation of reflective learning from the nursing student's point of view: A mixed method approach. *Nurse Education Today, 44*, 59–65. https://doi.org/10.1016/j.nedt.2016.05.005

Fulbright, S. (2018, October 18). Using rubrics as a defense against grade appeals. *Faculty Focus.* https://www.facultyfocus.com/articles/course-design-ideas/rubrics-as-a-defense-against-grade-appeals

Goh, H. S., Zhang, H., Lee, C. N., Wu, X. V., & Wang, W. (2019). Value of nursing objective structured clinical examinations: A scoping review. *Nurse Educator, 44*(5), E1–E6. https://doi.org/10.1097/nne.0000000000000620

Harris, M., Rhoads, S. J., Rooker, J. S., Kelly, M. A., Lefler, L., Lubin, S., Martel, I. L., & Beverly, C. J. (2020). Using virtual site visits in the clinical evaluation of nurse practitioner students: Student and faculty perspectives. *Nurse Educator, 45*(1), 17–20. https://doi.org/10.1097/nne.0000000000000693

Hwang, B., Choi, H., Kim, S., Kim, S., Ko, H., & Kim, J. (2018). Facilitating student learning with critical reflective journaling in psychiatric mental health nursing clinical education: A qualitative study. *Nurse Education Today, 69*, 159–164. https://doi.org/10.1016/j. nedt.2018.07.015

Johnson, C. E., Kimble, L. P., Gunby, S. S., & Davis, A. H. (2020). Using deliberate practice and simulation for psychomotor skill competency acquisition and retention: A mixed-methods study. *Nurse Educator, 45*(3), 150–154. https://doi.org/10.1097/nne.0000000000000713

Kardong-Edgren, S., Oermann, M. H., & Rizzolo, M. A. (2019). Emerging theories influencing the teaching of clinical nursing skills. *Journal of Continuing Education in Nursing, 50*(6), 257–262. https://doi.org/10.3928/00220124-20190516-05

Madson, M. (2017). Showing and telling! Screencasts for enhanced feedback on student writing. *Nurse Educator, 42*(5), 222–223. https://doi.org/10.1097/nne.0000000000000385

Melander, S., Hampton, D., Hardin-Pierce, M., & Ossege, J. (2018). Development of a rubric for evaluation of the DNP portfolio. *Nursing Education Perspectives, 39*(5), 312–314. https://doi.org/10.1097/01.Nep.0000000000000381

Minnich, M., Kirkpatrick, A. J., Goodman, J. T., Whittaker, A., Stanton Chapple, H., Schoening, A. M., & Khanna, M. M. (2018). Writing across the curriculum: Reliability testing of a standardized rubric. *Journal of Nursing Education*, *57*(6), 366–370. https://doi.org/10.3928/01484834-20180522-08

Oermann, M. H., Kardong-Edgren, S., & Rizzolo, M. A. (2016). Summative simulated-based assessment in nursing programs. *Journal of Nursing Education*, *55*(6), 323–328. https://doi.org/10.3928/01484834-20160516-04

Poorman, S. G., & Mastorovich, M. L. (2019). The meaning of grades: Stories of undergraduate, master's, and doctoral nursing students. *Nurse Educator*, *44*(6), 321–325. https://doi.org/10.1097/nne.0000000000000627

Willmarth-Stec, M., & Beery, T. (2015). Operationalizing the student electronic portfolio for doctoral nursing education. *Nurse Educator*, *40*(5), 263–265. https://doi.org/10.1097/nne.0000000000000161

Clinical Teaching at a Distance

Christine Lind Colella

The concept of learning at a distance can be defined in a variety of ways. At first glance it might be simply stated as the difference between learning on campus in a classroom or learning remotely. However, the multitude of methods that can be utilized make distance learning both fluid and confusing (Trexler, 2018). Terms such as online learning, distant or distance learning, or e-learning are often used interchangeably to identify a student learning in a setting that is different from the traditional classroom. The rigor and reputation for this type of a learning environment has shown continued growth, but the rigor is often dependent on the attributes of the course content, faculty, and student engagement (Wyse & Sonerl, 2018).

Across the distance learning landscape, there is often a difference in manner of delivery style. An educational institution may provide material as synchronous, which means the class is delivered at a specific time and the students must attend at that time. An alternative to this is an asynchronous approach: Offering this mode of content delivery means the student accesses the information within their own time frame, pace, and setting. Some institutions use a combination of both approaches called a hybrid approach. This hybrid approach can also be called blended learning (Hrastinski, 2019).

Distance learning will not fade away. There are more than 4.4 million learners enrolled in more than 2,497 programs at 27 open universities (Wotto, 2020), and distance learning will continue to evolve and change the landscape of education for the future. Students in registered nurse–bachelor of science in nursing, master of science in nursing, and doctor of nursing practice programs, as well as other types of nursing programs, will desire and have many opportunities for education delivered in this manner. However, the challenge for educators is to ensure that the student receives a quality education needed to meet the needs of the future of the healthcare system.

This chapter examines distance learning; clinical teaching in distance learning environments; developing partnerships with preceptors and clinical sites; and roles and responsibilities of the faculty member, preceptor, and student. Preceptors are important participants in clinical learning: They guide and evaluate student learning and performance and need to be well prepared for their role as educator. The faculty member also has responsibility for evaluating performance, and the chapter includes strategies for faculty to use such as site visits to clinical settings, on-campus intensives, and virtual site visits. Schools of nursing need to continually evaluate the quality of the clinical practicum in distance education courses. The chapter includes discussion about preceptor and site evaluation.

STUDENTS WHO SEEK DISTANCE LEARNING

It is understood that the desire and request for distance learning will continue to grow. The question one may ask is *why*: Why do students seek distance learning as their method of choice to further their education? Statistics show that this type of student is the largest growing community of learners (Wotto, 2020). The reasons for this growth are many, but the single most important reason is the expansion and availability of technology (Trexler, 2018). People and their relationship to their devices has exploded, and this access opens the door for students to learn at a distance. Through technology, reputable institutions can now offer high-quality education with flexibility for students. Students can now further their education while being able to maintain work and life commitments because they no longer have to drive to a campus. The ability to access information and further one's education without the geographical constraints is a driving factor for today's student.

Other reasons for choosing distance learning as an option along with time and flexibility is there may be no school where students live that offer them the program in which they are interested. Distance learning now gives students the opportunity to apply to a program that meets their passion and can be completed in an online setting. Therefore, availability, opportunity, technology, and passion are the foundation of why a student seeks distance learning.

However, the commitment to school is still needed, and this can become a challenge for students. Many prospective students may think that online learning is easier, but actually it takes self-direction, dedication, and superior time management skills. The work–life–school balance is often difficult for students new to distance learning to manage (Lee et al., 2019). This has to do with the many commitments that adult students carry related to other time constraints such as work, childcare, and family needs. Believing that they can commit to their education on top of all the other commitments can lead to burnout and progression issues (Lee et al., 2019). It is important that the academic institution understands this dilemma and has in place support for the students as they try and balance these competing forces.

MAKING A CONNECTION

Literature demonstrates that students who have a connection or a sense of belonging to their school, fellow students, and faculty perform better and are more likely to complete their education (Museus et al., 2017). This takes on new meaning with distance learning. Developing teaching strategies that give the student a sense of belonging and connectedness is an added challenge when the student is learning clinical practice at a distance. Strategies must be woven into all components of the education to highlight that students are part of a learning community and allow them to share their successes and challenges with peers and faculty. Identifying this as a cohesive component of the student's educational success will help faculty choose the appropriate teaching methods.

CLINICAL PRACTICE IN A DISTANCE LEARNING ENVIRONMENT

Understanding the components necessary for a successful clinical practicum offered at a distance from the nursing program will decrease faculty and student stress and increase satisfaction. These components include the role of the institution, faculty, student, and preceptor. The first element is the educational institution's role in committing to providing an outstanding clinical practice experience. This role includes state authorization, clinical partnerships (Albert et al., 2019), and the issuance of contracts.

State Authorization

State authorization is required and can be an involved and a major undertaking for any institution, but it must be in place if the student will be doing clinical practica in a different state (National Council for State Authorization Reciprocity Agreements [NC-SARA], 2021b). The NC-SARA is an agreement between member states and territories that establishes comparable national standards for interstate distance education (NC-SARA, 2021b). The NC-SARA website (nc-sara.org) provides resources on distance education including The State Authorization Guide, which is a tool for searching state authorization compliance information (NC-SARA, 2021a).

In addition, the requirements issued by the board of nursing vary from state to state but can involve items such as requiring all faculty to hold a license in that state, preceptor identification, an on-site presence, completion of forms regarding the educational expectations, syllabi, and more. To keep the educational institution in compliance, often one person is identified to monitor and manage compliance since requirements from each state board of nursing can change with minimal notice. Implementing a continual review should be in place so no changes occur without the institution's knowledge. Faculty and students must be aware of this process to avoid actions that inadvertently affect compliance. The consequences of not following a state board of nursing's requirements are many, including significant fines, preventing the school from having students in that state, and not issuing a graduate of a noncompliant program a license to practice in the state. Doing this vital board of nursing investigation before starting a distance learning program is imperative.

Clinical Partnerships

Developing clinical partnerships will ease preceptor and onboarding issues that are often cited as barriers to clinical practica (Albert et al., 2019). Having clinical partners requires preliminary groundwork that includes discussion on expectations, commitment, and ongoing evaluation of the partnership. This can be initiated at the dean or designee level and nourished by faculty members of the students directly involved.

Clinical Contracts

The next step is the development and tracking of clinical contracts. Most facilities require a written contract submitted by the educational institution and possibly adjusted by the clinical site. Corporate lawyers are often utilized by both sides, and this can be straightforward or require adjustments until it meets all the parties' interests. The contracts address liability, student insurance coverage, facility and institution responsibilities, and the role of the preceptor. At a setting such as a private clinical office, a more simple and straightforward type of contract is often used and signed by the office manager. Appendix C provides an example of a distance learning affiliation agreement.

FACULTY ROLE

The faculty role in supporting the student's clinical learning at a distance has many facets. The first component is often helping the student secure a preceptor and then vetting the preceptor and site as appropriate for the learning that needs to take place. Finding preceptors is an ongoing important issue. Schools of nursing continue to report difficulty in securing preceptor experiences with 95% of nurse practitioner (NP) programs stating that they are moderately or very concerned about the availability of clinical learning opportunities (American Association of Colleges of Nursing [AACN], 2015). Adding a program that is offered at a distance has increased challenges, and these are well known to schools of nursing that teach at a distance. When the student is local to the school, faculty may be able to solicit former graduates as preceptors, may have a cadre of preceptors who have taught previously for the school, or may have a clinical partner that can supply preceptors. Students may find a preceptor within their own network. However, it may be more difficult with clinical students at a distance since the Commission on Collegiate Nursing Education 2018 Executive Summary of Changes to Standard II, Key Element II-F, indicates that finding a preceptor is the ultimate responsibility of the school (AACN, 2018). This can be a significant burden for many distance education programs. Working with hospital systems in other states, looking for alumni in other states who might serve as preceptors, and advertising via free webinars may be possible ways to find preceptors.

Securing preceptors is a national problem, and there has been a rise in for-profit third-party companies attempting to meet the need (Murray, 2019). They offer to find preceptors at a cost to the student, and some schools are now charging a fee so the preceptor can be paid. This does not absolve the school from vetting the preceptor as appropriate—assessing the preceptor's education, license, certification, type of practice, and skill set. There have been instances in which one preceptor takes many students for the payment, but this scenario is not an appropriate learning environment for the student. The faculty member has the responsibility to identify this issue and intervene. The goal is to find a way that is equitable and safe for all who want to continue their education.

It is well documented that finding a preceptor is the singularly most stressful issue for many students (Doherty et al., 2020). There are many perceived barriers to securing preceptors. Preceptors may feel that they do not have the support of the faculty member or employer, may be unsure of expectations and role, and may not be rewarded for their efforts (Davis & Fathman, 2018; Jarrett et al., 2017). Many of these barriers can be overcome with a well thought out plan of support, frequent communication, and education. A key role for the faculty member, once the preceptor is found and vetted, is the interaction with the preceptor and student. This triad of communication is important to give both the preceptor and student the support they need. Preceptor communication has always been important but is vital to the success of a distance learning experience.

Communication should be initiated by the faculty member once the preceptor is committed to taking a student. This first contact should include:

- Faculty's warm welcome,
- Faculty contact information,
- Course syllabus,
- Plan for course/term: method of evaluation, conference, and visit, and
- Expectations of faculty, student, and preceptor.

It is important to set expectations from the beginning so preceptors know their role and what to do if they have questions or concerns. Setting out this plan and including the student brings the triad together, so all are aware of what is expected of each member. Student engagement is important to a successful clinical practicum. The student needs to be fully present and engaged in the learning. Oftentimes students are passive learners expecting to be "filled with knowledge" by the preceptor, but they must fully understand the importance of their questions and seeking out opportunities. Asking questions helps them formulate ideas and gives preceptors an opportunity to share their knowledge and passion for the topic. Assignments for students during their clinical courses can highlight items such as sharing their own clinical pearls discovered or their "aha" moments. Having the student share these moments through discussion boards or using a synchronous seminar option allows the connection to other students and for all students to learn from each other. Responsibilities of the faculty member, preceptor, and student are outlined in Exhibit 13.1.

EXHIBIT 13.1 Responsibilities of Faculty Member, Preceptor, and Student in Distance-Based Clinical Learning

RESPONSIBILITIES OF THE FACULTY MEMBER:

1. Provide a course syllabus and a letter of introduction to the preceptor.
2. Be available for consultation with the student or preceptor.
3. Share phone contact for texting or messaging.
4. Approve students' clinical objectives during the first week of the practicum.
5. Confer with the student and the preceptor at least twice during the practicum to guide students in achievement of clinical skills and course objectives.
6. Evaluate content of the clinical log and other course assignments.
7. Meet with students for scheduled clinical seminars to discuss role.
8. Provide preceptor the link to the evaluation tools used to assess student progress.
9. Provide final evaluation of student performance during the course.

RESPONSIBILITIES OF THE PRECEPTOR:

1. Communicate appropriate policies, procedures, expectations of the agency.
2. Assist the student to obtain appropriate identification required by the agency.
3. Prepare the agency/staff for the student's arrival and role in the care of clients.
4. Be present in the clinical area when students are seeing patients.
5. Orient student to the advanced nursing practice role.

(continued)

EXHIBIT 13.1 Responsibilities of Faculty Member, Preceptor, and Student in Distance-Based Clinical Learning (*continued*)

6. Review student objectives for the experience.
7. Provide opportunities to assess patients.
8. Review student assessments and validate findings. Cosign any documentation according to the policies of the agency.
9. Discuss the management of the client.
10. Guide the student in the performance of any intervention.
11. Guide the student in identifying ways to evaluate the plan of care.
12. Assist the student in learning the consultation process and the role of the advanced practice nurse on the healthcare team.
13. Guide the student in suggesting additional readings or other learning opportunities.
14. Confer with the faculty and student at least twice during the term about student progress. Reach out immediately with any concerns about the student's progress.
15. Expect students to perform only those functions appropriate for their level of graduate practicum.
16. Complete an evaluation form at mid-term and at the end of the practicum.

RESPONSIBILITIES OF THE STUDENT:

1. Prepare personal objectives for the clinical experience that complement the course outcomes. Gain approval of these objectives from the preceptor and faculty member.
2. Follow the dress code, policies, and procedures of the agency.
3. Demonstrate responsible professional behavior. Be on time for scheduled clinical practicum.
4. Know how to notify facility/preceptor if going to be late or absent.
5. Prepare for clinical experiences by planning ahead and reviewing most common diagnoses for the patient population.
6. Maintain confidentiality of patients, deidentify all patient materials.
7. Perform appropriate assessments of clients.
8. Interpret data obtained from labs, diagnostic tests, and monitoring devices to trend patient condition.
9. Prepare a differential diagnosis list.
10. Recognize emergency situations and make appropriate decisions regarding treatment and obtaining assistance of preceptor.
11. Provide appropriate health teaching for patients and families.
12. Perform new or advanced interventions only under the direction of the preceptor and according to agency policies.
13. Identify potential plans of care.
14. Identify measurable outcomes.
15. Ensure that the preceptor is informed of patient condition.
16. Recommend appropriate referrals.
17. Document patient encounters according to agency policy and identify self as a registered nurse NP student. Have documentation cosigned by preceptor.
18. Engage and communicate effectively with other members of the healthcare team.
19. Maintain a clinical log that is submitted to the faculty at required times (e.g., at least four times) during the course/term.
20. Confer with the faculty and preceptor at least twice during the term regarding progress toward meeting clinical and course objectives. This may be more often if any issues are identified.
21. Seek out learning opportunities.

Communication comes in many forms that may include email and text. These methods, though, can misconstrue tone, attitude, and perceptions, leading the way for communication errors. The faculty member should be sensitive to any misunderstanding and be willing to reach out and speak directly with the preceptor or student to minimize hurt feelings or incorrect information.

PRECEPTOR ROLE

The care of preceptors is critical to the success of a student's clinical experience. The utilization of a preceptor is the core way clinical experiences occur in many nursing programs. This means they are our greatest and our scarcest resource, and faculty need to nurture and appreciate their role so they will find it satisfying and precept again. The ways to mentor the preceptor is to give them the tools they need to fulfill their role. This may take many forms, but as mentioned earlier, communication is key. There are other needs as well. Understanding the preceptor's needs, whether novice or experienced, is foundational to their success. The school can offer:

1. Orientation to the role.
2. Instruction about how to complete an evaluation.
3. Tools such as how to manage or interact with a difficult student.
4. Signs of concern that the preceptor should share and when.
5. Assistance for preceptors to identify their expectations.
6. Preceptor incentives such as access to the school's library and continuing education, a title for preceptors to use and add to their curriculum vitae, and a formal thank you for precepting a student.

Developing or having a platform where preceptors may go to learn, ask questions, and reinforce their learning is also helpful. Faculty need to be cognizant and deliberate in their care and support of the preceptor.

EVALUATION

Evaluation is critical to successful clinical learning at a distance. The evaluation must encompass not only the student but also the preceptor and clinical site. There are a few ways that these evaluations may be accomplished.

Student Evaluation

The preceptor evaluation of the student should be developed by faculty and reflect the student learning outcomes, competencies, and behaviors that are to be accomplished in the experience (Altmiller & Dugan, 2020). Allowing for free text comments is helpful when trying to identify subtle components of the student's performance. The student evaluation tool should be explained and shared with the student and preceptor. The tool should be deployed at midterm and as a final evaluation to assess growth and progression toward successful completion of the learning outcomes. Examples of clinical evaluation tools for advanced practice nursing programs are provided in Appendix B.

The evaluation tool is often done electronically, possibly using a third-party system. It can also be done on paper and signed and uploaded or emailed by the preceptor to the faculty member. It is important to have as part of the evaluation process the requirement that the student and preceptor review the evaluation together so the student fully understands their progress or areas to improve. The evaluation should never be a surprise to the student or the faculty member.

When building the communication plan, the preceptor needs to know that if there are concerns about the student's performance, the preceptor should share these immediately with the faculty member and anytime throughout the course. The preceptor, faculty member, and student can then set limits or goals to meet. For example, if a student always arrives 10 minutes late to the clinical site, this may not seem monumental to the student, but it is disruptive to the clinical site and unprofessional. Early on the preceptor and faculty member need to identify this issue and, with the student, find out the cause and put in place a plan to remedy the situation. The faculty member should not learn at the end of the term that the student was always late. It is important to communicate with the preceptor that early intervention can make it a better experience for all.

Another important component that the faculty need to decide when developing the clinical experience is the weight of the preceptor evaluation in the overall grade and success of the student. Often in a clinical practicum there are other assignments or projects that are important and carry weight in the grade as well. Sometimes the preceptor evaluation can be the entire grade, or it may be a percentage of the overall grade for the student. Sharing this information with the preceptor is a vital part of the communication.

Another component of student evaluation can be an opportunity to assess actual skills the student needs to master before graduating from a nursing program. This may include completing a physical assessment, suturing, educating a patient, interacting with patients and other healthcare providers or students, or any skill that the student is expected to be able to perform. These competencies may be assessed via intensives. Intensives are skill-based interactions where the distance learning student may come to campus for the assessment, or it may be completed virtually via technology (Harris et al., 2020). These intensives can be completed at multiple times during the student's program, midway through it, or at the end of their program. Having students come to campus can be a wonderful experience but may be a problem if the program is fully online. It is also important to remember as faculty that managing, arranging, and communicating for an on-campus experience can be very time consuming for faculty engaged in other classes. It is important to identify the need for such support so the school can engage additional personnel to assist in the logistics. The expense and time to come to campus may be prohibitive for some students so a virtual experience is a possible alternative. If it is a specific skill, it can be shared live or recorded during clinical practice and uploaded for the faculty to review. Another option is to have the student gather the needed equipment and then do a live demonstration to the faculty as part of the class.

Making a site visit is an additional helpful strategy for evaluation. It gives the faculty member an insight to the physical environment as well as an opportunity to talk with the preceptor and student. It is important not to be intrusive and take up the valuable time of the preceptor during their care, but this is a way to establish communication and availability. A site visit can be done in person, but when the student is learning at a distance, the use of technology is fundamental. Skype, FaceTime, or a meeting program such as Zoom or Webex can be used. With technology, the student can bring the faculty member "into" the clinical setting for a tour, and the faculty member can even accompany the student into the patient's room to observe an assessment or care, with the patient's permission. A virtual site visit can give the faculty member an opportunity to see the clinical environment, meet with the student and preceptor, and establish a connection with them. It is recommended that this be done at least once in the clinical environment during the student's experience, but it can be done more frequently if there is any student issue or concern.

Preceptor and Site Evaluation

Another important evaluation is that of the preceptor and clinical site by the student. It is important to gather feedback from students about the clinical site and how they were treated by individuals in the setting. Just because a preceptor or site meet the qualifications for an experience, it may not be a good fit for the student. If there was an issue with the preceptor, the student should have reached out to the faculty member early on, but sometimes students do not want to lose a site or are fearful of retaliation and do not communicate their concerns until the end of the practicum. This is a concern when plans are to use the clinical site or preceptor again. It is important to listen to any negative experience shared by a student. The issues may be something that can be resolved using communication and a plan, or it may be a clinical site or preceptors that are no longer appropriate for use in the nursing program.

There may be times when the faculty member needs to remove a student from an experience because of personality conflicts, an unsafe learning environment, or educational needs that are not being met. This is never a good situation, but the student is always at the center of any decisions, and the faculty must care for students as their priority. This is where strong communication within the triad—faculty, student, and preceptor—is critical so all needs may be met, and students will have a successful clinical practicum.

An example of a form for student evaluation of the preceptor and clinical site is provided in Exhibit 13.2.

EXHIBIT 13.2 Student Evaluation of Preceptor and Clinical Setting

Preceptor/Setting _____ Semester: Fall Spring Summer Year_____
Practicum Course No._____ Title_____
Directions: This evaluation form is designed to provide you with the opportunity to evaluate the preceptor and clinical site. Please indicate your response in the appropriate column on the scoring sheet. Please provide us with additional written comments on the bottom or back of the page.

Items	Consis- tently				Never
Overall this preceptor stimulated my learning.	5	4	3	2	1
Clinical activity was presented at an appropriate pace.	5	4	3	2	1

(continued)

EXHIBIT 13.2 Student Evaluation of Preceptor and Clinical Setting (*continued*)

Items	Consis-tently				Never
The preceptor was well prepared for my visits and organized in guiding my experiences.	5	4	3	2	1
The preceptor used a variety of teaching methods to ensure that I learned the rationale for the management of patients.	5	4	3	2	1
I felt challenged to master the clinical practice.	5	4	3	2	1
The client population was appropriate to my learning goals.	5	4	3	2	1
The preceptor handled questions appropriately.	5	4	3	2	1
I felt respected as a student practitioner.	5	4	3	2	1
I had the opportunity to actively participate during clinical.	5	4	3	2	1
The preceptor offered feedback to guide my progress through the experience.	5	4	3	2	1
The preceptor specified the criteria for managing patients in that setting.	5	4	3	2	1
The preceptor related current research and professional issues to the practice experience.	5	4	3	2	1
The clinical setting offered rich experiences for the student.	5	4	3	2	1
The preceptor promoted an atmosphere that fostered critical thinking.	5	4	3	2	1
The preceptor provided opportunities to develop effective written and/or oral communication needed for practice.	5	4	3	2	1

Comments:

SUMMARY

Understanding the components necessary for a successful clinical practicum offered at a distance from the nursing program will decrease faculty and student stress and increase satisfaction. These components include the role of the institution, faculty, student, and preceptor. The first element is the educational institution's role in committing to providing an outstanding clinical practice experience. This role includes state authorization, clinical partnerships, and the issuance of contracts.

The faculty role in supporting clinical learning at a distance has many facets. The first component often is helping the student secure a preceptor and then vetting the preceptor and site as appropriate for the learning that needs to take place. Finding preceptors is an ongoing important issue.

Clinical learning at a distance seems insurmountable at first, but the same basic foundation needs to be in place whether the clinical practicum is offered locally or at a distant site. These include clinical expectations, communication, and relationship with the preceptor. If these are not in place no matter where the experience is occurring, it will not be successful. Identifying what the clinical expectations are for the student and preceptor will decrease anxiety, frustration, and a potential for clinical failure. Clearly communicating these expectations is also vital to success. The preceptor and student each need to know what is expected of them and what they can depend on from the faculty member. Communication should not be taken for granted: It is vital for the preceptor and student to feel supported and valued.

Evaluation is critical to successful clinical learning at a distance. The student evaluation tool should be explained and shared with the student and preceptor. Making a site visit is an additional helpful strategy for evaluation. It gives the faculty member an insight to the physical environment as well as an opportunity to talk with the preceptor and student. A site visit can be done in person, but when the student is learning at a distance, the use of technology is fundamental. The evaluation must encompass not only the student but also the preceptor and clinical site.

CNE® EXAMINATION TEST BLUEPRINT CORE COMPETENCIES

1. **Facilitate Learning**
   A. Implement a variety of teaching strategies appropriate to:
      2. setting (i.e., clinical versus classroom)
   M. Develop collegial working relationships with clinical agency personnel to promote positive learning environments
3. **Use Assessment and Evaluation Strategies**
   C. Use a variety of strategies to assess and evaluate learning in these domains
      1. cognitive
      2. psychomotor
      3. affective
   G. Use assessment instruments to evaluate outcomes
   H. Implement evaluation strategies that are appropriate to the learner and learning outcomes
   I. Analyze assessment and evaluation data
   J. Use assessment and evaluation data to enhance the teaching–learning process
   K. Advise learners regarding assessment and evaluation criteria
   L. Provide timely, constructive, and thoughtful feedback to learners

CNE®cl EXAMINATION TEST BLUEPRINT CORE COMPETENCIES

1. **Function within the Education and Health Care Environments**
   A. Function in the Clinical Educator Role
      1. Bridge the gap between theory and practice by helping learners to apply classroom learning to the clinical setting
      5. Act as a role model of professional nursing within the clinical learning environment
      6. Demonstrate inclusive excellence (e.g., student-centered learning, diversity)
   B. Operationalize the Curriculum
      1. Assess congruence of the clinical agency to curriculum, course goals, and learner needs when evaluating clinical sites
      2. Plan meaningful and relevant clinical learning assignments and activities
      5. Structure learner experiences within the learning environment to promote optimal learning
      8. Implement assigned models for clinical teaching (e.g., traditional, preceptor, simulation, dedicated education units)
   C. Abide by Legal Requirements, Ethical Guidelines, Agency Policies, and Guiding Framework
      3. Facilitate learning activities that support the mission, goals, and values of the academic institution and the clinical agency
      4. Inform others of program and clinical agency policies, procedures, and practices
      5. Adhere to program and clinical agency policies, procedures and practices when implementing clinical experiences
      6. Promote learner compliance with regulations and standards of practice
      7. Demonstrate ethical behaviors

2. **Facilitate Learning in the Health Care Environment**
   A. Implement a variety of clinical teaching strategies appropriate to learner needs, desired learner outcomes, content, and context
   C. Use technology (e.g., simulation, learning management systems, electronic health records) skillfully to support the teaching-learning process
   G. Develop collegial working relationships with learners, faculty colleagues, and clinical agency personnel

3. **Demonstrate Effective Interpersonal Communication and Collaborative Interprofessional Relationships**
   F. Use clear and effective communication in all interactions (e.g., written, electronic, verbal, non-verbal)
   N. Communicate performance expectations to learners and agency staff

6. **Implement Effective Clinical Assessment and Evaluation Strategies**
   B. Implement both formative and summative evaluation that is appropriate to the learner and learning outcomes
   C. Engage in timely communication with course faculty regarding learner clinical performance
   E. Provide timely, objective, constructive, and fair feedback to learners
   F. Use learner data to enhance the teaching-learning process in the clinical learning environment
   J. Document learner clinical performance, feedback, and progression
   K. Evaluate the quality of the clinical learning experiences and environment

REFERENCES

Albert, N. M., Chipps, E., Falkenberg Olson, A. C., Hand, L. L., Harmon, M., Heitschmidt, M. G., Klein, C. J., Lefaiver, C., & Wood, T. (2019). Fostering academic-clinical research partnerships. *Journal of Nursing Administration*, 49(5), 234–241. https://doi.org/10.1097/NNA.0000000000000744

Altmiller, G., & Dugan, M. (2020). Content validation of the quality and safety framed clinical evaluation for nurse practitioner students. *Nurse Educator*, 46(3), 159–163. https://doi.org/10.1097/nne.0000000000000936

American Association of Colleges of Nursing. (2015). *White paper: Re-envisioning the clinical education of advanced practice registered nurses*. https://www.aacnnursing.org/Portals/42/News/White-Papers/APRN-Clinical-Education.pdf

American Association of Colleges of Nursing. (2018). Executive summary of changes to the 2018 *Standards for Accreditation of Baccalaureate and Graduate Nursing Programs*. https://www.aacnnursing.org/Portals/42/CCNE/PDF/Summary-Major-Revisions-to-2018-Standards.pdf

Lee, K., Choi, H., & Cho, Y. (2019). Becoming a competent self: A developmental process of adult distance learning. *Internet and Higher Education*, 41, 25–33. https://doi.org/10.1016/j.iheduc.2018.12.001

Davis, L., & Fathman, A. (2018). Clinical education of nurse practitioner students: Identifying incentives, barriers, and working models to develop sustainable preceptorships. *Journal of Nursing Education and Practice*, 8(9), 18–24. https://doi.org/10.5430/jnep.v8n9p18

Doherty, C., Fogg, L, Bigley, M., Todd, B., & O'Sullivan, A. (2020). Nurse practitioner student clinical placement process: A national survey of nurse practitioner programs. *Nursing Outlook*. 68(1), 55–61. https://doi.org/10.1016/j.outlook.2019.07.005

Harris, M., Rhoads, S., Rooker, J., Kelly, M., Lefler, L., Lubin, S., Martel, I., & Beverly, C. (2020). Using virtual site visits in the clinical evaluation of nurse practitioner students. *Nurse Educator*, 45(1), 17–20. https://doi.org/10.1097/NNE.0000000000000693

Hrastinski, S. (2019). What do we mean by blended learning? *Tech Trends*, 63, 564–569. https://doi.org/10.1007/s11528-019-00375-5

Jarrett, A., Shreve, M., & Weymiller, A. (2017). Preceptor barriers and motivators. *International Journal of e-Healthcare Information Systems*, 4(1), 100–119.

Murray, T. (2019). Partnering with an online program management company: Heresy, innovative entrepreneurship, or an evolving mind-set? *Journal of Nursing Education*, 58(2), 67–68. https://doi.org/10.3928/01484834-20190122-01

Museus, S., Yi, V., & Saelua, N. (2017). The impact of culturally engaging campus environments sense of belonging. *The Review of Higher Education*, 40(2), 187–215. https://doi.org/10.1353/rhe.2017.0001

NC-SARA. (2021a). *The state authorization guide*. https://nc-sara.org/guide/state-authorization-guide

NC-SARA. (2021b). *What is SARA?* https://nc-sara.org/

Trexler, J. (2018). Distance learning—predictions and possibilities. *Education Sciences*, 8(1), 35. https://doi.org/10.3390/educsci8010035

Wotto, M. (2020). The future of high education distance learning in Canada, the United States, and France: Insights from before Covid-19 secondary data. *Journal of Education Technology*, 49(2), 262–228. https://doi.org/10.1177/0047239520940624

Wyse, S., & Sonerl, P. (2018). "Is this class hard?" Defining and analyzing academic rigor from a learner's perspective. *CBE-Life Sciences Education*, 17(4). https://doi.org/10.1187/cbe.17-12-0278

Appendices

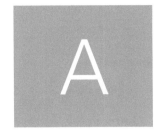

Resources for Nurse Educators

A.1. CERTIFICATIONS FOR NURSE EDUCATORS

The National League for Nursing recognizes the knowledge and expertise of nurse educators through certification as a Certified Nurse Educator (CNE®): www.nln.org/Certification-for-Nurse-Educators/cne

The National League for Nursing recognizes the knowledge and expertise of clinical educators through certification as a Certified Academic Clinical Nurse Educator (CNE®cl): www.nln.org/Certification-for-Nurse-Educators/cnecl

Certification for Nursing Professional Development

The American Nurses Credentialing Center provides certification to recognize the knowledge and skills of registered nurses in the Nursing Professional Development specialty. This credential is Registered Nurse-Board Certified (NPD-BC): www.nursingworld.org/our-certifications/nursing-professional-development/

A.2. SELECTED NURSING AND HIGHER EDUCATION ORGANIZATIONS

Organization	Mission	Website
American Academy of Nursing	Serves the public and nursing profession by advancing health policy and practice. Academy members, known as Fellows, are nursing's most accomplished leaders in education, practice, administration, and research.	www.aannet.org/about/about-the-academy
American Association of Colleges of Nursing	Represents baccalaureate and higher-degree nursing programs. Promotes quality nursing education. Offers faculty development programs and webinars. Collects data about nursing education programs, faculty, and students, and analyzes trends in nursing education. Publishes position papers.	www.aacnnursing.org/

(continued)

(continued)

Organization	Mission	Website
American Association of Community Colleges	Provides advocacy for community colleges at the national level. Works closely with states on policy.	https://www.aacc.nche.edu/
American Association of University Professors	Focuses on advancing academic freedom and shared governance. Defines fundamental professional values and standards for higher education and faculty.	www.aaup.org/
American Association of University Women	Promotes equity and education for women and girls. Advocates for fundamental educational, social, economic, and political issues.	www.aauw.org/
American Council on Education	Represents presidents of accredited, degree-granting institutions (2- and 4-year colleges, private and public universities, and nonprofit schools) in the United States. Focuses on higher education challenges, with the goal to improve access and better prepare students.	www.acenet.edu/Pages/default.aspx
American Nurses Credentialing Center (ANCC)	The ANCC provides a variety of services for practitioners, including certification in Nursing Professional Development.	https://www.nursingworld.org/ancc/ https://www.nursingworld.org/our-certifications/nursing-professional-development/
Association for Nurses in Professional Development (ANPD)	The ANPD's mission is to advance quality healthcare by promoting nursing professional development practice. The ANPD is the leading resource for nursing professional development and offers a variety of resources and education for nurses in this specialty.	www.anpd.org/page/about
Association of American Colleges and Universities	Focuses on promoting high-quality undergraduate liberal education. Website contains links to resources on liberal education, general education, curriculum, faculty work, assessment, diversity, and more.	www.aacu.org/about/index.cfm

(continued)

(continued)

Organization	Mission	Website
Association of Black Nursing Faculty, Inc.	Provides a group for Black professional nurses with similar interests and concerns to promote health-related issues and nursing education. Assists members in professional development and provides continuing education.	www.abnf.net/
Association of Community Health Nursing Educators	Focuses on promoting excellence in community and public health nursing education, research, and practice.	www.achne.org/ aws/ACHNE/pt/ sp/home-page
EDUCAUSE	Advances higher education through the use of information technology. Focuses on issues and emerging trends and technologies affecting higher education.	www.educause. edu/
Interprofessional Education Collaborative (IPEC)	Collaborative of schools of health professions to promote efforts that advance interprofessional learning experiences to prepare future health professionals for team-based care and improved population health outcomes. These organizations that represent higher education in medicine, dentistry, nursing, pharmacy, and public health created core competencies for interprofessional collaborative practice to guide curricula development across health professions schools.	https://www. ipecollaborative. org/
Multimedia Educational Resource for Learning and Online Teaching (MERLOT)	Includes repository of resources and information for faculty development and to download for use in teaching. Publishes *Journal of Online Learning and Teaching*.	www.merlot.org/ merlot/
National League for Nursing	Promotes excellence in nursing education at all levels. Offers faculty development programs, webinars, and annual educational conferences. Sponsors certifications for academic nurse educators and academic clinical nurse educators. Publishes position papers on nursing education and has a grant program for nursing education research. The Commission for Nursing Education Accreditation (CNEA) accredits nursing programs.	www.nln.org

(continued)

(continued)

Organization	Mission	Website
National Organization of Nurse Practitioner Faculties	Focuses on promoting quality nurse practitioner (NP) education at national and international levels. Leading organization for NP faculty in the United States and globally.	www.nonpf.org/?
National Student Nurses Association	Serves as an organization for nursing students with goal of enhancing their professional development and promoting transition into the profession.	www.nsna.org/
Organization for Associate Degree Nursing (OADN)	Is dedicated to enhancing the quality of Associate Degree (AD) nursing. Advocates for AD nursing and promotes academic progression of AD nursing graduates in furthering their education.	www.oadn.org/
Quality and Safety Education for Nurses (QSEN)	Collaborative of nurses and other healthcare professionals focused on education, practice, and scholarship to improve quality and safety of healthcare. Identified knowledge, skills, and attitudes (KSAs) necessary to continuously improve quality and safety of healthcare. Website is a central repository of information on core QSEN competencies, KSAs, teaching strategies, and faculty development resources.	www.qsen.org/about-qsen/
Sigma	Supports learning and professional development of nurses worldwide. Membership is by invitation to baccalaureate and graduate nursing students with excellence in scholarship and to nurse leaders with exceptional achievements in nursing. Offers conferences for sharing research and publishes *Journal of Nursing Scholarship*, among other resources.	www.sigmanursing.org/
United States Department of Education	Website includes links to legislation, regulations, guidance, and other policy documents related to education.	https://www2.ed.gov/policy/landing.jhtml?src=pn
	Family Educational Rights and Privacy Act (FERPA) is a federal law that protects the privacy of student education records.	https://www2.ed.gov/policy/gen/guid/fpco/ferpa/index.html

(continued)

(continued)

Organization	Mission	Website
United States Department of Justice, Civil Rights Division	Americans with Disabilities Act (ADA) website provides access to information about the ADA, regulations, and other resources.	www.ada.gov/
Vizient/AACN Nurse Residency Program™	Vizient and the American Association of Colleges of Nursing connect members to learn about and improve the Nurse Residency Program.	https://www.vizientinc.com/our-solutions/clinical-solutions/vizient-aacn-nurse-residency-program

A.3. Virtual Simulation Resources

Resource	URL
National League for Nursing Virtual Simulation Options for Undergraduate Nursing Students	http://www.nln.org/docs/default-source/professional-development-programs/virtual-simulation-undergraduate-students.pdf?sfvrsn=42
National League for Nursing Virtual Simulation Options for Nurse Practitioner Students	http://www.nln.org/docs/default-source/professional-development-programs/virtual-simulation-options-for-nurse-practitioner-students.pdf?sfvrsn=10
National League for Nursing vSIm for Nursing	http://www.nln.org/enterprise-development/nln-center-for-innovation-in-education-excellence/institute-for-simulation-and-technology/vsim-for-nursing-medical-surgical
Global Network for Simulation in Healthcare	www.gnsh.org/

Sample Clinical Evaluation Tools

B.1. EXAMPLES OF CLINICAL EVALUATION TOOLS IN PRELICENSURE NURSING PROGRAMS

B.1.1. At the Quality and Safety Innovation Center, The College of New Jersey, at https://qsicenter.tcnj.edu/resources/, QSEN-Based Clinical Evaluation Instruments are available for these courses:

Fundamentals of Nursing

Childbearing Family Nursing

Pediatric Nursing

Psychiatric/Mental Health Nursing

Med-Surg 1 Chronic Illness

Med-Surg 2 Adult Acute Illness.

Graduate Level Nurse Practitioner Clinical Evaluation instrument is also available at the website.

B.1.2. Bradley University Department of Nursing Practicum Evaluation Guidelines, Criteria, and Tool

Student Name/Date: _____

Instructor Name: _____

Bradley University Department of Nursing
Practicum Evaluation Criteria
NUR 315: Psychiatric/Mental Health Nursing - Practicum
Guidelines for Documentation of Student Performance on Tool

1. The practicum instructor will evaluate the student's performance in meeting each outcome in both written work and practicum performance. Students must achieve a grade of "Satisfactory" for the course in both written and performance evaluation areas.
2. If the written or performance outcome for the week is "Not Applicable" (per faculty discretion), an N/A will be awarded.
3. Both the student and the practicum instructor can make written entries in the anecdotal notes section. All items written in the anecdotal note section should be dated and initialed by the author. Once read by either the student or instructor, the entry should be initialed indicating that it has been reviewed. Entries should concisely, objectively, and accurately describe how the student did or did not meet the outcome(s).
4. Individual student conferences regarding practicum performance are to be documented in the anecdotal notes section. **Students receiving scores implying his or her performance is "Unsatisfactory" may be instructed to complete a remediation plan at the discretion of the faculty member. The student is responsible for developing his/her remediation plan. After agreement of the student's plan, the instructor and student will then sign the evaluation document.**
5. Observations by agency personnel regarding student performance may be recorded by the practicum instructor for use in evaluation when appropriate.
6. The practicum evaluation form will be filed as part of the student's record.
7. **Any practicum absence may hinder the student in meeting the course outcomes necessary for passing the nursing course and will result in "X" being recorded for the day in all outcomes.**

The foundation for the criteria are these critical behaviors required to successfully complete the course:

- Safe practice
- Confidentiality
- Respect for client rights
- Collaboration with client
- Consideration for all other healthcare team providers

Written Work Evaluation Criteria

E	EXEMPLARY	Outstanding effort and thought are obvious. All required areas are addressed in a complete and thorough manner. Information is accurate and presentation is professional in appearance. Assignments are turned in on or before due date.

(continued)

(*continued*)

S	SATISFACTORY	Considerable thought and effort are evident. Overall, written work is complete and accurate but lacks depth. Presentation is professional in appearance. Assignments are turned in on or before the due date.
U	UNSATISFACTORY	Little effort or thought is evident. Large or important pieces of information are missing and/or not factual. Presentation is non-professional. Assignments are late.
X	UNACCEPTABLE	No work is turned in or written worksheet is blank.

Performance Evaluation Criteria

Scale/Label	Standard Procedure	Performance Quality	Assistance
EXEMPLARY (E)	Safe and accurate Self-directed	Competent, skillful, confident. Expedient use of time. Consistently responsible. Thoroughly prepared.	Without direction unless appropriate
SATISFACTORY (S)	Safe and accurate with some supervision	Efficient, skillful, confident. Expedient use of time. Progressively responsible. Adequately prepared.	With occasional physical or verbal direction
UNSATISFACTORY (U)	Questionably safe and/or accurate, or Unsafe and/or inaccurate Dependent	Partial or no demonstration of skills. Inefficient or unskillful. Delayed or prolonged time expenditure. Lacks confidence. Does not maintain responsibility. Poorly prepared.	Frequent or continuous verbal and/or physical direction
UNACCEPTABLE (X)	Blatant safety violations Late, Absent, or Unprepared	Late, absent, or totally unprepared. Unsafe for presence in clinical area.	Instructor will communicate with student exactly what is unacceptable.

Weekly Practicum Performance Rating

Week	1	2	3	4	5	6	7	8	9	10	11	12
1. Apply critical thinking skills, principles, and concepts from the humanities, social sciences, physical sciences, biological sciences, mathematics, and prerequisite nursing coursework to meet the healthcare and mental health needs of the client, family, and community.												
2. Demonstrate active collaboration with members of the interprofessional team while implementing an individualized plan of care to maximize safety and quality outcomes in a mental health setting.												
3. Select articles from scholarly journals and use the current evidence to provide rationale for nursing interventions and to manage the care of clients in a mental health setting.												
4. Practice the roles of caregiver, support agent, colleague, advocate, collaborator, and client educator in a mental health setting.												
5. Analyze adequacy of care setting, potential system barriers, policies, nursing's role, and helpful strategies related to client needs and acuity in a mental health setting.												
6. Refine effective communication skills necessary when caring for clients with mental health needs and when actively participating as a member of the healthcare team to achieve positive client outcomes.												
7. Integrate client preferences in care planning and application of appropriate nursing strategies to promote health and wellness for clients in a mental health setting.												
8. Promote the image of nursing by modeling the values and articulating the knowledge, skills, and attitudes of the nursing profession while adhering to the professional standards of moral, ethical, and legal conduct in a mental health setting.												

(*continued*)

(continued)

Week	1	2	3	4	5	6	7	8	9	10	11	12
9. Employ the knowledge, skills, and attitudes essential to positive client outcomes and a culture of safety in the provision of care in a mental health setting.												
10. Demonstrate caring during interactions with clients in the mental health setting.												

Overall Weekly Written Work Rating

Week	1	2	3	4	5	6	7	8	9	10	11	12
Clinical Log Rating (E, S, U, or X) or Points Earned												

Anecdotal Notes

Date	Supporting Documentation (must be objective)

NUR 315: PSYCHIATRIC/MENTAL HEALTH NURSING: PRACTICUM EVALUATION FORM

Outcome 1: Apply critical thinking skills, principles and concepts from the humanities, social sciences, physical sciences, biological sciences, mathematics, and prerequisite nursing coursework to meet the healthcare and mental health needs of the client, family, and community. (Sample behaviors: Prepare a theoretically based plan of care, apply psychopharmacologic data to nursing actions, interpret lab data in terms of client's clinical status, share knowledge in pre and post conference, relate relevant clinical data, relate implications and consequences of nursing action, identify appropriate questions to solve clinical problems, and verbalize insight into own thoughts and feelings as they impact professional behavior and attitudes.)

Outcome 2: Demonstrate active collaboration with members of the interprofessional team while implementing an individualized plan of care to maximize safety and quality outcomes in a mental health setting. (Sample behaviors: Describe own strengths, limitations, and values in functioning as a member of an interprofessional team, initiate plan for self-development as a member of an interprofessional team, act with integrity, consistency and respect for differing views, function competently within own scope of practice as a member of the interprofessional team, and solicit input from other team members to improve client outcomes.)

(continued)

(continued)

Outcome 3: Select articles from scholarly journals and use the current evidence to provide rationale for nursing interventions and to manage the care of clients in a mental health setting. (Sample behaviors: Review research which impacts decisions of nursing care provision, demonstrate knowledge of basic scientific methods and processes, present reviewed literature to convey implications in evidence based practice, and discriminate between valid and invalid reasons for modifying clinical practice based on clinical expertise or patient/family preferences in light of scientific evidence.)

Outcome 4: Practice the roles of caregiver, support agent, colleague, advocate, collaborator, and client educator in a mental health setting. (Sample behaviors: Caregiver, support agent, colleague, advocate, collaborator, and client educator.)

Outcome 5: Analyze adequacy of care setting, potential system barriers, policies, nursing's role, and helpful strategies related to client needs and acuity in a mental health setting. (Sample behaviors: Examine common barriers to active involvement of clients, describe strategies to empower client systems, provide client with access to resources, discuss shared decision making with empowered clients even when conflicts are present, examine nursing roles in ensuring coordination, integration, and continuity of care via policies, discuss the tension between professional autonomy and system functioning, identify system barriers and facilitators within the setting, and identify gaps between local and best practices.)

Outcome 6: Refine effective communication skills necessary when caring for clients with mental health needs and when actively participating as a member of the healthcare team to achieve positive client outcomes. (Sample behaviors: Utilize principles of a helping relationship, demonstrate goal oriented communication, recognize effective and ineffective group process skills of clients, peers, and staff, use information technology effectively in communicating to the healthcare team when available, and verbalize insight into thoughts and feelings that impact communication with clients.)

Outcome 7: Integrate client preferences in care planning and application of appropriate nursing strategies to promote health and wellness for clients in a mental health setting. (Sample behaviors: Explain the influence of the environment on the health of the client, assess risk factors of the client, assess client teaching needs, analyze support systems of the client, and interpret available resources for clients.)

Outcome 8: Promote the image of nursing by modeling the values and articulating the knowledge, skills, and attitudes of the nursing profession while adhering to the professional standards of moral, ethical, and legal conduct in a mental health setting. (Sample behaviors: Exhibit professional appearance and behavior, assume responsibility for safety, participate in pre and post conferences, ask questions that reflect active awareness of situation, accept constructive criticism professionally, identify own strengths and weaknesses, demonstrate efforts to maintain strengths, and demonstrate efforts to overcome weaknesses.)

Outcome 9: Employ the knowledge, skills, and attitudes essential to positive client outcomes and a culture of safety in the provision of care in a mental health setting. (Sample behaviors: Assess the psychosocial status of the individual/family, assess the physiological status of the individual/family, complete a mental status exam, interpret data in terms of implications for nursing actions, identify appropriate nursing diagnoses, complete nursing interventions, examine client outcomes, discuss effective use of strategies to reduce risk of harm to self or others, and communicate observations or concerns related to hazards to instructor and the healthcare team.)

(continued)

(continued)

Outcome 10: Demonstrate caring during interactions with clients in the mental health setting. (Sample behaviors: Receptive to assigned clients, able to grasp the perspectives of assigned clients, available to assigned clients, work to bring about the best outcomes for assigned clients, energy focus is toward assigned clients, and treat assigned clients as individuals.)

Student Comments:

Midterm Final

Faculty Comments:

Midterm Final

Summarize Midterm Evaluation Findings and Midterm Practicum Grade

_____ Satisfactory
_____ Unsatisfactory

Student Signature & Date: _____
Faculty Signature & Date: _____

Summarize Final Evaluation Findings and Final Practicum Grade

_____ Satisfactory
_____ Unsatisfactory

Student Signature & Date: _____
Faculty Signature & Date: _____

Illinois State University
Mennonite College of Nursing

Clinical Performance Evaluation Tool (CPET) Guidelines

Tool Guidelines
- Each student will fill out an evaluation at (1) midterm and (2) final.
- Each faculty member will fill out an evaluation at (1) midterm and (2) final.
- Each outcome must be evaluated as "Satisfactory (S)," "Needs Improvement (NI)," or "Unsatisfactory (U)."
- A passing grade will only be assigned if all the items are checked "S" at the time of the final evaluation.

Grading Guidelines, Entire Course
- The final grade for each student in the course will be the numeric grade received for the course based on all of the didactic work required in the syllabus.
- Clinical performance will be evaluated with a CPET and will be scored either "pass" or "fail."
- Every student must receive a score of "pass" on the CPET to pass the course.
- If a student passes the didactic portion of the course and fails the CPET, the student fails the entire course.
- If a student receives a "fail" on the CPET the student will receive a grade of "F" for the course.

NUR 229 Adult Nursing I
Clinical Performance Evaluation Tool (CPET)

Student Name_____   ULID_____

Clinical Site_____   Semester/Year_____

Faculty Name_____   NSL Date _____

Patient Centered Care
Recognize the patient or designee as the source of control and full partner in providing compassionate and coordinated care based on respect for patient's preferences, values, and needs (QSEN.org)

NUR 229 Objectives
Objective 5: Utilize the nursing process as a systematic method of providing nursing care for adult patients across the lifespan

Specific Knowledge, Skills, & Attitudes (KSAs)	Student Midterm S/NI/U	Faculty Midterm S/NI/U	Student Final S/U	Faculty Final S/U
A. Demonstrates compassion in caring for individuals and families				
B. Treats patients, staff, peers, and faculty with respect regardless of varying cultural backgrounds, lifestyles, and value systems				
C. Seeks knowledge and understanding on how to provide culturally and spiritually competent care using the nursing process				
D. Utilizes critical thinking and clinical reasoning skills throughout the nursing process to provide client centered care				
E. Uses principles and theories from nursing, and biological, psychological, and social sciences as a foundation for nursing practice				
F. Identifies relationships between, and significance of, client's bio-psycho-social status, culture, and underlying pathologies				
G. Establishes priorities according to client/resident need				
H. Implements established routine, therapeutic nursing interventions for the client/resident				
I. Evaluates client response to interventions in care plan				
J. Evaluates goals/outcome criteria of care plan				
K. Adjusts priorities for therapeutic nursing interventions as client/resident's situation changes to care plan				
Comments				

Teamwork and Collaboration

Function effectively within nursing and inter-professional teams, fostering open communication, mutual respect, and shared decision making to achieve quality patient care (QSEN, 2014)

NUR 229 Objectives

Objective 1: Identify the need for effective communication and collaboration with patients, families, and other members of the healthcare team to advocate for improved health capacities

Specific KSAs	Student Midterm S/NI/U	Faculty Midterm S/NI/U	Student Final S/U	Faculty Final S/U
A. Informs staff/faculty in a timely manner of significant changes in client/resident status				
B. Utilizes appropriate channels of communication				
C. Demonstrates effective, goal-oriented verbal and written communication skills incorporating concepts of adult life span considerations, patient privacy, confidentiality, and advocacy				
D. Demonstrates appropriate effective group process skills:				
■ actively participates with the weekly clinical group				
■ actively participates in simulation day				
■ contributes to the development of the adult teaching project				
■ evaluates the group process				
E. Supports peers and staff in delivery of client/resident care				
F. Recognizes the role of the nurse in collaborating with the interdisciplinary team to improve client outcomes				
G. Identifies principles and various modes of communication (including health information technology) in effective collaboration				
H. Identifies the roles of client, family, significant others, and healthcare team in planning outcomes and evidence-based nursing interventions				
Comments				

Evidence-Based Practice
Integrate best current evidence with clinical expertise and patient/family preference and values
for delivery of optimal healthcare (QSEN.org)

NUR 229 Objectives
Objective 2: Define evidence-based practice for clinical decision making in the delivery of
nursing care

Specific KSAs	Student Midterm S/NI/U	Faculty Midterm S/NI/U	Student Final S/U	Faculty Final S/U
A. Identifies nursing problems that incorporate evidence-based practice				
B. Incorporates evidence-based interventions (including client teaching) into practice				
C. Provides safe, competent care in compliance with best practices				
Comments				

Quality Improvement
Use data to monitor the outcomes of care processes and use improvement methods to design and
test changes to continuously improve the quality and safety of healthcare systems (QSEN, 2014)

NUR 229 Objectives
Objective 3: Examine health promotion strategies that contribute to safe, quality care
Objective 4: Discuss concepts of accountability and responsibility in the management of
professional nursing care

Specific KSAs	Student Midterm S/NI/U	Faculty Midterm S/NI/U	Student Final S/U	Faculty Final S/U
A. Analyzes factors affecting health of clients in nursing homes and hospitals				
B. Discusses legal, ethical, political issues that influence professional nursing practice				
C. Alters nursing practice according to constructive feedback and suggestions for improvement				
D. Identifies how the professional nurse delivers care within the parameters of the Nurse Practice Act, Nursing Standards of Care, and the Nursing Code of Ethics				
Comments				

Safety
Minimizes risk of harm to patients and providers through both system effectiveness and individual performance (QSEN.org)

NUR 229 Objectives
Objective 3: Examine health promotion strategies that contribute to safe, quality care

Specific KSAs	Student Midterm S/NI/U	Faculty Midterm S/NI/U	Student Final S/U	Faculty Final S/U
A. Identifies components of the nursing process in delivery of safe and responsible healthcare				
B. Describes environmental and healthcare facility safety concerns for the resident/client				
C. Differentiates normal from abnormal physiological and psychosocial processes in adult clients				
D. Safely administers medications according to the Nine Rights				
E. Verbalizes understanding of medication purpose, action, side effects, nursing implications and method of determining effectiveness				
F. Recognizes limitations of self and seeks help when necessary				
G. Recognizes changes in client's condition and takes appropriate, timely action				
H. Incorporates systems thinking in the development of nursing interventions that support illness prevention and health promotion				
I. Selects appropriate nursing diagnosis based on assessment				
J. Performs physical assessment using appropriate technique				
K. Serves as a client/resident advocate				
L. Identifies the role of the nurse in assisting clients in the management of their protection, comfort, physiological, safety, and situational needs				

(continued)

(continued)

	Student Midterm S/NI/U	Faculty Midterm S/NI/U	Student Final S/U	Faculty Final S/U
M. Explains concepts and rationales for nursing skills as discussed in the nursing skills course				
N. Identifies factors and corresponding interventions which affect an individual's ability for self-protection				
O. Recognizes clients/residents at risk for complications				
Comments				

Informatics
Use information and technology to communicate, manage knowledge, mitigate error, and support decision making (QSEN.org)

NUR 229 Objectives
Identify the need for effective communication and collaboration with patients, families, and other members of the healthcare team to advocate for improved health capacities.

Specific KSAs	Student Midterm S/NI/U	Faculty Midterm S/NI/U	Student Final S/U	Faculty Final S/U
A. Communicates in writing completely and concisely				
B. Navigates the electronic medical record through:				
▪ Finding interdisciplinary notes				
▪ Finding test results				
▪ Finding patient care plan				
C. Documents within the electronic medical record:				
▪ Assessments				
▪ Notes				
▪ Interventions				
D. Utilizes informatics to support patient care:				
▪ Obtain pertinent policy/procedure guidelines				
▪ Obtain appropriate patient education material				
Comments				

Professionalism

Demonstrates a commitment to professional nursing and "Applies principles of altruism, excellence, caring, ethics, respect, civility, communication, and accountability in one's self and nursing practice." (American Association of Colleges of Nursing [AACN], 2008)

NUR 229

Discuss concepts of accountability and responsibility in the management of professional nursing care

Specific KSAs	Student Midterm S/NI/U	Faculty Midterm S/NI/U	Student Final S/U	Faculty Final S/U
A. Demonstrates an awareness of how personal and professional values impact nursing care				
B. Demonstrates an awareness of self by:				
■ Examining own ideas, feelings, and behavior				
■ Evaluating own performance through written reflection (Clinical Objective Tool/Reflective Journals)				
C. Demonstrates personal and professional responsibility for:				
■ Maintaining confidentiality of information				
■ Interacting in a collegial manner				
■ Accepting responsibility for own preparation, learning, and behavior				
■ Completing Lab and Success Plan requirements satisfactorily and on time				
■ Uses resources for continuous learning and development				
■ Arriving on time; informing faculty of absence				
■ Adhering to school policies regarding dress code				
■ Coming to clinical prepared; submitting all assignments correctly, on time, using own work, and crediting resources appropriately				
■ Demonstrating truthfulness and honesty				
Comments				

Midterm Assessment

Midterm Faculty Assessment
(Strengths, goals, opportunities for improvement)

Midterm Student Goals
(Provide a minimum of three goals mutually decided upon by student and faculty)

1.
2.
3.
Additional Goals

I will work with my faculty in meeting these goals.
Student Signature _____   Date _____
Printed Student Name (Legible) _____

I agree and will support this growth.
Faculty Signature _____   Date _____
Printed Faulty Name (Legible) _____

NSL Remediation Date _____   Absences _____
Makeup Plan _____

Final Assessment

*Faculty: Please provide a copy of this Final Assessment for the student after completion of this course

*Students: Please retain a copy of this Final Assessment and share with your clinical faculty next semester

Final Student Assessment
(strengths, attainment of goals, and opportunities for improvement next semester)
What opportunities do you see are needed next semester to improve you as a nurse?

Final Faculty Assessment
(strengths, attainment of goals, and opportunities for improvement next semester)
What areas or opportunities are needed to continue or improve for next semester?

I will work with my faculty in meeting these goals.

Student Signature _____ Date _____

Printed Student Name (Legible) _____

I agree and will support this growth.

Faculty Signature _____ Date _____

Printed Faulty Name (Legible) _____

NSL Remediation Date _____ Absences _____

Makeup Plan _____

This CPET is based on the Quality and Safety Education for Nurses (QSEN) competencies, https://qsen.org/; American Association of Colleges of Nursing. (2008). *The essentials of baccalaureate education for professional nursing practice.* Author; Cronenwett, L., Sherwood, G., Barnsteiner, J., Disch, J., Johnson, J., Mitchell, P., Taylor, D., & Warren, J. (2007). Quality and safety education for nurses. *Nursing Outlook, 55*(3), 122–131. https://doi.org/10.1016/j.outlook.2007.02.006

B.2. EXAMPLES OF CLINICAL EVALUATION TOOLS IN ADVANCED PRACTICE NURSING PROGRAMS

B.2.1. University of Cincinnati College of Nursing

Final Student Evaluation

Directions: The preceptor is asked to evaluate the student's performance through Chart Review, Direct Observation, Case Discussion, and Performance Characteristics. Evaluation criteria are provided for the preceptor's convenience. However, additional comments are helpful and appreciated. Please evaluate the performance of the student you precepted using the following scale:

6 = Always performed this behavior without prompting or reminders

5 = Usually performed this behavior (76–99% of the time)

4 = Frequently performed this behavior (51–75% of the time)

3 = Occasionally performed this behavior (26–50% of the time)

2 = Rarely performed this behavior when given the opportunity (<25% of the time)

1 = Never performed this behavior when given the opportunity

N/A = Not observed or experience not available in your setting

Assessment

1. Obtains appropriate and complete information for full histories.
2. Obtains appropriate and complete information for focused histories.
3. Uses correct technique in performing a physical exam.
4. Identifies pertinent abnormal findings.
5. Records history and physical exam findings in an organized and thorough manner.

Differential Diagnosis

1. Demonstrates critical thinking skills.
2. Identifies appropriate differential diagnoses.
3. Recommends/orders appropriate lab and diagnostic tests for the patient.
4. Correctly interprets lab and di agnostic test results.

Developing a Plan of Care

1. Develops an appropriate plan of care for the patient including medications and treatments.
2. Personalizes the plan of care and teaching.
3. Teaches patients/families appropriate health promotion and risk reduction regimens.
4. Identifies appropriate follow up.

Evaluation

1. Identifies desired outcomes for patients.
2. Evaluates plan of care for patients.
3. Assesses ongoing educational needs.

Collaboration

1. Demonstrates collaboration with other members of the healthcare team.
2. Suggests appropriate referrals to colleagues.

Interpersonal and Professional skills

1. Communicates clearly and effectively.
2. Builds trusting relationship with patients.
3. Demonstrates respect for patients and families.
4. Sets mutual goals with patients and families.
5. Acts in a responsible manner and adheres to policies and procedures of the institution.
6. Is on time for clinical and meets commitments to preceptor.

Please comment on student's strengths and potential areas for improvement:

B.2.2. Carlow University Department of Nursing, MSN—Family (Individual Across Lifespan) Nurse Practitioner Program

On-site Family Nurse Practitioner Student Clinical Evaluation Form NU7501

- ▪ The Nurse Practitioner Student must perform and obtain a history and physical with subsequent information, with the clinical faculty member present.
- ▪ Clinical faculty will circle the point value that best matches the student performance level for each portion of the evaluation and provide constructive feedback.
  - ▪ *If a student doesn't achieve a minimum total score of 28 out of 32 points, arrangements must be made to revisit the student after remediation to reassess student performance.*
  - ▪ *If a student receives a score of 1 in any area, arrangements must be made to revisit the student after remediation to reassess student performance.*

Please Note: Once completed, clinical faculty should provide feedback to the student and this evaluation form needs to be emailed directly to the student for signature and for student to upload to Typhon.

STUDENT NAME:		DATE:	
CLINICAL FACULTY:		COURSE NUMBER:	
PRECEPTOR NAME:			
PRECEPTOR ADDRESS:			

SUMMARY OF STUDENT PERFORMANCE
(Please see the evaluation point value summary for more detail regarding grading of each section)

SECTION DESCRIPTION	SCORE				COMMENTS
Subjective History Taking Skills Score	1 ☐	2 ☐	3 ☐	4 ☐	
Objective Physical Examination	1 ☐	2 ☐	3 ☐	4 ☐	
Assessment Skills	1 ☐	2 ☐	3 ☐	4 ☐	
Oral Presentation Skills	1 ☐	2 ☐	3 ☐	4 ☐	
Communication Skills	1 ☐	2 ☐	3 ☐	4 ☐	
Management Planning	1 ☐	2 ☐	3 ☐	4 ☐	
Implementation of Management Plan	1 ☐	2 ☐	3 ☐	4 ☐	
Record Keeping Skills	1 ☐	2 ☐	3 ☐	4 ☐	
TOTAL SCORE					

MAJOR STRENGTHS OF STUDENT	
PRINCIPAL DIFFICULTIES OF STUDENT	
PROFESSIONALISM	Students must consistently demonstrate all of the characteristics listed below throughout the semester to "Pass." Extraordinary circumstances that interfere with the student's clinical progress during the semester must be discussed with the clinical faculty member (Initial Each Below)
FACULTY INITIAL	
	—Aware of own professional strengths and areas for future growth
	—Possess a strong sense of responsibility for own learning and willingness to take initiative in pursuing achievement of learning goals
	—Display a positive attitude and accept constructive feedback
	—Interact in a collegial respectful manner with clinical preceptor, staff, faculty, and other students
	—Present self in a professional manner, including appropriate dress, by being punctual, cooperative, and dependable when scheduled to be in a clinical setting. Uphold contract with preceptor to complete clinical hours on a regular basis by the end of the designated time.
Please Check PASS or NOT PASS to Indicate if Student Successfully Completed the On-Site Evaluation	**PASS ☐** / **NOT PASS ☐**
Faculty Signature:	**Date:**
Student Signature:	**Date:**

NU7501 EVALUATION POINT VALUE SUMMARY—Use this as a guide to determine the appropriate score for a student based on the student's demonstrated clinical performance

	Unacceptable	Below Average	Acceptable	Superior
	1 point	**2 points**	**3 points**	**4 points**
SUBJECTIVE HISTORY TAKING SKILLS	Misses much critical information, which leads to incomplete or incorrect assessment	Misses some basic history, which could lead to incomplete or incorrect assessment	Reasonable complete history, missing some basic history, not likely to lead to missed diagnosis	Elicits thorough history relevant to patient's problems, complete as per data base. May miss some sharpness of focus or detail relevant to differential diagnosis
	1 point	**2 points**	**3 points**	**4 points**
OBJECTIVE PHYSICAL EXAMINATION SKILLS	Poor technique, likely to miss significant findings; Fails to note abnormalities	Awkward skills, disruptive use of notes; does not select areas for patient's problems. Technique might miss significant findings	Fairly good technique. Misses minor steps, but not likely to miss diagnosis or injured patient	Complete, smooth exam focused to patient's problems
	1 point	**2 points**	**3 points**	**4 points**
ASSESSMENT SKILLS	Assessment dangerously over or understated; grossly inadequate problem list	Assessment incomplete. Unable to state major differential diagnoses. Significantly incomplete problem list	Reasonable assessment. Identifies most major differential diagnoses. Problem list may be incomplete	Correct assessment, but may miss minor differential diagnoses or minor items from problem list

(continued)

(continued)

	1 point	2 points	3 points	4 points
ORAL PRESENTATION SKILLS	Dangerously unclear incomplete and/or incorrect presentation of patient data	Unclear, incomplete and/or incorrect presentation of patient data	Presents basic data clearly. Minor errors or omits some major pieces of data. Order may be mixed	Presents patient as a person. Clearly organized; includes most major issues from problem list. May be less succinct and may not include all problems
COMMUNICATION SKILLS	Inappropriate communication; lacks sensitivity to patient's position. Unable to acknowledge own feelings or problems with faculty or preceptor	Frequently awkward communication. Appears ill at ease. Poor use of communication techniques. Does not recognize patient's emotional signals. (Use of notes or note taking inhibits dialogue). Guarded or incomplete communication with faculty or preceptor regarding patient's role and development and professional growth	Generally clear, fairly smooth communication. Reasonably comfortable with patient. Aware of and reports delicate problems, but does not fully pursue or then provide support. Usually communicates openly and constructively with preceptor and faculty	Smooth, clear communication. Recognizes and openly acknowledges patient's stated feelings. Pursues "red flags." Communicates openly and constructively with preceptor and faculty
MANAGEMENT PLANNING	Plan dangerously incomplete or inappropriate. Inadequate or inappropriate use of preceptor given student's skill level or patient's problem(s)	Plan incomplete and may be unsafe. Inadequate use of preceptor for identifying management options needed for patient's problems(s)	Plan incomplete, but safe. Options and rationale incomplete, but includes basic management needed for patient's problems(s)	Appropriate plan for most problems, most areas. Options chosen and their rationale may be insignificantly incomplete

(continued)

(continued)

	1 point	2 points	3 points	4 points
IMPLEMENTATION OF MANAGEMENT PLAN	Omits initiation of all basic elements of the treatment plan and clearly unsafe; lack of any effort to promote patient self-responsibility for health	Omits initiation of some basic elements of the treatment plan and may be unsafe. Insufficient effort to promote patient self-responsibility for health	Able to initiate basic elements of the treatment plan essential for safe care in all three areas while promoting patient self-responsibility for health to a limited extent	Able to initiate most aspects of the treatment plan in all three areas (diagnostic, therapeutic, and patient education) in consultation with preceptor while promoting patient self-responsibility for health to a moderate extent
RECORD KEEPING SKILLS	Much important information missing; very hard to follow, dangerous to patient follow-up, and/or illegible	Some important information missing which might compromise adequate follow-up. Not clearly organized; laborious to read	Major areas clear, minor ones may not be; some mixing of categories in SOAP format. Problem list includes major but not all minor health issues	Clear and logically organized in SOAP format with all sections appropriate; includes most pertinent positives and negatives; may mix problems. Complete problem list

Clinical Faculty Final Grading Checklist	
Student Name	
Course Number/Name	
Semester/Year	
Clinical Faculty Name	
Date	

—This form MUST be submitted to the FNP Clinical Coordinator by the Wednesday of the final week of the term.
—If a student has failed to meet clinical requirements, please contact the clinical coordinator by the last day of clinical rotations (The Friday before the end of the term)

	As clinical faculty, I have …	YES	NO	COMMENTS
1	Verified in Typhon that student's compliance documents (health for, clearances, etc.) are current	☐	☐	
2	Reviewed, commented, and signed off on SOAP #1 assignment in Typhon	☐	☐	
3	Reviewed, commented, and signed off on SOAP #2 assignment in Typhon	☐	☐	
4	Reviewed, commented, and signed off on SOAP #3 assignment in Typhon	☐	☐	
5	Reviewed, commented, and signed off on H&P assignment in Typhon	☐	☐	
6	Reviewed the students case logs and verified they have completed 50 appropriate case logs for each 75-hour clinical practicum course or 75 case logs for NU7921 Integration course	☐	☐	

(continued)

(*continued*)

Clinical Faculty Final Grading Checklist					
7	Conducted an onsite evaluation to assess the student's clinical performance and progress toward assimilation, reviewed the evaluation form with the student, and provided a copy of the evaluation to the student	☐	☐	DATE OF ONSITE EVALUATION	
8	Met with the preceptor to discuss student's performance	☐	☐		
9	Shared recommendations or concerns from the preceptor with the student	☐	☐		
10	Reviewed the accuracy of clinical hours in the student's time log in Typhon	☐	☐		
11	I have verified that the student has uploaded the following documents to Typhon external documents:	☐	☐		
	Preceptor Signed Time Log	☐	☐		
	Student Signed On-site Evaluation	☐	☐		
	Preceptor Evaluation of Student	☐	☐		
	Student Evaluation of Preceptor/ Facility	☐	☐		
STUDENT FINAL CLINICAL GRADE				*PASS* ☐	*FAIL* ☐
ADDITIONAL COMMENTS/SUGGESTIONS					

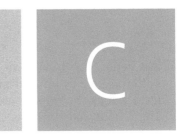

Sample Distance Learning Affiliation Agreement

THIS AGREEMENT, entered into between the **University** on behalf of the **School of Nursing**, hereinafter referred to as the **"School,"** and hereinafter referred to as the **"Agency,"** shall govern the use of the Agency's facilities by the faculty and students of the School.

WHEREAS, it is to the mutual benefit of the **Agency** and the **School** to cooperate in educational programs using the facilities of the **Agency**, and WHEREAS, it is in the best interests of the parties to jointly plan for the organization, administration, and operation of the educational programs.

NOW, THEREFORE, in consideration of the mutual covenants by each party to be kept and performed, it is agreed as follows:

ARTICLE I—SCHOOL RESPONSIBILITIES

A. The School agrees to assign only students who are in good standing and for whom the School has on record:
1. documentation that the student is free of communicable diseases, including results of a 2-step Mantoux tuberculin test;
2. current immunizations; and
3. evidence of at least basic life support certification in cardiopulmonary resuscitation. The certification card must show inclusive dates.
B. Students of the School will not be reimbursed for services rendered to the Agency during the course of the educational program and will not be considered as employees of the Agency while participating in the program.
C. The standards and philosophy of education, the instruction, and preparation of all instructional schedules and plans, including hours of clinical experience, shall be the responsibility of the School. These standards and plans shall be made available to the authorized Agency personnel.
D. The School shall insure the School and its employees, students, agents, and volunteers while acting on the School's behalf through a comprehensive program of self-insurance. Evidence of this insurance shall be provided to the Agency upon the Agency's request. If employees of the School will be in the Agency with students during the affiliation experience, the School shall provide, upon request, evidence of Workers' Compensation insurance covering its employees.

E. The School shall make all reasonable effort to assure that the students comply with the Agency policies and procedures; provided that the Agency first orients the School's students in such policies and procedures.

F. The School shall inform students that Agency requires access to students' education, training, prior experience, levels of competency, and such other information. The School shall make reasonable efforts to obtain from students authorization to release such records.

G. The School shall ensure that all students involved in the educational program at the Agency will receive training regarding the privacy rules of the Health Insurance Portability and Accountability Act (HIPAA) prior to entering the facilities of the Agency. The School will present proof of such training to the Agency upon request.

H. Conducting criminal background checks on students assigned to Agency:

1. If requested by Agency, the student shall be responsible for completion of a criminal background check conforming to specific criteria Agency provides to School. The student will submit the results of the criminal background check to School.

2. Upon receipt of the student's criminal background check results, School will: (a) provide the results of the criminal background check to Agency after School obtains student's consent to do so, or (b) compare the criminal background check results against a list, provided by Agency, of specific crimes that would prevent a student from being placed with Agency. School will not send to the Agency any student whose criminal background check shows the student has been convicted of, pled guilty to, or pled no contest to any crime on the provided list. If the University has any question regarding whether a crime listed on a student's criminal background check would prevent the student from working in the Agency, the background check will be submitted to the Agency for its review after the University obtains student's consent to do so.

ARTICLE II—AGENCY RESPONSIBILITIES

A. The Agency controls the Agency's administrative and professional operations and the direct or indirect care of the Agency's patients.

B. The School shall be informed regarding changes in clinical facilities, which may affect the clinical experience of the School's students.

C. The Agency shall ensure emergency care is provided to students for any accident, injury or illness. The student's health insurance shall be billed for any emergency service, and the balance billed to the student. Responsibility for follow-up care remains the responsibility of the student.

D. The Agency shall provide information regarding each student's performance in the clinical setting if so requested by the School.

E. When in the opinion of the Agency, a student's conduct or performance adversely affects patient care, disrupts the operations of the Agency, or violates the policies and procedures of the Agency, the Agency shall notify the School and the School and the Agency shall together determine whether the student should be removed from the clinical rotation at the Agency.

F. The Agency shall provide access at reasonable times and with reasonable advance notice to representatives of the School and to representatives of the School's accrediting bodies.

G. The Agency will protect student confidential information and education records from disclosure and agrees to abide by all applicable law, including but not limited to, the Federal Family Education and Privacy Rights Act (FERPA), 20 U.S.C. & 1232 (g), and the Health Insurance Portability and Accountability Act (HIPAA), Codified at 42 U.S.C. § 300 gg and 29 U.S.C § 1181 et seq. and 42 USC 1320d et seq. Agency further agrees to be liable for and report any breach of such confidential student information or educational records to the College within five (5) days of determining such a breach.

H. Agency shall develop, implement, maintain and use appropriate administrative, technical and physical security measures to preserve the confidentiality, integrity, and availability of all electronically maintained or transmitted student education records received from, or on behalf of School or its students. The procedures will be documented and available for School to review upon request. Upon termination, cancellation, expiration, or other conclusion of the agreement, Agency shall securely store or destroy student education records in accordance with its own human resource retention policies.

I. Agency will be responsible for enforcement of its HIPAA policies and procedures and compliance by School's students. School's students will be functioning as part of the Agency's workforce pursuant to 45 C.F.R. §160.103 and will be subject to the Agency's HIPAA policies and procedures.

J. The Agency shall insure itself and its employees through a fiscally sound program of self-insurance or commercial insurance or a combination thereof, for professional and general liability.

ARTICLE III—JOINT RESPONSIBILITIES

A. Both the Agency and the School shall designate liaison personnel to assure systematic planning and the exchange of information regarding the students' clinical experience.

B. The School and the Agency agree that in the event that either becomes aware of a claim asserted by any person arising out of this agreement or any activity carried out under this agreement, the parties shall cooperate in defending the claim, securing evidence, and obtaining the cooperation of witnesses.

C. The maximum number of students assigned to the Agency during any instructional period shall be established by mutual agreement thirty (30) days in advance of any student's clinical affiliation with the Agency. The Agency reserves the right to limit the number of students it accepts for affiliation.

D. When Agency staff serve as preceptors supervising students' clinical experiences the preceptors: (1) May not supervise more than two students at any one time and (2) will implement the clinical education plan at the direction of a faculty member participating in the course in which the student is enrolled. Preceptors and roles and responsibilities of the preceptors and faculty are mutually agreed upon by the Agency and the School.

E. Where areas of difference exist or occur in rules, regulations, or questions of nursing, clinical, medical or other Agency practices, the Agency rules, regulation or practices shall prevail and such conflict shall be referred to School and Agency liaison personnel.

F. The parties agree that there shall be no discrimination based on race, color, religion, national origin, sex, sex orientation, age, physical or mental handicap or status as a disabled veteran or veteran of the Vietnam era.

G. This agreement shall become effective as of _____ and shall continue in effect for five years from the effective date with the understanding that this agreement may be reviewed annually and revised, if necessary. The contract can be terminated at the will of either party hereto upon giving the other party no less than ninety (90) days written notice of the party's intention to terminate. All students involved in the clinical experience at the time of termination shall be permitted to complete the current term.

ARTICLE IV—NOTICES

Notice to School shall be in writing and sent by United States regular mail, postage prepaid, to:

ARTICLE V—PRECEPTOR RESPONSIBILITIES

1. Orient the student to the agency's physical facilities, policies, procedures, and the role the student will assume.
2. Provide supervision for an assigned student in the clinical area.
3. Implement the clinical education plan at the direction of the faculty member responsible for the course in which the student is enrolled.
4. Facilitate and guide the clinical experiences of the student (i.e., assess learning experiences available, arrange for alternative experiences or use of resources, assess student's preparation for clinical assignment, including medications, pathophysiology or diagnoses, and so forth).
5. Maintain communication with the assigned faculty member. Notify faculty immediately of any concerns regarding the student's performance.
6. Meet frequently for informal conferences with the student. Provide students and faculty with feedback related to performance.
7. Provide ongoing and final evaluations of clinical performance to both the student and the faculty advisor.
8. Participate in an overall evaluation of the preceptor guided experience.
9. Serve as a professional role model immediately available to the student within the clinical setting.
10. The preceptor may not supervise any more than two students at any one time.

IN WITNESS WHEREOF, we have hereunto set our hands.

UNIVERSITY

By:

Name, Title:

Date:

AGENCY

By:

Name, Title:

Date:

Index

notes about performance, 232, 235, 252
nursing care plan, 148–149
nursing curriculum, 3, 4, 6, 9–11

objective structured clinical examinations
(OSCE), 46, 240, 251
observing performance, 87
organizational skills, 30
orientation, 62, 64, 65, 72-74
outcomes of clinical teaching
intended outcomes, 17–28
unintended outcomes, 28–29

part-time teachers, 65–66
partnership model, 94–96
patient assignment, 8
patient privacy laws, 122
patient care, 8, 9, 13, 68
patient-centered care competencies, 26
patient simulators, 168
perfection, standard of, 111
philosophical context of clinical
teaching, 5–12
positive unintended outcomes, 28
postclinical conferences, 143
preceptor-student teaching method, 36
preceptors and preceptorship
accreditation requirements, 208
advantages and disadvantages of,
206–208
attributes of effective, 209
defined, 205
evaluation of outcomes, 218–219
implementation, 213–218
in distance education delivery, 211,
262-265
mentoring model, 94
payment of, 210-211
preparation of, 211–213
regulation of, 208, 209, 211
rewarding, 219–220
role model behaviors, 213-214
selecting, 208–211
site visits, 217-218
student preparation for, 213
uses of, 206
preclinical conferences, 143
prelicensure curriculum, 10
privacy
patient right to, 103-107, 121–122
student right to, 109–110, 112
problem solving, 155, 161–162, 168
process of clinical teaching, 82–89

psychomotor domain outcomes, 22–24
psychomotor preparation for clinical
practice, 71
psychomotor skills, 30, 168

Quality improvement (QI), 26–27
quality and patient safety outcomes, 26–28
Quality and Safety Education for Nurses
(QSEN)
QSEN competencies, 26–28
QSEN Institute, 19
QSEN-based clinical evaluation tools, 235
questioning students, 88

rating scales, 235–239
reflective journals, 150–151
role model, 25, 28, 31, 62, 206, 213–214, 219

safety
competencies, 27
safe clinical practice policy and
standards, 118–120
self-assessment, 248
self-confidence, 215
self-efficacy, 215
service learning, 42–43, 137–138
short written assignments, 148
Simulation. *See* clinical simulation
simulation-based experience (SBE), 167
simulation-based pedagogy, 168
Simulation Innovation Resource Center
(SIRC), 168
skill acquisition, 8, 13
social determinants of health, 37
social media use, 103–106, 191–192
students
distance learning, 260
with disabilities, 112–115
individual characteristics of, 84-85
interpersonal relationships with, 107-108
preparation of, for clinical learning, 68–73
privacy rights, 109–110
role and responsibilities of
in discussions, 139
in preceptorships, 215
stresses in clinical practice, 91
student–teacher conferences, 121
summative evaluation, 68, 88

teacher and student discussion
assessment of own learning, 142